Artificial Intelligence Strategies for Analyzing COVID-19 Pneumonia Lung Imaging, Volume 1

Characterization approaches

Artificial Intelligence Strategies for Analyzing COVID-19 Pneumonia Lung Imaging, Volume 1

Characterization approaches

Edited by
Ayman El-Baz
University of Louisville, Louisville, KY, USA
and
University of Louisville at AlAlamein International University (UofL-AIU), New Alamein City, Egypt

Jasjit S Suri
AtheroPoint LLC, Roseville, CA, USA

IOP Publishing, Bristol, UK

ISBN 978-0-7503-3795-3 (ebook)
ISBN 978-0-7503-3793-9 (print)
ISBN 978-0-7503-3796-0 (myPrint)
ISBN 978-0-7503-3794-6 (mobi)

DOI 10.1088/978-0-7503-3795-3

Version: 20220401

IOP ebooks

British Library Cataloguing-in-Publication Data: A catalogue record for this book is available from the British Library.

Published by IOP Publishing, wholly owned by The Institute of Physics, London

IOP Publishing, Temple Circus, Temple Way, Bristol, BS1 6HG, UK

US Office: IOP Publishing, Inc., 190 North Independence Mall West, Suite 601, Philadelphia, PA 19106, USA

With love and affection to my mother and father, whose loving spirit sustains me still.

—Ayman El-Baz

To my late loving parents, immediate family, and children.

—Jasjit S Suri

Contents

Preface

The book covers state-of-the-art artificial intelligence techniques for analyzing Coronavirus disease 2019 (COVID-19) lung infections. COVID-19 was initially detected in Wuhan, China, and is believed to have been transmitted to humans through an intermediate mammalian host from bats before undergoing human-to-human transmission. The clinical diagnosis of COVID-19 depends on different symptoms, which include fever in most cases. Although the severity of the symptoms varies between patients, early detection significantly increases patients' chances of survival. Recently, artificial intelligence, in particular, deep learning has shown significant ability to perform this task. This book focuses on the use of artificial intelligence to develop accurate and reliable techniques for the early detection of COVID-19. Among the topics discussed in the book are the detection of COVID-19 from chest radiographs using convolutional neural networks (CNNs), automatic lung infection segmentation from CT images, radiology smartphone applications, the detection of COVID-19 from cough sounds, the diagnosis of COVID-19 from among eight other lung respiratory diseases, and post-analysis of COVID-19 pneumonia from a clinical perspective.

In summary, the main aim of this book is to help advance scientific research within the broad field of COVID-19 detection. This book focuses on major trends and challenges in this area, and it presents work that aims to identify new techniques and their use in biomedical analysis.

Ayman El-Baz
Jasjit S Suri

Acknowledgement

The completion of this book could not have been possible without the participation and assistance of so many people whose names may not all be enumerated. Their contributions are sincerely appreciated and gratefully acknowledged. However, the editors would like to express their deep appreciation and indebtedness particularly to Dr Ali H Mahmoud and Ebrahim Farahat for their endless support.

Ayman El-Baz
Jasjit S Suri

Editor biographies

Ayman El-Baz

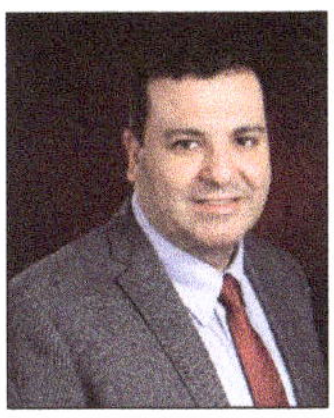

Ayman El-Baz is a Distinguished Professor at the University of Louisville, Kentucky, United States and the University of Louisville at AlAlamein International University (UofL-AIU), New Alamein City, Egypt. Dr El-Baz earned his BSc and MSc degrees in electrical engineering in 1997 and 2001, respectively. He earned his PhD in electrical engineering from the University of Louisville in 2006. Dr El-Baz has been named as a Fellow of Coulter, AIMBE, and NAI for his contributions to the field of biomedical translational research. Dr El-Baz has almost two decades of hands-on experience in the fields of bio-imaging, modeling, and non-invasive computer-assisted diagnosis systems. He has authored or co-authored more than 500 technical articles (182 journals, 44 books, 95 book chapters, 253 refereed-conference papers, 215 abstracts, and 38 US patents and Disclosures).

Jasjit S Suri

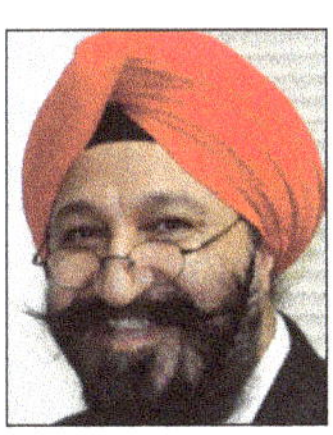

Jasjit S Suri, PhD, MBA is a Fellow of IEEE, AIMBE, SVM, AIUM, and APVS. He is currently the Chairman of AtheroPoint, Roseville, CA, USA, dedicated to imaging technologies for cardiovascular and stroke. He has nearly ~ 22,000 citations, coauthored 50 books, and has an H-index of 72.

List of contributors

Hala M Abd El-Kader

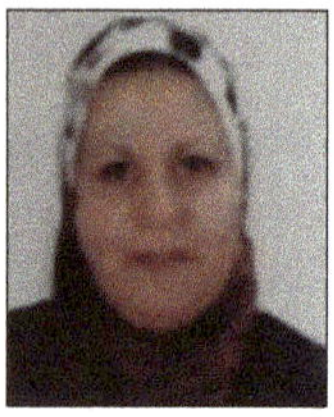

Hala Mohamed Abd El-Kader is Professor and Head of the Electronics and Communication Session, Electrical Engineering Department, Faculty of Engineering, Benha University, where she has been since 1980. Currently, she is Head of the Communication and Computer Engineering Program—Credit Hours, Faculty of Engineering (Shoubra), Benha University. She has completed many investigations in the field of optical wireless communications. She has more than 110 published papers.

Dairi Abdelkader

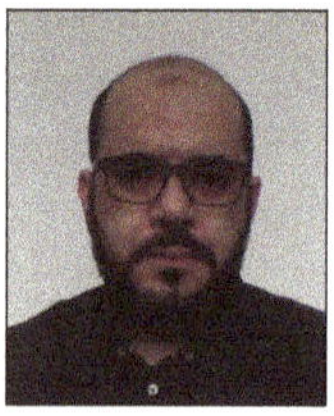

University of Science and Technology of Oran Mohamed Boudiaf (USTO-MB), Bir El Djir, Algeria and Laboratoire des Technologies de l'Environnement LTE, BP 1523 Al M'naouar ENP Oran, 31000, Oran, Algeria

Dairi Abdelkader is an Assistant professor of the Department of Computer Science at the University of Science and Technology of Oran Mohamed-Boudiaf. He received his Engineering degree in computer science from the University of Oran 1 Ahmed Ben Bella, Algeria, and his Magister's degree in computer science from the National Polytechnic School of Oran, Algeria. In 2018, he obtained his PhD degree in computer science from Ben Bella Oran1 University, Algeria. From 2007 to 2013, he was a senior Oracle database administrator (DBA) and enterprise resource planning (ERP) manager. He has over 20 years of programming experience in different languages and environments. His research interests include programming languages, artificial intelligence, computer vision, machine learning, and deep learning.

Hamid Abdollahi

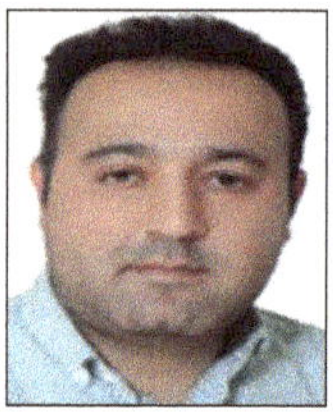

Department of Radiologic Sciences and Medical Physics, Faculty of Allied Medicine, Kerman University of Medical Sciences, Kerman, Iran

Hamid Abdollahi received his PhD degrees in Medical Physics at the Iran University of Medical Sciences (IUMS) and currently works at the Department of Radiologic Sciences and Medical Physics, Faculty of Allied Medicine, Kerman University of Medical Sciences, Kerman, Iran

Maryam Ahmadi

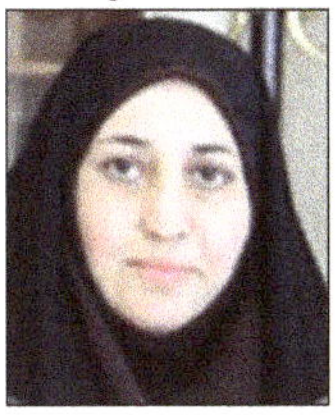

Department of Health Information Management, School of Health Management and Information Sciences, Iran University of Medical Sciences, Tehran, Iran

Maryam Ahmadi received her MS and PhD degrees in Health Information Technology at the Iran University of Medical Sciences (IUMS) and is currently a faculty member at the Department of Health Information Management, School of Health Management and Information Sciences, Iran University of Medical Sciences, Tehran, Iran

Mugahed A Al-antari

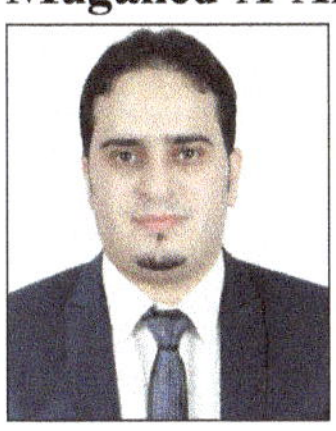

Department of Computer Science and Engineering, College of Software, Kyung Hee University, Gyeonggi-do 17104, Republic of Korea
Department of Biomedical Engineering, Sana'a Community College, Sana'a, Republic of Yemen

Mugahed A Al-antari received his PhD degree from the Department of Biomedical Engineering, Kyung Hee University, Republic of Korea. Now, Al-antari is a postdoctoral researcher in the Ubiquitous Computing Laboratory (UCLab), Department of Computer Science and Engineering, Kyung Hee University, Republic of Korea. Since 2010, Al-antari has been a lecturer in the Department of Biomedical Engineering at Sana'a Community College, Republic of Yemen. Al-antari has more than five years of professional industrial experience (Executive Engineering Director) developing mini- and whole-body dual-energy X-ray absorptiometry (DXA) machines using dual x-ray pencil and fan beams at the YOZMA BMTech Group, Seoul, Republic of Korea. He has been a member of IEEE Engineering in Medicine and Biology Society since 2014. His current research interests include deep learning, machine learning, artificial intelligence (AI), pattern recognition, medical signal and image processing, and medical imaging using DXA. His recent AI-based publications have earned a lot of attention from researchers as well as international journal editorials and have been selected to represent a cornerstone of modern medicine.

Annesya Banerjee

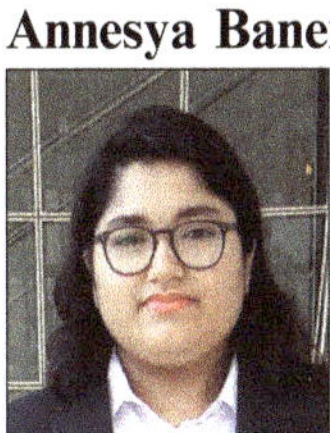

Department of Electronics and Telecommunication Engineering, Jadavpur University, Kolkata, India

Annesya Banerjee received her Bachelor of Engineering (BE) degree in Electronics and Telecommunication Engineering from Jadavpur University, Kolkata, India in 2021 and has recently joined the Speech and Hearing Biosciences and Technology program at Harvard University, Cambridge, MA, USA, to pursue her Doctor of Philosophy (PhD) degree. She served as an Undergraduate Researcher in the Texas Instruments (TI) Innovation Lab at Jadavpur University from 2018 to 2021. Her research interests include biomedical signal (audio) processing, speech analysis, and computational audition and its application in advanced hearing device development. Ms Banerjee has been awarded the Jagadish Bose National Science Talent Search Senior Fellowship and the IEEE Best Outgoing Student (Runner Up) award and is a co-recipient of multiple research grants from the University of California (UC) Berkeley, WeRobotics, and the Department of Telecommunications, Government of India. She also holds the position of co-founder of Jadavpur University (JU) UAV Innovators' Lab.

Geng Chen

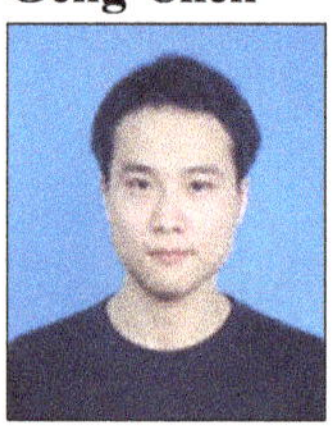

School of Computer Science and Engineering, Northwestern Polytechnical University, China

Geng Chen is a professor at School of Computer Science and Engineering, Northwestern Polytechnical University, China. He received his PhD from Northwestern Polytechnical University, China, in 2016. He was a postdoctoral research associate at the University of North Carolina at Chapel Hill, USA, from 2016 to 2019. He has published more than 50 papers in peer-reviewed international conference proceedings and journals, such as Medical Image Analysis, IEEE Transactions on Medical Imaging, the International Conference on Medical Image Computing and Computer Assisted Intervention (MICCAI), the International Conference on Information Processing In Medical Imaging (IPMI), etc.

Barakat Adeyinka Dawood

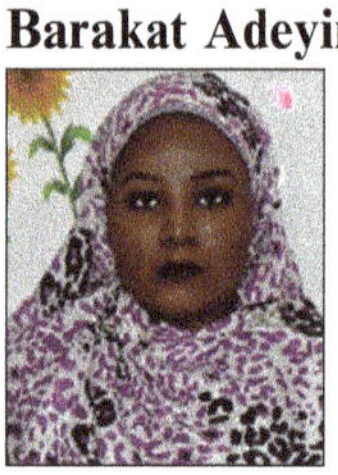

Computer Engineering Department, Research Centre for AI and IoT, Near East University, Nicosia, Mersin 10, Turkey

Barakat Adeyinka Dawood is currently a MSc student at Near East University in the Turkish Republic of Northern Cyprus. She holds a BSc degree in Computer Engineering from Near East University, Turkish Republic of Northern Cyprus, awarded in 2019. She has taken part in several projects and research works. She holds several certifications. She is also a member of the Research Centre for AI and IoT at Near East University in the Turkish Republic of Northern Cyprus.

M Parimala Devi

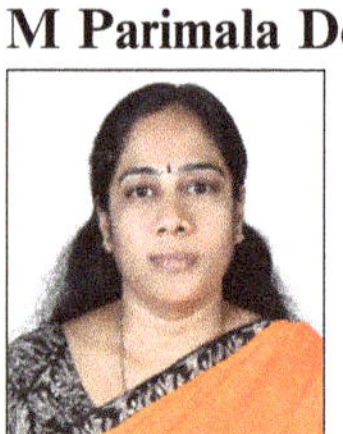

Department of ECE, Velalar College of Engineering and Technology, Erode, Tamil Nadu, India

Dr Parimala Devi M has received a BE (Electronics and Communication) from Bharathiyar University, Coimbatore, an ME (VLSI Design) from Anna University, Chennai, an MBA (Human Resource Management) from Anna University and a PhD (Information and Communication Engineering) from Anna University, Chennai. Currently, she is an Associate Professor in the Velalar College of Engineering and Technology, Erode. She has published 25 papers in national and international journals and conferences. She has been a reviewer for many

SCOPUS-indexed journals and has received Best Paper awards at international conferences. She has published a book 'Advanced Microprocessors and Microcontrollers' via University Science Press, New Delhi. She is a lifetime member of the IETE. Her research interests include VLSI, SoC, IoT, microprocessor-based system design and nanoelectronics.

Deng-ping Fan

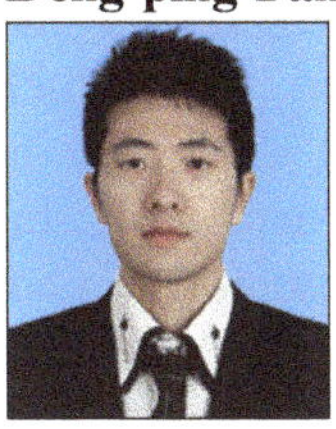

Nankai University, China

Deng-Ping Fan received his PhD degree from Nankai University in 2019. He joined the Inception Institute of AI (IIAI) in 2019. He has about 30 published papers in top journals and conferences, such as CVPR, ICCV, ECCV, etc. His research interests include computer vision and visual attention, in particular, RGB salient object detection (SOD), RGB-D SOD, Video SOD, and Co-SOD. He won the Best Paper Finalist award at IEEE CVPR 2019 and was the Best Paper award nominee at IEEE CVPR 2020.

Huazhu Fu

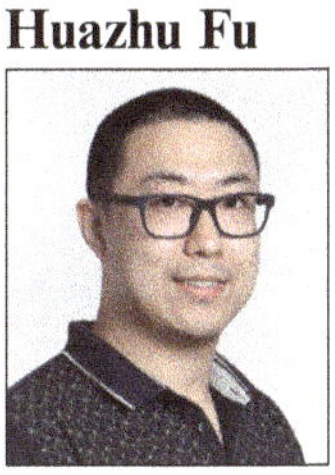

Institute of High Performance Computing, Agency for Science, Technology and Research, Singapore

Huazhu Fu is a Senior Scientist at the Institute of High Performance Computing, Agency for Science, Technology and Research, Singapore. He received his PhD from Tianjin University in 2013, and was a Research Fellow at Nanyang Technological University for two years. From 2015 to 2018, he was a Research Scientist in the Institute for Infocomm Research at the Agency for Science, Technology and Research, Singapore. His research interests include computer vision, machine learning, and medical image analysis. He currently serves as an Associate Editor of IEEE Transactions on Medical Imaging, the IEEE Journal of Biomedical and Health Informatics, and IEEE Access.

V Gowrishankar

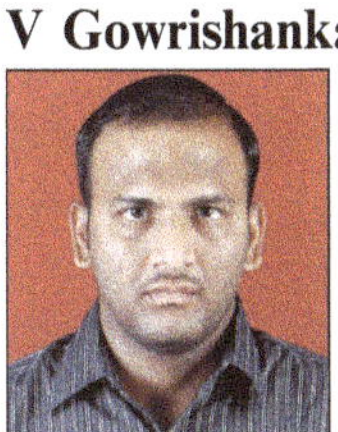

Gowrishankar V received a bachelor degree (BE) in Electronics and Communication Engineering from Anna University, Chennai and a postgraduate degree (ME) in VLSI Design from Anna University, Chennai in 2008 and 2010, respectively. He is now pursuing a PhD at Anna University, Chennai. He has been an Associate Professor at the Department of Electronics and Communication Engineering, Velalar College of Engineering and Technology, Erode, since 2010. His research areas of interest are low-power embedded devices, open-source hardware, the internet of things, wireless sensor networks, low-power systems on a chip, and the optimization of analog-to-digital conversion in deep-submicron technologies. He has authored or co-authored more than 30 journal articles (mostly Scopus-indexed journals) and conference proceedings. He is a lifetime member of the Institution of Electronics and Telecommunication Engineers and Indian Society for Technical Education.

Fouzi Harrou

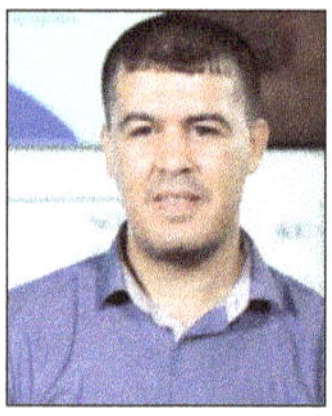

King Abdullah University of Science and Technology (KAUST), Thuwal, Saudi Arabia

Fouzi Harrou received an MSc degree in Telecommunications and Networking from the University of Paris VI, France, and a PhD degree in Systems Optimization and Security from the University of Technology of Troyes (UTT), France. He was an Assistant Professor at UTT for one year and at the Institute of Automotive and Transport Engineering, Nevers, France, for one year. He was also a Postdoctoral Research Associate at the Systems Modeling and Dependability Laboratory, UTT, for one year. He was a Research Scientist at the Chemical Engineering Department, Texas A&M University at Qatar, Doha, Qatar, for three years. He is currently a Research Scientist at the Division of Computer, Electrical and Mathematical Sciences and Engineering, King Abdullah University of Science and Technology, Saudi Arabia. He is a coauthor of the book 'Statistical Process Monitoring Using Advanced Data-Driven and Deep Learning Approaches: Theory and Practical Applications' (Elsevier, 2020). His current research interests include statistical decision theory and its applications, fault detection and diagnosis, and deep learning.

Amira M Hasan

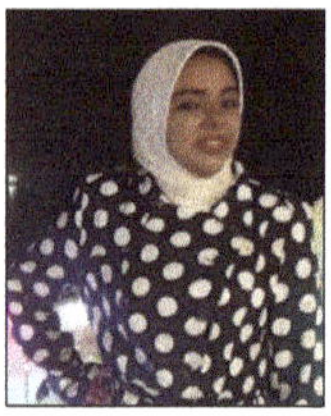

Amira Mohamed Hasan received a BS degree in Electronics and Communications Engineering from Alexandria University, Alexandria, Egypt in 2009. She is an Engineer of Electronics and Communications at the Alexandria Higher Institute of Engineering Technology (AIET), Alexandria, Egypt. Her research interests include signal processing, image processing, data mining, and artificial intelligence.

Mohammad Heydari

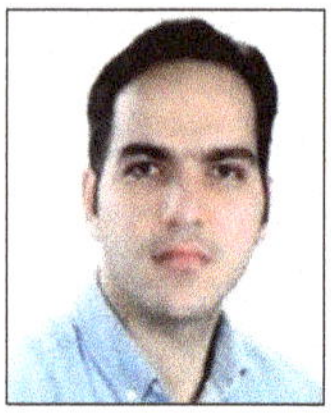

Department of Health Information Technology, Khalkhal University of Medical Sciences, Khalkhal, Iran
Student Research Committee, School of Health Management and Information Sciences Branch, Iran University of Medical Sciences, Tehran, Iran

Mohammad Heydari is currently a faculty member at the Khalkhal University of Medical Science, Department of Health Information Technology. He earned his Bachelor of Computer Engineering degree at the Hamedan University of Technology (HUT) and his Master's degree in Health Information Technology at the Iran University of Medical Sciences (IUMS). For his thesis, he worked on a mobile-based education application for parents of autistic children.

Aya Hossam

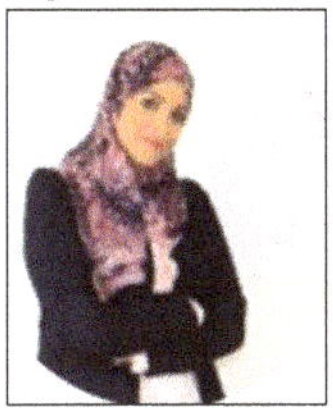

Aya Hossam received BS, MS, and PhD degrees in electronics engineering from Benha University, Cairo, Egypt in 2012, 2015, and 2019, respectively. She is currently an Assistant Professor at the Electronics Branch of the Electrical Engineering Department, Benha University, Cairo, Egypt. Her research interests include the internet of things, signal processing, image processing, acoustic devices, sensor networks, and AI. She received the Best Student award from the President, the Best Student award from the Minister of Higher Education, and the Best Engineer award from the President of the Egyptian Engineers Syndicate.

Cam-Hao Hua

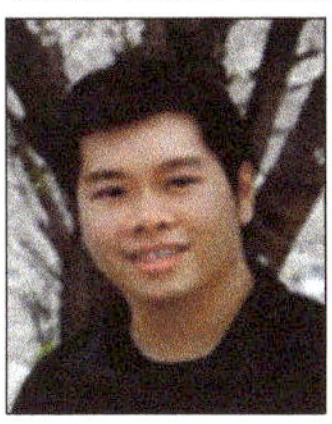

Department of Computer Science and Engineering, College of Software, Kyung Hee University, Gyeonggi-do 17104, Republic of Korea

Cam-Hao Hua received the BS degree in Electrical and Electronic Engineering from Bach Khoa University, Ho Chi Minh City, Vietnam, in 2016. He is currently pursuing a PhD degree at the Department of Computer Science and Engineering, Kyung Hee University, Gyeonggi, Republic of Korea. His research interests are computer vision and deep learning.

Adedoyin Ahmed Hussain

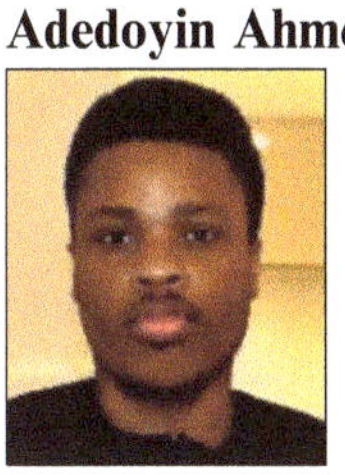

Adedoyin Ahmed Hussain is doing his Ph.D. at Near East University in the Turkish Republic of Northern Cyprus. He holds an MSc. degree in Computer Engineering from Near East University, Turkish Republic of Northern Cyprus, in 2019. He is serving as a reviewer in several notable journals. He is also a member of several notable organizations and journals. He has written several books in various fields of engineering. He has several publications in top journals, conferences, and book chapters, in addition to numerous keynotes talks at flagship venues. He has partaken in several projects and research works. He holds several certifications. He is also a member of the Research Centre for AI and IoT at Near East University in the Turkish Republic of Northern Cyprus and a member of several notable venues.

Meerja Akhil Jabbar

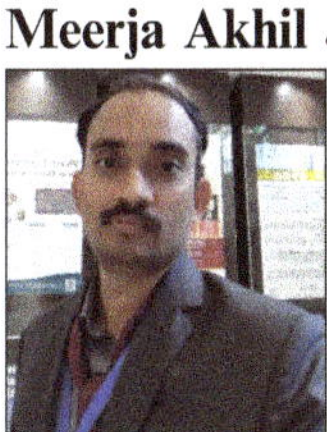

Vardhaman College of Engineering, Hyderabad, India

Dr M A Jabbar is a Professor and Head of the Department of Artificial Intelligence and Machine Learning, Vardhaman College of Engineering, Hyderabad, Telangana, India. He obtained a PhD from Jawaharlal Nehru Technological University, Hyderabad, and Telangana, India. He has been teaching for more than 20 years. His research interests include artificial intelligence, big data analytics, bioinformatics, cyber security, machine learning, attack graphs, and intrusion detection sstems.

He is a senior member of the IEEE, and a lifetime member of professional bodies such as the Computer Society of India (CSI) and the Indian Science Congress Association (ISCA). He is currently serving as the chair of the IEEE CS chapter, Hyderabad section. He is also a member of the Machine Intelligence Research Labs (MIRLABS, USA), USERN (Iran), the Asia Pacific Institute of Science and Engineering (APISE) (Hong Kong), the Internet Society (USA), the Data Science Society (USA), and the Artificial Intelligence and Machine Learning Society of India (AIML), Bangalore.

He has received the Best Faculty Researcher award from the CSI's Mumbai chapter and Fossee Labs IIT Bombay, and has been recognized as an outstanding reviewer by Elsevier; he has also received the Outstanding Leadership award from the IEEE's Hyderabad section. He has published five patents (Indian) in machine learning and allied areas and a book 'Heart Disease Data Classification using Data Mining Techniques', with Lambert Academic Publishing, Mauritius in 2019.

Mohammad (Behdad) Jamshidi

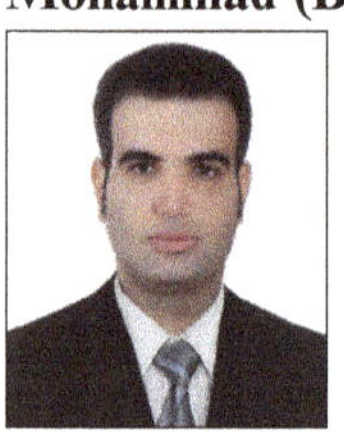

Research and Innovation Centre for Electrical engineering (RICE), University of West Bohemia, Pilsen, Czech Republic

Mohammad (Behdad) Jamshidi received the Associate degree in Electronics from the Shamsipour Technical and Vocational College (former American College), Tehran, Iran, in 2005, the BSc degree in Telecommunication Engineering from the University of Applied Science and Technology, Shiraz, Iran, in 2008, and the MSc degree in Mechatronics Engineering, for which he graduated as the Third Best Student, from Islamic Azad University (IAU), South-Tehran Branch, Tehran, in 2011. He is currently pursuing a PhD at the University of West Bohemia (UWB) in Pilsen, Czech Republic. From 2011 to 2019, he was a Senior Researcher with the Young Researchers and Elite Club, IAU. From 2012 to 2017, he was also a full-time faculty member of the Department of Electrical Engineering, IAU. He has published and presented more than 30 papers in international journals and IEEE conferences. His research interests include complex systems, big data, computational intelligence, artificial intelligence, machine learning, and deep learning. Furthermore, he has received several prestigious awards, such as the Distinguished Researcher Award for the Best Researcher of Engineering Departments at IAU (Kermanshah), second place at the 6th International Robotic Competitions of the International Federation of Robot Sports Association (FIRA), and first place at the National Robotics Open Competition of Kurdistan. He has also taken part in international collaborations with the University of California at Berkeley; Waseda University, Tokyo; Macquarie University, Sydney; and Seoul National University.

Ge-Peng Ji

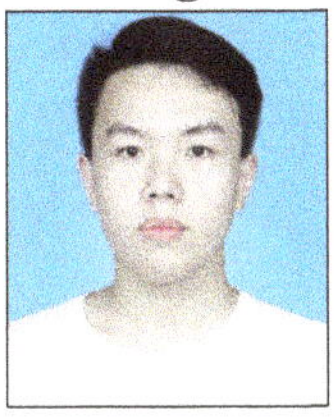

Ge-Peng Ji was born in 1996. He is currently an MS student of Communication and Information Systems at the School of Computer Science, Wuhan University. His research interests lie in the design of deep neural networks and the application of deep learning to various fields of low-level vision, such as RGB salient object detection, RGB-D salient object detection, video salient object detection (VSOD), camouflaged object detection (COD), and medical image segmentation.

Amirali Karimi

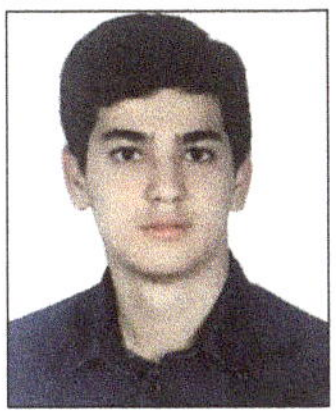

School of medicine, Tehran University of Medical Sciences, Tehran, Iran

Sofiane Khadraoui

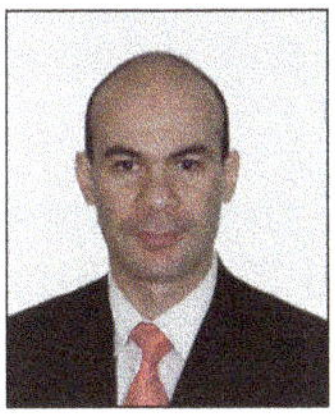

University of Sharjah, Department of Electrical Engineering, Sharjah, UAE

Sofiane Khadraoui received Engineering and Magister degrees in Automatic Control from Abou Bekr Belkaïd University, Algeria, in 2004 and 2007, respectively. In 2012, he was awarded a PhD degree in Automatic Control by the University of Franche-Comté, France. From 2012 to 2015, he was a Postdoctoral Research Associate at Texas A&M University at Qatar. In 2015, he joined the Electrical Engineering department at the University of Sharjah, UAE, where he is currently an assistant Professor. His main research interests include robust control design for uncertain systems, active disturbance rejection control, data-based control design for unknown systems, process monitoring/fault detection and deep learning, compensation for nonlinearities, the modeling of uncertainties, optimization, and interval computation.

Mukesh Kumar

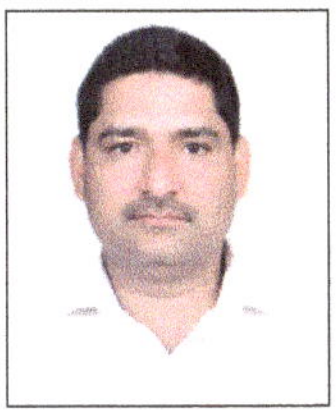

Department of Physics, Swami Shraddhanand College, University of Delhi, New Delhi, India

Dr Mukesh Kumar is an Assistant Professor at the Department of Physics of Swami Shraddhanand College, University of Delhi (SSNC). He has been a CSIR fellow at the University of Delhi. He is actively involved in the fields of science and society, energy and waste, and computational physics. He has published more that 30 research papers and organized various workshop, conferences, and short-term courses. He has been awarded the 'Best Teacher' award by the Government of the National Capital Territory of Delhi. He has also held various administrative positions, such as Examination Supervisor, Solar Project nodal officer, student admission nodal officer, NCC and NSS, etc. Mukesh is not only involved in teaching Physics to his students but is also well-known in the college for his active participation in the organisation of science awareness programs.

David Lee

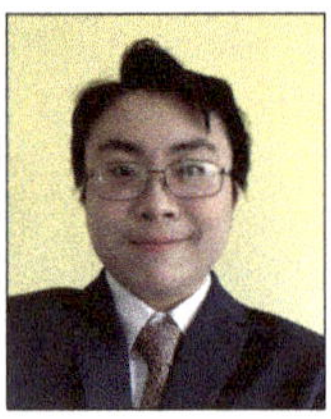

David Lee is a student of the class of 2025 at Boston University and is planning to major in computer science. As an artificial intelligence enthusiast, he is curious about exploring how machine learning can benefit society and how to solve related ethics issues. In 2020, he attended the MIT Beaver Works Summer Institute to study the applications of machine learning and data science in health and medicine. He is a National Merit Finalist and a member of his high school's Student Advisory Committee. Since David was seven, he has been selling his own children's science fiction books and visiting libraries and bookstores to help local young writers achieve their goals. For more information about his community involvement, please visit his website at https://infomages.square.site/

Sungyoung Lee

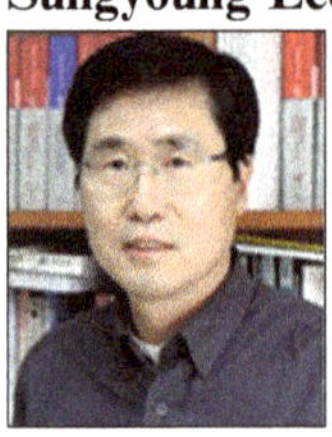

Department of Computer Science and Engineering, College of Software, Kyung Hee University, Gyeonggi-do 17104, Republic of Korea

Sungyoung Lee (M'89) received the BS degree from Korea University, Seoul, Republic of Korea, and the MS and PhD degrees in Computer Science from the Illinois Institute of Technology, Chicago, IL, USA, in 1987 and 1991, respectively. He was an Assistant Professor at the Department of Computer Science, Governors State University, University Park, IL, USA, from 1992 to 1993. He has been a Professor at the Department of Computer Engineering, Kyung Hee University, Republic of Korea, since 1993, where he has been the Director of the Neo Medical ubiquitous-Life Care Information Technology Research Center since 2006. He is currently the Founding Director of the Ubiquitous Computing Laboratory. His current research interests include ubiquitous computing and applications, sensor and ad-hoc wireless networks, context-aware middleware, sensor operating systems, real-time systems, embedded systems, and activity and emotion recognition. He is a member of the ACM.

Andrew Li

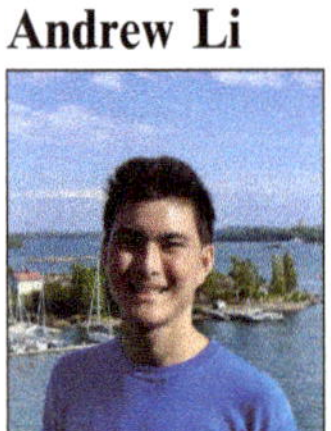

Andrew Li is a student at Harvard College and is interested in economics, computer science, and the life sciences. He attended the Beaver Works Summer Institute of the MIT Lincoln Laboratory to study the application of machine learning to health data and researched the use of digital smartphone contact tracing as a part of the Privated Automated Contact Tracing project. He is a Presidential Scholars candidate and a recipient of the Massachusetts Association of School Superintendents' award for academic excellence. His main interest lies in the intersections and applications of economics, artificial intelligence, and biochemistry to the development of innovative solutions to address critical challenges.

Lakshna Mahajan

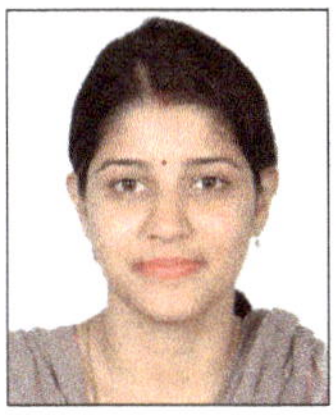

Department of Microbiology, Swami Shraddhanand College, University of Delhi, New Delhi, India

Dr Lakshna Mahajan is a microbiologist working as Assistant Professor at the Swami Shraddhanand College, Delhi University, with research experience in microbiology and cell biology. She has been a Department of Biotechnology (DBT, Govt. of India) Post-Doctorate Fellow at the National Institute of Immunology and holds a PhD from the Institute of Genomics and Integrative Biology, Delhi and M.S. University of Baroda, Vadodara. She is a Review Editor in Molecular Innate Immunity, part of the journal 'Frontiers in Immunology'. She has authored many national and international research publications in refereed journals and chapters of books. Dr Lakshna has also published an international U.S. Patent Cooperation Treaty (PCT) patent as a part of her research work.

Esmaeil Mehraeen

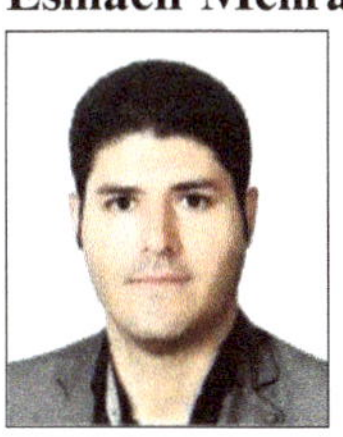

Department of Health Information Technology, Khalkhal University of Medical Sciences, Khalkhal, Iran

Esmaeil Mehraeen received his MS and PhD degrees in Health Information Technology at the Tehran University of Medical Sciences (TUMS). His thesis was on the subject of the design and development of an intelligent mobile-based self-management system for people living with HIV. Dr Mehraeen is currently a faculty member at the Department of Health Information Technology, Khalkhal University of Medical Sciences, Khalkhal, Iran

Kristoff Misquitta

Kristoff Misquitta is an incoming freshman at MIT who blends a strong passion for aerospace with a molecular biology expertise. He has presented research into zero-gravity fluid flow and morphing wing architectures at two national conferences, and inspired by his work at the Beaver Works Institute, he hopes to continue using artificial intelligence to contribute to cutting-edge efforts in the field. Currently, as the winner of the National Genes in Space Contest, he is developing an experiment to test a novel fluorescence-based approach for analyzing drug metabolism in astronauts; it will be launched to the International Space Station in the summer of 2021.

Achal Nilhani

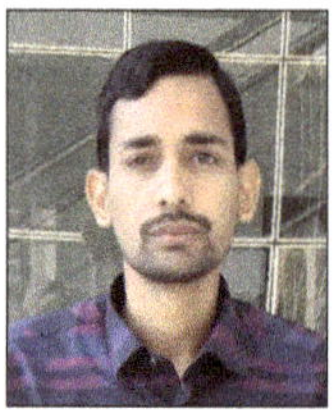

Department of Electronics and Telecommunication Engineering, Jadavpur University, Kolkata, India

Achal Nilhani received his Bachelor of Engineering (BE) degree in Electronics and Telecommunication Engineering from Jadavpur University, Kolkata, India in 2021 and has recently joined the Music and Acoustics Engineering program at Politecnico di Milano, Milan, Italy, to pursue his Master of Science (MS) degree. He has served as an Undergraduate Researcher in the Texas Instruments (TI) Innovation Lab at Jadavpur University from 2018 to 2021. His research interests include spatial audio processing, computational music analysis, machine learning and AI for audio applications, and robot audition. Mr Nilhani is a co-recipient of multiple research Grants from the University of California (UC) Berkeley, WeRobotics, and the Department of Telecommunications, Government of India. He also holds the position of co-founder of Jadavpur University (JU) UAV Innovators' Lab.

Zdeněk Peroutka

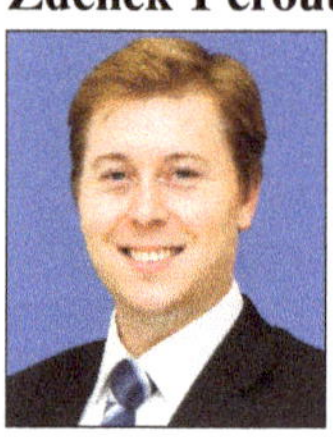

Research and Innovation Centre for Electrical engineering (RICE), University of West Bohemia, Pilsen, Czech Republic
Student Research Committee, School of Health Management and Information Sciences Branch, Iran University of Medical Sciences, Tehran, Iran

Zdeněk Peroutka (Member, IEEE) received his master's and PhD degrees in Electrical Engineering from the University of West Bohemia (UWB), Pilsen, Czech Republic, in 2000 and 2004, respectively. From October 2010 to June 2016, he was the Scientific Director and a Principal Investigator of the Research and Development Center, RICE, UWB. He is currently a full Professor of power electronics and drives and the Dean of the Faculty of Electrical Engineering, UWB. Since July 2016, he has been the CEO and a Principal Investigator of the Research and Development Center, RICE. He has published more than 200 papers in international journals and conference proceedings. He is the owner of three international patents and three utility models. His main research interests include power electronics and drives for modern transport systems and power engineering. He is a member of the European Power Electronics and Drives (EPE) Association. He has received several national and international awards, for example, the Best Paper awards from the EPE Power Electronics and Motion Control (PEMC) 2006, Electrical Drives and Power Electronics 2007, and EPE-PEMC 2010 conferences.

Nitin K Puri

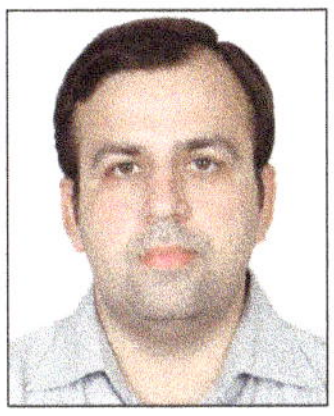

Department of Applied Physics, Delhi Technological University, New Delhi, India

Dr Nitin Kumar Puri is Professor in the Department of Applied Physics at Delhi Technological University (DTU). His research work includes accelerator-based atomic physics and experimental materials science (nanotechnology, sensors, and biosensors). Dr Nitin has more than 100 published research articles in various journals and in conferences of national and international repute. He has been granted sponsorship for research projects by the SERB, Department of Science and Technology (DST), Govt. of India; DAE-BRNS, Govt of India; and the Inter-University Accelerator Centre (IUAC), UGC Delhi. Dr Nitin has held the positions of Chairman and Vice Chairman of the International Nuclear Security Education Network (INSEN) at the International Atomic Energy Authority (IAEA), Vienna. He has been awarded Radiological Officer Level 1 by the Atomic Energy Regulatory Board, Bhabha Atomic Research Centre.

G Boothpathi Raja

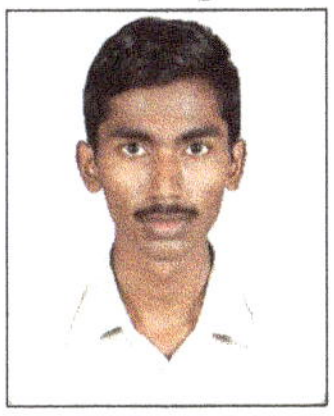

Mr Raha G Boopathi received his BE (Electronics and Communication Engineering) from the Anna University of Technology, Coimbatore, and his ME (Applied Electronics) from Anna University, Chennai. Currently, he is an Assistant Professor in the Velalar College of Engineering and Technology, Erode. He has published ten papers in national and international journals and conferences. He is a lifetime member of the Institution of Electronics and Telecommunication Engineers. His research interests include VLSI design, medical electronics and signal processing.

Syed Saba Raoof

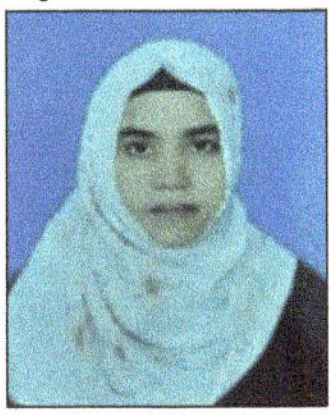

Vellore Institute of Technology, Vellore, India

Syed Saba Raoof is a Research Scholar in Computer Science and Engineering at the Vellore Institute of Technology, Vellore, India. Her research interests include machine learning, medical imaging, the internet of things, and artificial intelligence.

T Sathya

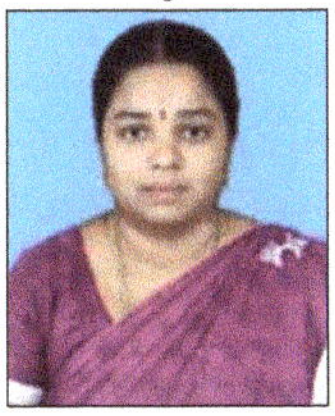

Ms T Sathya received her BE (Electronics and Instrumentation Engineering) and ME (Applied Electronics) from Anna University, Chennai. She is currently an Assistant Professor in the Department of Electronics and Communication Engineering, Velalar College of Engineering and Technology, Erode. She has published six papers in national and international journals and conferences. She has received Best Paper awards at international conferences. She is a lifetime member of the ISSE. She authored a book titled Fundamentals of Electric Circuits and Electronic Devices, which was published in 2018. Her areas of interest include circuit theory, signal and image processing, and sensor measurements and instrumentation.

Ling Shao

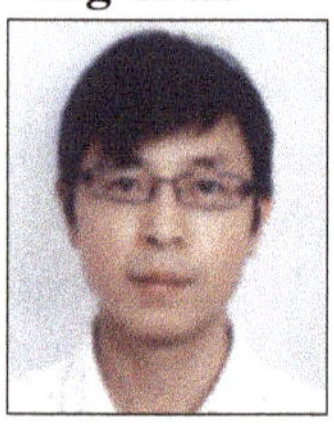

Inception Institute of Artificial Intelligence (IIAI), Abu Dhabi, United Arab Emirates

Ling Shao is currently the CEO and the Chief Scientist of the Inception Institute of Artificial Intelligence, Abu Dhabi, United Arab Emirates. His current research interests include computer vision, machine learning, and medical imaging. Dr Shao is a fellow of the IAPR, the IET, and the BCS. He is an Associate Editor of IEEE Transactions on Image Processing, IEEE Transactions on Neural Networks and Learning Systems, and several other top journals.

Sonia Sharma

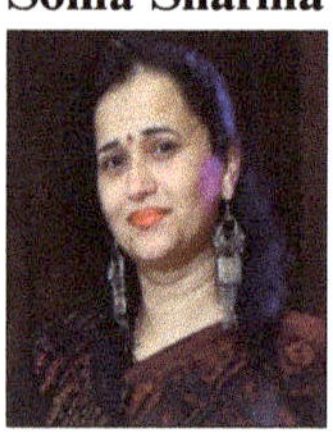

Ms Sonia Sharma is presently working as an Assistant Professor of Computer Science at Hindu Girls College, Jagadhri, Haryana (India). She has presented research papers at national and international conferences and has also chaired sessions at conferences and seminars. Her research interests include: data mining, ICT, and e-governance. Her competency is reflected by the books she has authored and co-authored. She has been the editor of a book on ubiquitous computing and more recently the author of a book on e-commerce for undergraduate and postgraduate students. She is often invited to attend different colleges and universities to give motivational and subject-related talks. She has successfully organized six DGHE/UGC/ICSSR-sponsored national seminars and motivational and technical workshops.

Ying Sun

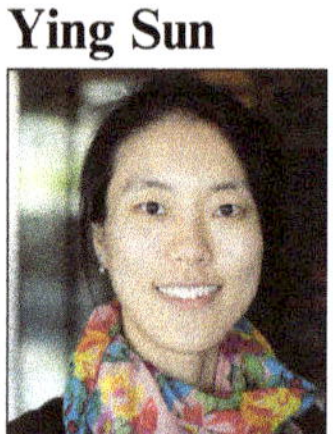

King Abdullah University of Science and Technology (KAUST), Thuwal, Saudi Arabia

Ying Sun received a PhD degree in statistics from Texas A&M, in 2011. She held a two-year postdoctoral research position at the Statistical and Applied Mathematical Sciences Institute and the University of Chicago. She was an Assistant Professor with Ohio State University for a year before joining KAUST in 2014. At KAUST, she established and leads the Environmental Statistics research group, which develops statistical models and methods for complex data to address important environmental problems. She has made original contributions to environmental statistics, in particular, in the areas of spatiotemporal statistics, functional data analysis, visualization, and computational statistics using an exceptionally broad array of applications. She has received two prestigious awards: the Early Investigator Award in Environmental Statistics presented by the American Statistical Association and the Abdel El-Shaarawi Young Research Award from The International Environmetrics Society.

Jakub Talla

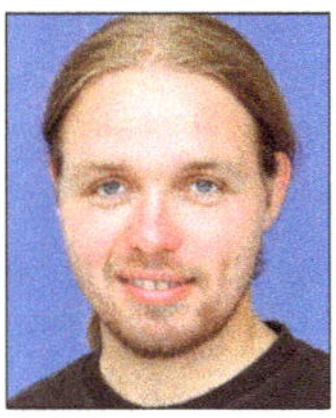

Research and Innovation Centre for Electrical engineering (RICE), University of West Bohemia, Pilsen, Czech Republic

Jakub Talla received his MS and PhD degrees in Electrical Engineering from the University of West Bohemia (UWB), Pilsen, Czech Republic, in 2006 and 2013, respectively. Since October 2010, he has been a Research and Development Engineer with the Regional Innovation Centre for Electrical Engineering (RICE), UWB. His main research interests include the control of AC drives and grid-connected converters, predictive control, power management methods, and soft computing techniques.

Kaiji Uno

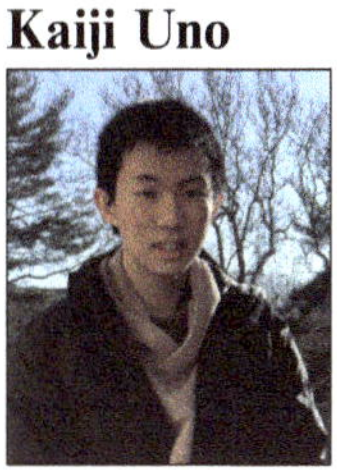

Kaiji Uno is a student at Brookline High School with an interest in mathematics. His curiosity extends to many fields of applied math, such as finance, blockchain technology, and machine learning. He conducts passion projects in algorithmic trading, coding and testing various strategies to make profits on a market simulator. He attended the Beaver Works Summer Institute of the MIT Lincoln Laboratory to study the applications of artificial intelligence and data science in health and medicine. In the future, he wishes to combine his interests to develop products that can create disruptive innovations.

Sasha Wald

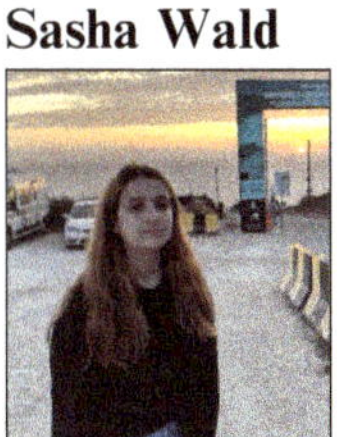

Sasha Wald is a student at the School of Computer Science at Carnegie Mellon University, class of 2025. She is interested in machine learning and computational biology. She attended the Beaver Works Summer Institute in 2020 to study applications of machine learning and data science in medicine. She is a National Merit Finalist and is an active leader in her school's chapter of the American Red Cross. In the future, she hopes to continue exploring the interactions between computer science and medical technology, and hopes to major in computational biology.

Tao Zhou

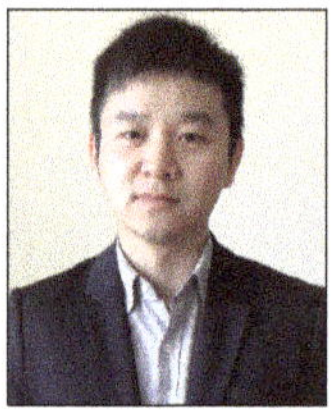

School of Computer Science and Engineering, Nanjing University of Science and Technology, China

Tao Zhou is currently a Professor at the School of Computer Science and Engineering, Nanjing University of Science and Technology, China. He received a PhD degree in Pattern Recognition and Intelligent Systems from the Institute of Image Processing and Pattern Recognition, Shanghai Jiao Tong University, in 2016. From 2016 to 2018, he was a Postdoctoral Fellow at the BRIC and IDEA labs, University of North Carolina at Chapel Hill (UNC-CH), USA. From 2018 to 2020, he was a Research Scientist at the Inception Institute of Artificial Intelligence (IIAI), Abu Dhabi, UAE. His research interests include machine learning, computer vision, and medical image analysis.

IOP Publishing

Artificial Intelligence Strategies for Analyzing COVID-19 Pneumonia Lung Imaging, Volume 1
Characterization approaches
Ayman El-Baz and Jasjit S Suri

Chapter 1

Applying deep learning and emerging technologies in combating COVID-19

Adedoyin A Hussain and Barakat A Dawood

COVID-19 has caused remarkable emergencies in the fields of health and finance. Innovative responses have been basic, given restricted assets and the urgent requirement for clinical supplies, medical services, and therapies. As the world continues to experience the COVID-19 pandemic, deep learning and emerging technologies have a significant task, which is to create an efficient solution. The point of this review is to provide an overview and to summarise and classify the utilization of deep learning and emerging technologies used to help study, diagnose, and combat COVID-19. From the dissemination of data about COVID-19 to infection protection, infection location, and treatment, emerging technologies have been of enormous support and assistance. The primary spotlight is on the uses of deep learning and its techniques and the utilization of emerging technologies, such as 'the cloud', 5G, and big data. These help in the battle against COVID-19 and offer ways to progress this fight. We further offer a point-by-point discussion of how the utilization of these innovations can be of great assistance in battling diverse related diseases. We also survey the difficulties, features, and identified issues with finding lasting solutions. This survey concludes by discussing the requirement for coordinated effort in mainstream research using open information sharing, expertise, and tools. This book will give trained professionals and analysts new information about the way in which deep learning and emerging technologies can be used to improve the COVID-19 situation and drive further assessments with the objective of ending the flare-up of the infection. The investigated techniques described allow clinical information to be examined with an accuracy of up to 90%.

doi:10.1088/978-0-7503-3795-3ch1

1.1 Introduction

A few viral pandemics, for example, SARS-CoV and H1N1 flu have emerged in recent years. Viral infections continue to emerge and represent a critical general medical issue recognised by the World Health Organization (WHO), as shown in figure 1.1. Fairly recently, Middle East respiratory syndrome coronavirus (MERS-CoV) in the Middle East was first recognized in Saudi Arabia [1]. Severe acute respiratory syndrome coronavirus 2 (SARS-CoV-2) assaults the respiratory framework in a similar way to a flu infection, causing symptoms of, for example, fever and breathlessness. COVID-19 is a respiratory illness brought about by SARS-CoV-2, an infectious disease that is a member of a group of positive-sense, single-stranded RNA infections known as Coronaviridae. In spite of the fact that the specific origin of the infection is debatable, researchers have mapped the SARS-CoV-2 genome and classified it as one from the CoV genera which are generally spread by bats and rodents [2]. COVID-19 has propagated quickly everywhere in the world, appearing in almost all nations and states [3]. In December 2019, COVID-19 was first recorded as affecting human existence in Wuhan, a city in China. Coronavirus is an irresistible disease. While it was first found in China, it is currently a pandemic [4, 5]. The known signs and manifestations of an infected patient are respiratory problems which might actually prompt deadly conditions like SARS [6]. It moves from one individual to another by means of patient coughs [7]. As a novel disease, there is still much that medical science does not know about this infection. At the moment, there is no specific antibody or medication that can be used for COVID-19 treatment. Up until this point, millions have been infected worldwide; some have recuperated, while others have passed on. The early detection of the infection and a fast reaction are the correct actions agreed on so far to keep the infection from spreading and to address the cases. Steady medical care has been the essential treatment, and it has kept a few patients from complications and demise [8].

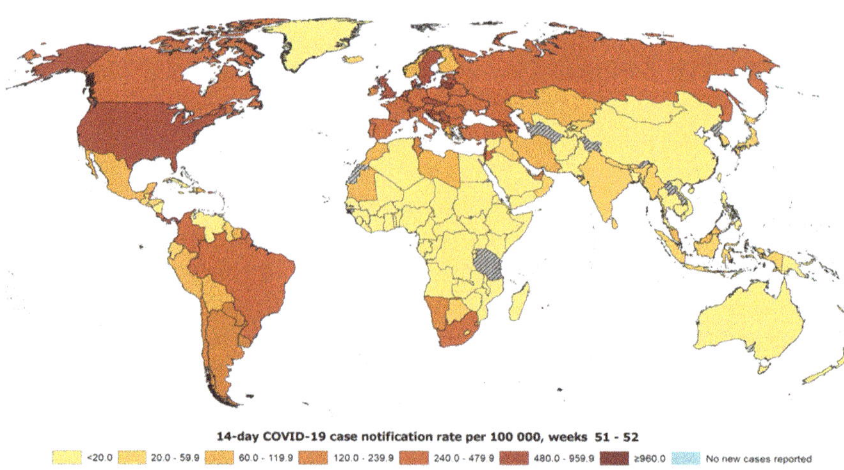

Figure 1.1. Worldwide statistics for COVID-19 cases [10]. Copyright ECDC (2005–2021).

At the pinnacle of the emergency, to all intents and purposes, the administration of each country forced a lockdown. The pandemic has influenced all parts of daily life, causing a phenomenal worldwide financial decline. Lockdown was the strategy adopted to stop the spread of the infection and to contain it. Lockdown and physical containment functioned admirably in forestalling the spread of the infection, yet there is a cost to pay. It was not palatable for billions of individuals, but they were required to remain inside, practice physical separating, and innovate to adjust to the 'new normal'. The world economy will endure, on the grounds that lockdown will not just prompt a worldwide downturn, as experienced in the past; it could, however, cause a worldwide monetary loss of momentum. The continuation of lockdown implies keeping numerous individuals out of their occupations and leaving them with almost no income for themselves and their families. Because of this turn of events, we have two choices: either to proceed with lockdown and starve to death or to open up the economy and face the pandemic. The day the infection was proclaimed a pandemic, the WHO's director-general plotted four key zones for urgent global activities against infection: plan and be prepared, ensure and treat, and develop and learn [9]. Indeed, no country will proceed with lockdown due to its serious impacts on the general public; however, the recovery of any economy will critically rely on mass testing for infection, tracing people who have had contact with infected patients, and treating them. Coronavirus has come to stay. We should simply acknowledge its reality in our midst as an undetectable adversary and battle and contain it by utilizing smart innovations. We have no other choice than to acknowledge it and live with it, in much the same way as for other known infections that were present before COVID-19.

At the pinnacle of the worldwide lockdown and in keeping with physical separation, individuals had no other option than to resort to computerized innovation for the entirety of their human communications. We became inseparable from our cell phones, cushions, PCs, and TVs for our communication with the rest of the world. Innovation remained in the frame and assumed an essential role. Applications that offer video gatherings, such as Skype, Facebook, and WhatsApp became our mode of communication. Robots were utilized by law enforcement offices for checking. Self-driving vehicles became the means through which things were conveyed to individuals. As certain nations and locales open for human activity in a return to routine, our typical lifestyle will now not be the same as before, as this irresistible infection will completely modify our standard lifestyle. This chapter discusses the advanced mechanical methodology being used to combat this harmful and profoundly infectious disease. The pandemic has brought a defining moment that will accelerate disruptive technology.

1.1.1 Comparison to other surveys

In the months after the COVID-19 flare-up, a few papers were published that analyzed the different roles of the internet of things (IoT) in the battle against COVID-19 [11]. Coronavirus' exceptional pandemic has caused various researchers, clinicians, labs, and associations around the globe to engage with an enormous scope of work to help in the creation of antibodies and different treatment techniques. The insight provided by the Determination and Treatment Assistant Program (nCapp) helped in the treatment and management of patients suffering from COVID-19; nCapp knowledge helped self-prevention, and applying nCapp knowledge helped organization in finding and treatment of COVID-19.

The authors of study [12] identified the different uses of COVID-19 intelligence. The authors of [13] recognized the effect of the pandemic on the worldwide economy in their exploration; they identified its effects in numerous financial areas, for example, oil and gas, flight, cars, medical care, media transmission, and others. The authors of [14] created ongoing gauges and evaluated the danger of novel Covid cases. Likewise, the authors of [15] discussed the effects of IoT usage in diminishing medical care cost and improving the therapy results for infected patients and portrayed the utilization of 'industry 4.0' advances and the utilization of blockchain innovation in the battle against COVID-19. They evaluated the danger of the novel COVID-19 for certain profoundly affected nations by displaying explicit specific segment attributes of these nations alongside different qualities of the sickness. The authors' forecast of things to come proposes the utilization of IoT gadgets as an early warning framework to support the precise allocation of medical care assets. The authors of [16] discuss an intelligent damp-observing framework for pernicious infection prevention. The authors present a crossover approach that depends on an autoregressive incorporated moving-normal model and a wavelet-based gauging model to tackle the primary issue of producing transient figures for the quantity of cases revealed daily for several nations. The air conditioning is likewise constrained by the framework and the humidifier in the space keeps the ideal degree of humidity somewhere in the range between 45 and 55%. The creators thought about the valuable impacts of damp protection, and a sensor-based IoT module was created which monitors the relative room temperature and the status changes of occupants of the room.

This underlines the need to discover the difficulties experienced and create proposals for development. In this chapter, we also attempt to recognize solutions crafted by certain nations that have used the IoT in the battle against COVID-19. Table 1.1 shows a comparison between this work and other published works.

Table 1.1. Comparison to other works.

Reference	Big data	AI	Deep learning	Durability	Robustness	Scalability
[11]		✓		✓	✓	
[12]		✓		✓	✓	
[13]	✓	✓	✓		✓	
[14]			✓	✓		
[15]	✓	✓		✓	✓	
[16]		✓	✓		✓	✓
Our survey	✓	✓	✓	✓	✓	✓

1.1.2 Scope of the survey

The scope of the survey addresses the way in which advanced innovation and the IoT have been used in the battle against irresistible illnesses. This study audits past examinations of the utilization of emerging innovations in the medical care framework. It assesses how intelligent frameworks can be used to address the WHO's four key activity zones for containing SARS-CoV-2, the infection that causes COVID-19 [17], as shown in figure 1.2. As it is a profoundly infectious disease, physical separation is fundamental; however, medical care workers have to care for infected patients. This part plots and completely reveals the essential ways to deal with, battle, and contain the pandemic. This is the place where an intelligent and connected public health framework assumes a significant role. This section inspects the different emerging advancements that can be utilized to battle and contain the irresistible sickness and furthermore examines their rapidity and organisation. These are helpful in health services due to their adaptability of use, high accuracy, and their ability to perform nonstop patient checking.

Healthcare workers are overextended due to the inundation of individuals looking for clinical care. The COVID-19 pandemic has overloaded emergency clinics. How might they adapt to different patients who were under their consideration before the pandemic, and whose ailments cannot tolerate this novel infection? Deep learning and emerging technologies proffer arrangements that will take the heat off exhausted medical care providers. Must people with medical issues really be present in clinics before they will be taken care of? This survey researches the deep learning and emerging technologies that can be applied in dialling down the work strain on clinical professionals. This issue is addressed by the use of different intelligent frameworks, which require remote wellbeing checking, in-home help, intelligent nursing homes, wireless body area networks (WBANs), and telemedicine

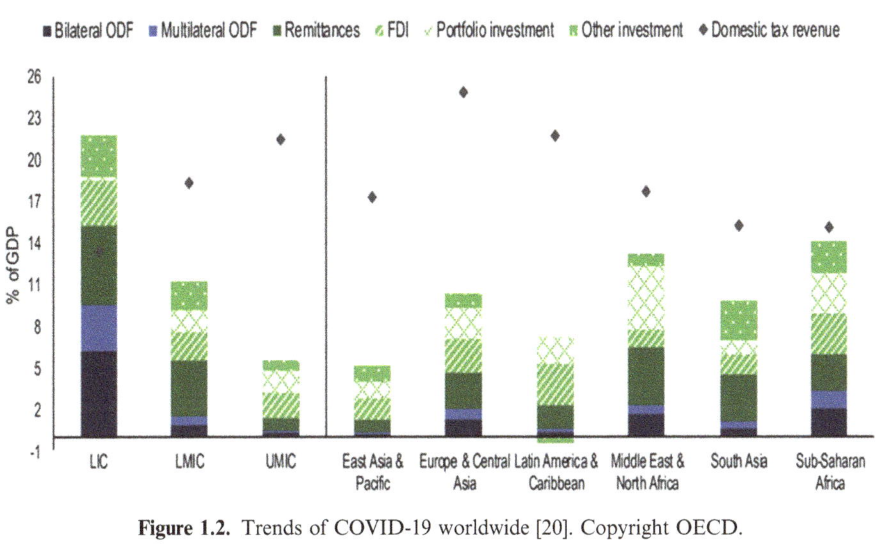

Figure 1.2. Trends of COVID-19 worldwide [20]. Copyright OECD.

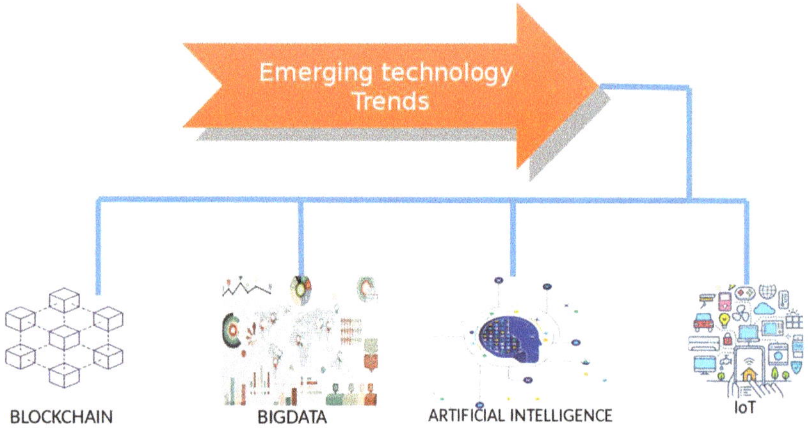

Figure 1.3. Emerging technology trends.

[18, 19]. Several emerging technologies are portrayed in figure 1.3. The emerging technologies we will discuss are 'the cloud', 5G, and big data.

In a similar way, our commitment can be depicted as follows:

- This study outlines a wide and fruitful review of deep learning and emerging technologies used to fight COVID-19.
- We propose suitable strategies for the use of these technologies against COVID-19.
- The progress of these advances against COVID-19 is described.
- The motivations for utilizing these technologies against COVID-19 are discussed.
- The identified issues and challenges of deep learning and emerging technologies are discussed.
- Finally, we discuss open research issues and challenges.

This chapter is organised as follows. In section 1.2, we present vital data on battling COVID-19 with deep learning and discuss the fundamental motivations driving the use of deep learning. The use of deep learning strategies, 'the cloud', 5G, and big data in engaging the COVID-19 pandemic, for instance, in detecting infected patients, following the COVID-19 progression, performing drug investigations, and improving clinical treatment, are assessed and summarized in sections 1.3, 1.4, 1.5, and 1.6 in like manner. Section 1.7 highlights the issues and proposals acquired from this chapter, including challenges that will be clarified later on. Ultimately, section 1.8 offers conclusions. Table 1.2 gives a summary of the abbreviations used and their importance.

1.2 Deep learning and COVID-19

Since the rise of the pandemic, there has been a scramble to use and examine deep learning and other data insight techniques [21]. The use of deep learning can be

Table 1.2. Abbreviations used.

Terms	Meaning
PC	Personal computer
NN	Neural networks
WHO	World Health Organisation
SNN	Siamese neural system
CDC	Centers for Disease Control
ML	Machine learning
IoMT	Internet of medical things
CNN	Convolutional neural system
CT	Computed tomography
DL	Deep learning
WBAN	Wireless body area network
AI	Artificial intelligence
IoT	Internet of things
NHIA	National Health Insurance Administration
CNN	Convolutional neural network

important to see, analyse, predict, and explain COVID-19, and to help to establish the financial impacts. It allows conclusions to be drawn from a rapidly expanding discussion and it also allows a huge assortment of information to be amassed for research, clinical strategy, and clinical assessment. Improving deep learning, quite possibly the most promising logical data apparatus, to help decrease its weaknesses, is of great interest at the moment. The cost of the COVID-19 pandemic, notwithstanding lives and monetary damage, will be horrendous if deep learning is not eventually realized. Reassuringly, data analysts have reacted to the call. The use of deep learning is hampered by a lack of data, and by an excess of erroneous and irregular data. In fact, deep learning has not yet been a viable for use against COVID-19. It is unthinkable that these techniques would, in general, be of much help during the current pandemic. Achieving these goals requires a mindful coexistence between data security and overall clinical concerns and progressively more intensive deep learning. The correlation of logical data on overwhelming infections may be central to saving lives and restricting the financial damage inflicted by lockdown guidelines. Or maybe, deep learning may assist with the pandemic. The authors of [21] prescribed deep learning to follow and to anticipate how the COVID-19 illness can spread after some time and over space. Models, for instance, ought to be rearranged using data from the COVID-19 pandemic. For example, following a previous pandemic similar to the Zika virus, an incredible neural framework was made to visualize its spread. Various institutions proposed the use of computation to foresee an intermittent pipe, which are today being rearranged to use new data from COVID-19. This is apparently happening now. The authors of [21] state that the deep learning system can quickly and consistently classify chest x-rays of COVID-19 patients by identifying sporadic pneumonia, which could help to quicken investigations in the midst of an advancing pandemic. Such systems are, moreover, precise 92% of the time, rather than the 90% rate achieved by trained human professionals. In any case, these learning structures have characterized the disease precisely 87% of the time it appeared differently, compared to human specialists. The authors of [22] proposed an advantageous examination and triaging approach for patients under investigation that can be fundamental to the control of increasing powerful infections, for example, the current COVID-19. In this examination approach, the creators had the option of developing a deep learning program by analysing specialist computed tomography (CT) images using a deep-learning-based procedure. Due to the limitation of nucleic-destruction-based examinations, there is a pressing need to look for rapid elective strategies that can be used by front-line human administration personnel to quickly and decisively diagnose the disease. In the following paragraphs, we sum up the application regions in which deep learning can add to the battle against COVID-19:

- Early treatment and medicines.
- Early COVID-19 expectations and follow up.
- Early alarms and warnings against COVID-19.
- Early predictions and findings.
- Social control.

In the examination of clinical images, deep learning calculations can sort, recognize, and list the attributes of sicknesses. This is based on deep learning calculations using large information sets. It additionally permits the expansion of hypothetical targets and makes predictive treatment plans for patients. A representation of the utilization of deep learning is depicted in figure 1.4. By applying a deep learning calculation, for example, a CNN can help the experts to select the best treatment plan. In the area of clinical tasks, the total utilization of these big data innovations would fundamentally

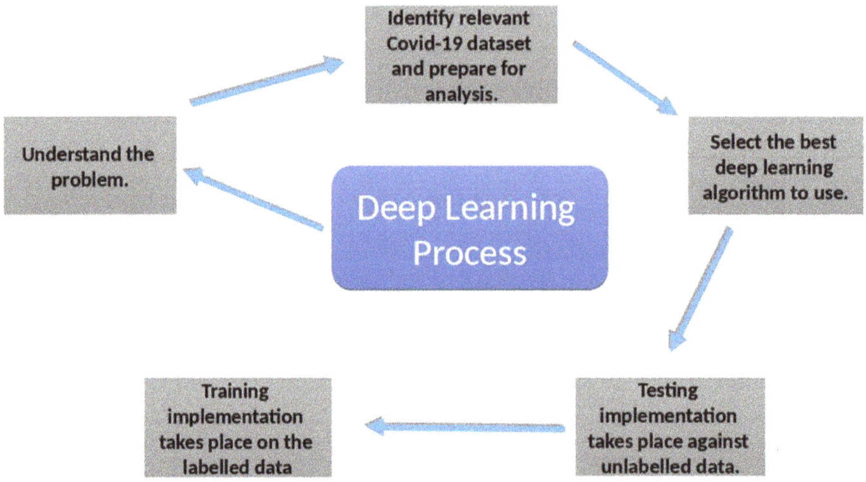

Figure 1.4. Deep learning working process.

decrease current clinical costs. The authors in [22] described their discoveries for the location of strabismus utilizing CNNs. Following preparation with a few gaze deviation (GaDe) pictures, the CNN model was effective in distinguishing strabismus. A CNN model has been prepared that depends on an assortment of information assembled by an eye-movement tracker, including visual information from both ordinary and strabismus dreams while considering deviations in viewing (GaDe). The rising IoMT worldview, which depends on intelligent clinical frameworks, can likewise consistently detect huge human medical problems. Scourge infections can likewise be followed and avoided by incorporating the information gathered with the IoMT sensors and the data acquired from the related wellbeing framework [22]. In this worldview, robots can give assistance to older and impaired individuals by means of their intelligent homes and mechanical helpers.

1.3 Deep learning methods used for the detection of COVID-19

The rapid improvement of present-day detection offers an opening for deep learning to provide a way to create neural frameworks with a colossal number of fragmented layers, which can be infeasible for old-style neural frameworks. This procedure is a high-level expansion of the old-style neural framework strategy. One can consider it to be a neural framework with various layers. In that limit, this methodology analyses logically complex nonlinear models in the data. Also, a bigger piece of this strategy is actualized in image examination, which appears promising, considering that photos normally require huge capacity. Another reason for the noticeable progress in the quality of the procedure results from an increase in the volume and the multifaceted nature of data [23]. Convolutional neural networks are often used in a clinical setting, but in addition neural discontinuous frameworks, deep neural frameworks, and even deep convection frameworks are also used. An interesting observation concerning the old-style neural framework is that its learning utilizes progressively covered layers; therefore its assessments may overlook convoluted information comprising different structures [24]. Usually, deep learning estimations are expected to explore data for which the number of characteristics is nearly zero. This model was developed after considering the insufficiency of the customary AI estimations when dealing with high-dimensional data, in other words, data containing a colossal number of characteristics. Image data are regularly high-dimensional, considering the fact that each image usually contains a considerable number of pixels which are the qualities. However, heuristic ‘component decision’ techniques may miss information in the photos. One of the possible courses of action is to perform an estimation reduction. First, make a preselection of a subset of the pixels as features; then, play out the deep learning counts with the resulting lower-dimensional features. The CNN model was first advanced and upheld for a high-dimensional image examination by the authors of [25]. This model now moves the considered pixel in regards to the image by weighting the convolution sections and likewise reviewing the subsampling fragments. The requirements for the model are normalized proper pixel views with respect to the picture. At long last, the yield will reach a recursive limit due to the weighted data views. The use of this model has been associated with notable programming groups [26] and TensorFlow [27]. Heaps are set up to restrict the ordinary errors in the midst of the results and assumptions. Starting recently, this respected model has been viably used in clinical areas to assist in disease detection. The model yields a precision of more than 91% in detection and proposing medicines. In [28], it was used to investigate intrinsic cascade infirmity by learning visual images. Its abilities to successfully detect underlying wounds and benign bruises are both over 90%, which justify the predominant introduction of this model. In [29], it was used to detect skin sickness using clinical images. In [30], it was applied to recognize diabetic referable retinopathy using an immense volume of fundus retinal photographs. The performance of this model compared to that of experienced specialists with respect to its precision in distinguishing both normal and diseased cases justifies referring to all of these uses. In terms of affectability, the distinction made by the estimation is likewise also more than 90%; this shows the feasibility of using this framework on diabetes. The use of deep learning for the COVID-19 pandemic has been of substantial interest recently. Clinical affiliations are a critical prerequisite for dynamic advances in the management of this virus and they help them to get suitable and logical proposals to contain the spread. This development requires a critical task, which is to distinguish a collection of cases, to foresee where this infection may have a later impact due to social mixing, and to analyse each and every piece of existing data. Deep learning has the ability to imitate parts of human knowledge. CT has now become a fast technique for deciding which patients have COVID-19. It can, moreover, include a basic task of viewing and suggesting the progression of a vaccine for COVID-19 [31]. However, the introduction of radiologists into the battle against COVID-19 has been moderate. An exploratory community test is the current mechanical assembly; it requires time, it drives critical costs, and needs a reliable and available lab for assessment [32]. In the same way, additional assessments are required to improve the initial diagnosis of COVID-19. Table 1.3 shows the usage of these models in the battle against the coronavirus. The subsections beneath the table discuss the related AI techniques which help to overcome the previously mentioned difficulties.

Table 1.3. Deep learning performance in the detection of COVID-19.

Model	ACC	Data size
3D UNet++	99.1%	Rotation
ResNet-50	99.1%	CT
SqueezeNet	98.3%	Random clipping
Bayesian Optimization	98.3%	
DenseNet121	85%	
Randiomic features	82%	
FPN	85%	
CNN	99%	31%

1.3.1 Feature-based deep learning methods

The authors of [33] incorporated extraction and later arranged these characteristics using support vector machines with architectures such as AlexNet and VGGNet. This assessment shows that merged features for sore assumptions beat the characteristics of all of the deep learning models. In a similar way, the makers consolidated isolated features for skin sore affirmation. The results demonstrated that interweaving manual processes and deep learning features gave higher accuracy in the images. In [34], the same process was used with different parts of images to demonstrate highlights of CT imaging of the novel coronavirus. The procedure divided the skin image into seven directional Gabor bands and subsequently showed all of the depictions using deep learning approaches such as AlexNet. In [35], to provide a way to see dangerous melanomas and seborrheic keratosis skin wounds, the creators proposed deep learning that depended on Gabor wavelets. Their assessment demonstrated that COVID-19 generally shows up on CT images as separate ground-glass and consolidative aspiratory opacities. The experts similarly saw that lung cavitation, discrete pneumonic handles, pleural discharges, and lymphadenopathy were commonly absent in occurrences of COVID-19. Nodular opacities, disordered clearing plans, and a periphery dispersal of sickness may be additional features in the early stages.

1.3.2 Ensemble deep learning strategies

This system was proposed in order to create a couple of deep learning models for ResNet. The authors of [36] used a collection of convolutional neural framework devices called ResNet to see fever, such as that encountered as part of COVID-19. This architecture develops different extension data. They merged all of the model probabilities into a distinctive confirmation of melanoma and seborrheic keratosis classes per skin class. Four definitive methodologies led to the last probabilistic polymerase chain estimate. The authors of [37] used the AlexNet approach, Google devices for convolutional neural frameworks, and a joint model to yield probabilities for melanoma; this can likewise be proposed for the fluorescence polymerase chain response for COVID-19. This model outperforms single deep learning techniques, such as GoogLeNet, AlexNet, and VGGNet. The mixed frameworks offer the best probabilities when it comes to analyzing the virus. The authors of [38] used convolutional neural frameworks to characterise skin sores using approaches such as ResNet, DenseNet, and Inception V3. Their assessment presents two planning frameworks. They predicted skin wounds using all of these neural models, and again surveyed sore types by combining the yield assessments of all of the models. One planning framework was to set up the models using altered skin pictures around the area of interest. The other was to set up the models using exceptional pictures. The researchers' blend approaches a higher precision of conjecture than those of single neural organization models. The authors of [39] delivered deep learning models and consolidated these models to anticipate skin injury using approaches such as Inception V3, DenseNet, and ResNet. In [40], for chest registered tomography, a combination of two ResNet models was used as a result of considering the above technique. The authors eventually evaluated the chest pictures using joint-yield saliency maps. The authors defined a strategy for convolving pictures using a three-dimensional model and later combining the saliency guides of the two models. Similarly to the case of [41], in which melanoma was detected among seborrheic keratosis and nevus, they used techniques such as dual ResNet models. The published results showed that the two ResNet models outperformed all of the single ResNet models. In any case, they used all of the ResNet models when predicting melanoma.

1.3.3 Single deep learning strategies

The authors of [42] used a Google deep learning device called Commencement v3 for the characterization of skin injury, while retaining a primary concern for the use of these strategies for other potential sicknesses. The authors of [43] described an alternate kind of strategy for the order of procedures for COVID-19. A profound learning model was prepared using around 129,450 clinical pictures to see non-cancerous skin developments called carcinoma basal cells, seborrheic keratosis, keratinocytes, and nevi tumours as well as harmful tumours. The developed strategy allows the characterization of pneumonia and other expressed conditions, as mentioned above. They defined a strategy that used a deep learning calibrated ResNet-152 model. The authors saw different qualities of pneumonia in their discoveries. They used a couple of external data sets to make deep learning models. In [44], they described a deep learning strategy to identify COVID-2019 using ResNet-101 and Inception-v4. In [45], they additionally used Google devices to portray skin sores using a convolutional neural strategy. In the first place, this methodology collected unsafe and non-destructive kinds of skin wound. In a similar way, they further segregated each wound into more subcategories. Furthermore, the strategy further apportioned compromising and benign types into epithelial and melanocytic states. Hence, they could see skin wounds in up to 21 classes. These models recognized basal cell carcinoma and chest illnesses like the one described previously. The authors of [46], with the assistance of the previously mentioned procedure, used profound convolutional neural frameworks to characterize CT filters using algorithms such as Inception v3, ResNet-152, and DenseNet-210. The ResNet-152 models outperformed various models used to distinguish melanomas and melanocytic nevi. DenseNet-210 gave the best results for basal cell carcinoma and dermatofibroma. The Inception v3 model beats various models for actinic keratosis and positive CT filter plans. Most of these approaches have been used in the fight against COVID-19 but are, as yet, unsuccessful due to the absence of a huge data set.

1.4 'The cloud' and COVID-19

The recent months have been ones of isolation, both physical and social. In response, our virtual lives have woken up in abundance, as we attempt to replace our physicality using virtual gadgets that make a mechanical difference to our social affiliations and regular daily existence. In an attempt to prevent COVID-19 from spreading, our actual universes have become geofenced and surround our homes and localities. If one development had the possibility to provide encouragement in the midst of office closures, detachment, social partition, and disquiet, it is ‘the cloud’. Many cloud providers are helping in the fight against COVID-19 in an assortment of ways. Cloud organizations have allowed us to continue our high-level lives using various applications. At a late stage, a business affiliation pushed its first Salesforce Care solution for Healthcare Systems, organized expressly for human administration providers experiencing a deluge of requests due to COVID-19 [47, 48]. Courses of action to support ideas can be developed expeditiously and set up quickly. They have also expanded arrangements with additional free features to aid associations in any industry related to colleagues, even when everyone is working remotely. A depiction of the cloud model is shown in figure 1.5. A huge company has offered an AI-controlled dispersed registering stage and an unlimited supercomputing pack to research establishments to animate viral quality sequencing, protein screening, and other explorations in treating or hindering the coronavirus.

The first-class Computing Consortium has decided to join workplaces around the world and academic pioneers to offer access to the world’s most exceptional computing resources for COVID-19 exploration [49]. In like manner, with this structure, it licenses researchers to run colossal amounts of calculations in the course of investigating sickness transmission, bioinformatics, and nuclear imaging. The consortium will provide a remarkable amount of power to research establishments, consisting of the speediest supercomputer on earth. This makes tests possible that would otherwise be set aside due to the long effort required to complete them at some future point. New organizations have been steadfast customers of cloud providers [50]. Bleeding-edge developments are most likely to receive the most endorsements, especially from the media. They should be supported in their undertakings so that they can remain viable. Their ability to continue supporting their customer base, which uses cloud organizations, will be an essential part of their

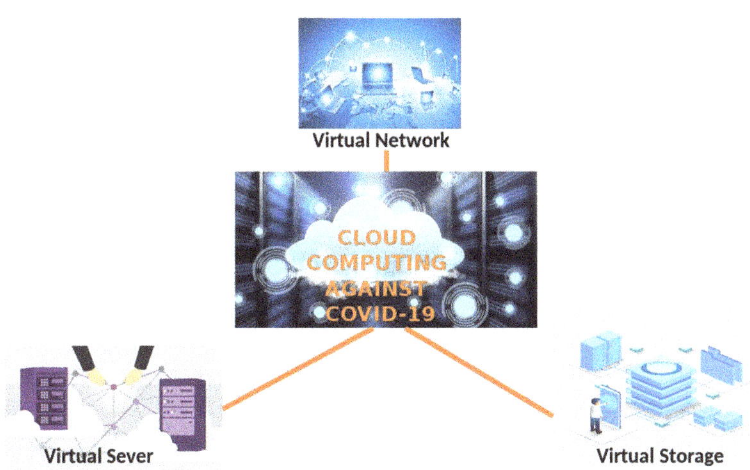

Figure 1.5. Illustration of the cloud computing resources available to help fight COVID-19.

recovery. They may not all be as attractive as supercomputers, but they provide vocations and organization to their local economies. Some of the cloud administrations are discussed below [51]. We are witnessing a marvellous event in general and this is an open entryway for high technology to step forward and support their clients and lead the way in assisting businesses to persevere.

1.4.1 Virtual storage

As we know, virtual storage is a staple component of 'the cloud' and is generally available as an internet service. Virtual storage suggests a virtualised kind of limited medium; as such, it exists as a feature inside a virtual space. Virtual storage used to be inseparable from virtual memory, which was a growth of central memory through discretionary storage. However, with the presence of 'the cloud', the term has continued to become more demanding, which is significant, as it is created in a virtual area. This is generally an intermediate layer between the customer and the real storage hardware. A virtual machine appears to the customer as an actual PC with a working operating system and all the additional miscellaneous items, and clearly with its own personal limited drive [52, 53]. A virtual device is commonly also associated with a virtual machine.

Using this strategy, customers do not need to worried about the specific location of their data, which can be seen if it is used in a reasonable way. Storage virtualization is a system association practice that permits the decoupling of the actual state of the equipment from its visible depiction. Storage virtualization allows us to harness a wide range of storage areas and address them using a singular real record structure. This model uses frameworks for devices that are accessible through ultra-high speed relationships, which offer storage areas [54]. There are different frameworks for capacity virtualization; perhaps the most well-known of which is framework-based virtualization that uses techniques for capacity-region frameworks.

1.4.2 Virtual servers

The amount of models a given actual server can support is limited by its capacity. Most services are hosted on a virtual machine; this is a kind of virtualization in 'the cloud' that emulates an actual server, and which is overseen by cloud providers that offer identical servers to different cloud purchasers, which gives cloud buyers a single simulated virtual server. Each virtual server can have different IT resources, cloud-based strategies, and other distinctive published processing frameworks. As a crucial framework, the virtual server is the most focal structure of the cloud. The allocation of a virtual server for image reports is a resource appropriation measure that can be performed rapidly and on demand. Be that as it may, a virtual service duplicates and provides service functionalities. Cloud customers who pay for the administration of virtual services may choose to re-try their current workload using a different cloud resource that might utilize a virtual server that provides the equivalent essential actual service [55].

Instead of a totally dedicated server, a few virtual servers might support a single service. A virtual server that is used for web engagement, page headers, or internet service provider (ISP) may have separate name spaces, IP addresses, records, and evaluation. Likewise, security systems and passwords are maintained as if they were under normal operational conditions. An individual virtual server represents a commitment to another operating system (OS), its own programming, and self-sufficient reboot provisioning. Likewise, to reduce the costs of enabling the web, basic programming reduces a huge piece of the time. Today, the 'virtual' part denotes that the server is anything but a dedicated server; that is, the whole PC cannot run the worker programming. A flood of virtual servers in an actual machine may cause the asset to be fully committed and if one virtual server utilizes a larger number of central focuses than another, its performance may need to be considered. Virtual web servers are an outstanding methodology for creating effortless web-empowering servers. If all else fails, each site functions as if it is being served by a dedicated server. Rather than requiring a separate PC for every server, various virtual servers can coexist on a practically identical PC. If an absurd number of virtual servers is present on a similar PC, or in the event that one virtual server begins to reserve assets, web pages will gradually start to be significantly delayed [56].

1.4.3 Virtual networks

This module creates a structure that gives a cloud infrastructure substance. As we presumably know, a virtual framework partner's organizations and resources such as virtual machines and information-based applications communicate with each other and the rest of the web through a safe, encoded, and private framework. The centralization of control reduces the expense and uncommonness of working, keeps equipment and programming separated, and controls distinct separate hardware in generally limited geographical regions. Virtual system association supports the relationships required by fluctuating associations and hardware on a single piece of equipment called a virtual association switch. Maintenance staff and managers can introduce hardware drivers, perform tests, and resolve issues on remote machines from a single zone. A couple of vendors offer virtual framework affiliation programming. It may very well be necessary to present virtual framework affiliation programming on remote PCs or services to support this movement. With this, experts can arrange their thoughts about battling COVID-19 issues with the help of a virtual framework [57]. A few vendors offer broad virtual structure affiliations, allowing organizations to allocate staff to rearrange work and resources for the seller.

The main limitation of virtual systems association is the way in which specific issues can undeniably be settled without direct actual contact with the equipment being alluded to. So often, virtual structure associations may make it possible to avoid inconvenience by taking elective assets out of service until a specialist can fix or replace them. Models join broken wires and repair drives and flawed chips. Virtual framework organization relies upon actual PC arrangement guidelines.

However, its abilities are, for the most part, programming driven. Basically, a virtual area is created by software-based virtual switches that offer a correspondence between all virtual and related machines. The virtual machines (VMs) can be accessed using the predefined internet protocol (IP) address of each objective virtual machine. The organization framework may also be executed on virtual machines that are presented or sent on Internet-enabled machines [58].

1.5 5G and COVID-19

Versatile 5G applications are a stage in the improvement of both patient considerations and the doctor's abilities, but also diminish asset use, which might actually decrease costs. 5G organizational innovation can possibly bring about a transformation of medical care areas by better helping staff and encouraging improved infection-distinguishing proof, administration, information collection, and examination. 5G has amazingly high speed, versatility, energy effectiveness, and low inactivity compared to 4G [59].

5G offers fast information movement capacity, for example, the transmission of enormous imaging clinical information records or the control of a remote medical procedure that benefits from rapid innovation as a result of immensely upgraded picture quality and continuous video contact [60]. For a virtual facility, the information available by 5G will be as acceptable or better than face-to-face contact, making virtual centers, interdisciplinary conferencing, and remote patient checking a reality. The medical care industry is likewise anticipating investigating the expected use of 5G-powered robots in conveying immunizations, drugs, and blood tests to their destinations as fast as could be expected under the circumstances, which can save numerous lives lost because of the absence of clinical buildings, especially in remote regions [61]. Artificial consciousness can develop an acculturated clinical climate in cases requiring serious consideration. 5G telephony has an ultra-high-speed goal and a 3D camera arrangement which allows specialists to oversee activities. Despite the fact that it is valuable, its unfavourable fundamental impacts related to its use ought to likewise be recalled.

The zones in which we can apply 5G innovation to combat current pandemics may include:

- Diagnosis.
- Trauma and medical procedure applications.
- Thermal imaging.
- Education and preparation.
- Counselling.
- 5G robots.
- Patient checking.
- 5G telemedicine.

1.5.1 Telemedicine

To increase the availability of telemedicine, innovations in 5G organization are required. Telemedicine alludes to the act of treating patients distantly. To this end,

5G, with its attributes and fast information transmission, would require versatile organizational handling in regard to these issues [62]. Likewise, 4G LTE networks regularly block IoMT gadgets from associating with cloud devices, rendering them useless. Additionally, 5G may take into consideration vivid virtual and expanded reality applications that may prompt intelligent telemedicine encounters and give parental figures rapid advice about potential inconveniences and treatment procedures [63].

1.5.2 Thermal imaging

5G systems administration permitted 5G-powered heat-imaging frameworks to be improved and to have numerous security and medical services applications. First produced for antiaircraft protection, the heat-imaging innovation has now discovered its way into a few spaces, including medical care, where it has be shown to be especially helpful [64]. This element will mean that public temperatures can be taken nonstop for COVID-19 flare-up monitoring [65]. Utilizing 5G organization, the information the equipment gathers would then be able to be communicated to the focal control framework with ultralow inactivity.

1.5.3 Monitoring

The Global Positioning System (GPS) can recognize exact areas, and the closeness of infected persons can likewise be distinguished by cell phones using the Bluetooth innovation [66]. Knowing precisely where infected individuals are is fundamental. Cell phone information can enable the production of populace gauges and other versatile data that can be utilized by different areas to comprehend and follow up on their patterns [67].

1.5.4 Robots

A few endeavors have been made since the appearance of COVID-19 to construct and send robots across the globe to reduce the load on first-line staff. In addition, noncontact surface purification strategies for 5G robots may likewise be utilized to restrict the transmission of sickness via contaminated surfaces. As 5G-powered robots and other robots obtain more functionality, they become more proficient in the performance of their tasks [68]. In contrast with the manual cleansing practices, which require the transport of cleaning staff, hence putting them in danger of being infected, self-governing purification robots can perform quick and successful sanitization [69].

1.5.5 Education, preparation, and advice

Educational institutions were closed, and online talks were held by instructors [70]. COVID-19 has had a critical effect on instruction and preparation. Classes, workshops, nearly all planned gatherings, and the quantity of online courses have expanded immensely, and other scholarly exercises that have been dropped are now effectively accessible using 5G. With the assistance of cell phones, students can access talks on the web. For wellbeing guidance and exercise, institutions planned to use ZOOM and Facetime, to which a network of individuals can be directed. Such specialized arrangements help to set up social distancing rules, but additionally give coherent treatment [71].

1.6 Big data and COVID-19

Big data has been demonstrated to be a valuable device for quick ongoing assessments [72]. Big data analytics can possibly assume a critical role in forestalling COVID-19-related emergency clinic flare-ups. With the creation of big data for examination, an abundance of data from around the globe can be made accessible to researchers, specialists, disease transmission experts, and policymakers. The capacity to store and arrange exact individual travel and contact histories permits infections to be followed and screening to be directed for all patients and guests before they enter a clinical office. This has given current data to the outside isolation stations of every emergency clinic and center. In Taiwan, the public authority has incorporated and investigated a few big data sets from the National Health Insurance Administration (NHIA), the National Immigration Agency (NIA), and the Taiwan Centers for Disease Control. All guests have subsequently been screened by means of individual recognizable proof cards and any suspected carrier is additionally inspected prior to entering the building [73]. An equivalent system can be applied to allow quicker movement through air terminals and ports. This model could provide an approach for addressing possible disease transmission. For instance, in Taiwan, the NHIA and the NIA created the Entry Quarantine System. Travel history information is obtained at the hour of departing from or landing at a Taiwanese airport. This framework utilizes the previous 14-day travel history of an individual and their NHIA distinguishing proof card information to screen them for COVID-19. Today, travellers have to finish a wellbeing assertion process by checking a QR code. This framework has provided a quicker migration process for those with negligible risk [74]. A versatile wellbeing presentation pass is then sent by means of SMS to telephones utilizing a nearby telecoms provider. In the subsections below, we will discuss the application of big data in the fight against the pandemic.

1.6.1 Treatment, diagnosis, and prognosis

Despite the rise and spread of conjecture, large data sets can support COVID-19 assurance and treatment structures. In the fields of discovery and treatment, big data has offered various courses of action, as reported above. The ability of big data to diagnose overpowering infections such as COVID-19 has been demonstrated using late prognosis, early discovery [75], the prediction of therapeutic results, and the building of consistent instruments for an operation. An assessment in [76] introduced a good, sensitive, unequivocal, and significantly quantitative course of action that relies on multiplex polymerase chain reactions which could dissect SARS-CoV-2. The proposed multiplex PCR plot is shown to be a beneficial and simple strategy for breaking down *Plasmodium* falciparum infections, with a high incorporation of up to 99%. This model contains various included arrangements of express preparations identified with the genome of the SARS-CoV-2 which could be assembled from the National Center for Biological information in China. This examination had critical encounters with viral infection and it supported COVID-19 discovery in domains lacking genomic data.

Even more expressly, the data contain a large number of proteins for human cells with the infection. Meanwhile, the authors of [77] used proteomics cells which were infected for investigation. Given that, with the supportive assessment of viable preliminiary research, a framework examination could be constructed to separate the data collected in the Kyoto genetic encyclopedia. In light of the data set required for COVID-19 research and drugs, preliminary data is provided in [78], in which six epitopes can incite the body to start working on antibodies, producing express humoral immunity. A comparative course of action in [79] used straightforward opened rats and primates for a non-neural explanation of the SARS-CoV-2 entry characteristics. Thus, the authors based their philosophy on an estimation of the 3D model of the checked protein and an assumption for the cell conformational epitopes of a stamped protein of SARS-CoV-2 joined with an assessment of epitope protection.

It contains a standard procedure in the study of disease transmission, detection, and treatment of COVID-19 illness. Unusually, the progressing research in [80] gave a thorough principle of significant mechanical assemblies to help in the elimination and treatment of COVID-19. An assortment of clinical analyses were performed using a huge information base, from atypical and typical x/CT-bar imaging signs to hematology evaluation and the presence of a catalyst in the respiratory framework. As a starter, a huge amount of data from Wuhan was researched, obtained from a variety of systems used to screen a great many individuals; hundreds were perceived as theoretical overwhelming setbacks, and others were analysed.

1.6.2 Predicting flare-ups

Big data has a critical role in engaging COVID-19 through its capacity to predict a scenario from a large-scale data assessment. As opposed to using a clear and deterministic strategy, the authors of [81] have developed progressively more complex techniques that could correctly detail the components of the infection that rely on various protein strands. For example, the work in [82] used data sets assembled from the COVID-19 pandemic in a locale in Europe to assess the eruption likelihood, which is of fundamental importance to configuring convincing disease control frameworks. Another data hotspot for eruption assumptions is an open data set that can be used to picture the topographical zones with possible scenarios [83]. Meanwhile, the work described in [84] used COVID-19 scenario-related data from authoritative sources. A first primer is an assessment in China, which hoped to screen personal movement to and from Chinese urban communities so that workplaces could foresee the part of general population infected with COVID-19 for segregation. Furthermore, this permits us to perform experiments to predict the development of a COVID-19 scenario, for instance, perceiving the domains at critical risk of infection and recognizing the general population with a growing level of infection; all of these add to the achievements in the fight against infection. This enormous data source can help us to interpret the numbers of infected people and recovered cases in territories in China.

Huge data moreover engages assumptions to an overall degree. Its accuracy could depend upon the quantity of elements contributed, extrapolation from infected cases, people, everyday conditions, circumstances, etc. From the data assessment viewpoint, the scenario is foreseen using available data centers, which puts the precision of the circumstances for reliable appraisals in jeopardy in the light of complete assessments. Spurred on by this, an assessment in [85] used a huge data set from various areas and countries to measure the pandemic using a determined technique which may articulate the steadfast nature of the measurement. This variety of data sources can help us to imagine the eruption tendency and check the possible scenarios. A comparison of the fundamentals in [86] used Trends from Google as a data-building device to accumulate Covid-related information for a few nations. The organizational reports accumulated from the Covid pandemics in those nations were in like manner assembled and examined by [87] using a data improvement model, which proposed the creation of an exact assumption for the cases, which may allow long-term estimates of future scenarios. Another data explanatory strategy described in [88] was inspected in America using the colossal extension data sets accumulated by US metropolitan networks. The primer was executed in Asia, indicating that the proposed data analysis can check transient ranges. The critical purpose behind the study was to acquire continuous data to smooth out the data display strategy to improve the concept of the approaching result; this could conceivably be used for comparable pandemics.

1.6.3 Discovery of antibodies and medications

Developing a novel inoculation is fundamental to shield the population from the rapid relentless overall burden of the COVID-19 pandemic. Very few undertakings have been made to develop a suitable vaccination for COVID-19 using big data within this short period of time. Big data can obtain pieces of information relating to vaccination against the COVID-19 pandemic. The work in [89] used the GISAID information that has been used to isolate amino-destructive stores. A comparable effort for improving counteracting agents is described in [90], which focused on investigating the protein spike of SARS-CoV-2, including four diverse earlier outbreaks of human covid strains. The investigation is required to search for incredible concentrations that can make future antibodies against the pandemic. This study could enable the essential discovery of collections and structures from SARS-CoV-2, which could help in the development of a proper neutralizer.

The SARS-CoV-2 strain has been picked by inspecting different sections of information from the National Center for Biotechnology Information, though the web Immune Epitope Database was utilized for the B-cell and T-cell epitope figures. The techniques of inverse vaccinology and safe informatics can be useful to make subunit antibodies against the infection [91]. An assortment of stages may be used to extract information from the created information base, which includes antigenicity, allergenicity, and physicochemical trademark assessment, which means the perception of the possible vaccination. Different peptides were proposed to develop another immune response to COVID-19 in two phases. The whole COVID-19 genome was dismembered by a comparative genomic approach to manage the recognition of a normal antigenic goal. A gigantic information base has been furthermore assembled through the National Center of Biotechnology Information to empower neutralizers in [92]. The use of an Artemis comparative tool to separate Covid reference courses of action allows us to encode the four critical assistant proteins in the infection.

For example, an answer subject to atomic docking was proposed in [93] for lesser red flagged viruses. Big data moreover offers systems to ease data access for fighting COVID-19. More than a few little particles in the FDA-attested cure data set were first discovered and endorsed by a nuclear docking program known as Glide. The critical inspiration driving this endeavour is the use of machine learning (ML) to join both data graphs and compose the vaccination improvement. This is a significant data-driven medicine repositioning plan that was moreover introduced in [94].

1.7 Challenges and discussion

Medical services is perhaps the most energizing IoT change innovation. Advances going from information security to patient security may impede IoT activities in medical services. Medical care pioneers can unquestionably push forward into the New Year. Some of the difficulties are described and a discussion is offered in the subsections below.

1.7.1 Security and protection

Each and every IoT gadget could represent a possible danger, either hurting end clients or imperilling their security. Furthermore, this may create risks for individual security. On the off chance that IoT security is undermined, data belonging to end clients could be accessed by unapproved actors. The security and protection of the IoT's electronic health (eHealth) spans the whole lifecycle of the framework, from creating particulars to execution and organization. These issues should be addressed to drive the IoT's eHealth. Safeguarding IoT eHealth biological systems is an unpredictable and complex task.

1.7.2 Data management

The eHealth information, however, comes from human-attached clinical sensors. The executive challenges of the IoT's eHealth information are are similar to those confronting other areas. The human body is a dynamic framework, continually changing its state. The costs of sensors and computing are declining, and as a result, gathering a huge amount of information in a brief timeframe has become less expensive. As can be seen from the IoT and big data eHealth applications, information from edge sensors will continually stream through cloud computing hubs. Information volume and speed difficulties are more connected with the capacity of cloud hub equipment to obtain, cycle, store, and convey high-consistency, highly ambitious information from clinical gadgets that may be accessible to patients, medical clinics, or centers. At the end of the day, IoT eHealth needs to manage the details of the information in terms of its variety, volume, and speed. As a result, cloud managers will be needed to screen the information moving around the cloud and distributed computing. An estimate suggests that medical services will be responsible for creating most of their information from other areas. Likewise, medical care will create an enormous volume of information. Also, as indicated by government and state laws, the wellbeing business should be especially diligent in taking care of patient information from IoT gadgets. The present moment offers an ideal opportunity for organizations to comprehend that if they keep on utilizing IoT innovation, information storage needs are probably going to increase.

1.7.3 Standardization and administrative undertakings

All manufacturers, specialist organizations, and end clients are expecting to see the principles of operability applied both inside and between IoT application-focused spaces. The IoT has commonly raised concerns about standardisation. The test of standardisation lies in the way that the IoT tries to include a wide assortment of information which is ordinarily managed by different administrations. Before IoT eHealth items start to become available, eHealth will have to explore an overwhelming multiagency administrative structure. Because of IoT eHealth, the intricacy will even increase because of the strict guidelines imposed by clinical principles. IoT eHealth and emerging technologies will be confronted by comparable patterns in all parts of the world.

1.8 Conclusions

Technologies have been utilized in the examination, determination, and treatment of COVID-19. Deep learning and recent innovations can be viably used to help clinical networks to quickly react to the expanded requests and magnitude of COVID-19. Recent advancements have demonstrated that cooperation between clinical analysts and architects is fundamental to the improvement of rapid and more affordable methods of dealing with the pandemic. We have examined the use of deep learning and emerging technologies ('the cloud', 5G, and big data) to distinguish proof and assurance, follow up, predict, and battle the COVID-19 cases. Our study has revealed the mystery parts of advancements which will eventually help to control the pandemic. In a similar way, the deep learning technique has been used to gather information about the protein in the patient body from clinical notes. This study has found that methodologies utilizing potential advances could yield better advantages and that these mechanical techniques can be used either to control the pandemic or to help society's repression during a pandemic, therefore helping to manage the spread of disease. Thus, a short period of time later, the patient results were beneficial, achieving a precision of more than 91%. In addition, this relates to the quick surge that happened during the pandemic and its effect on the environment and society. A discussion of these various advancements was presented. Notwithstanding the advancements actualized, this work additionally addresses undiscovered possible innovations with forthcoming applications in controlling pandemic conditions. Medicines developed that use recent innovations should likewise be subjected to standard clinical preliminaries. With regards to the quick and broad spread of infection, open access to information, apparatus, and innovation is fundamental to an appropriate reaction. The researched strategies propose clinical data assessments with precisions of up to 90%. There is a need to maintain all these wellbeing principles to guarantee the best results for patients. Logical future studies will need to be finished to guarantee that everybody gives and participates in a manner that is likely not to miss the fundamental interests of any center. Thus, it it will be fundamental to zero in on quiet voices. We should join a conversation among all parties, in any case. Further work will subsequently have to address their needs, bearing in mind that the improvement of these advances is to serve patients and not ignore them. Future developments can be considered after the emergency of COVID-19 at various scales.

References

[1] Chesbrough H 2020 To recover faster from Covid-19, open up: managerial implications from an open innovation perspective *Ind. Mark. Manag.* **88** 410–13

[2] Madurai Elavarasan R and Pugazhendhi R 2020 Restructured society and environment: a review on potential technological strategies to control the COVID-19 pandemic *Sci. Total Environ.* **725** 138858

[3] Rahman M S, Peeri N C, Shrestha N, Zaki R, Haque U and Hamid S H A 2020 Defending against the novel coronavirus (COVID-19) outbreak: how can the internet of things (IoT) help to save the world? Heal *Policy Technol.* **9** 136–38

[4] Waheed A, Goyal M, Gupta D, Khanna A, Al-Turjman F and Pinheiro P R 2020 CovidGAN: data augmentation using auxiliary classifier GAN for improved Covid-19 detection *IEEE Access.* **8** 91916–23

[5] Halgurd S M, Ghafoor K Z, Sadiq A S, Curran K and Rabie K 2020 A novel AI-enabled framework to diagnose coronavirus COVID-19 using smartphone embedded sensors: design study arXiv:2003.07434

[6] Song Y, Jiang J, Wang X, Yang D and Bai C 2020 Prospect and application of internet of things technology for prevention of SARIs *Clin. eHealth.* **3** 1–4

[7] WHO May 2020 Contact tracing in the context of COVID-19, interim guidance https://who.int/publications/i/item/contact-tracing-in-the-context-of-covid-19

[8] WHO 2020 Clinical management of severe acute respiratory infection when novel coronavirus (nCoV) infection is suspected https://who.int/publications-detail/clinical-managementof-severe-acuterespiratory-infection-when-novel-coronavirus-(ncov)-infection-is-suspected

[9] Carter L J, Garner L V, Smoot J W, Li Y and Zhou Q *et al* 2020 Assay techniques and test development for COVID-19 diagnosis *ACS Cent. Sci.* **6** 591–605

[10] ECDC 2020 COVID-19 situation update worldwide, as of week 52 https://ecdc.europa.eu/en/geographical-distribution-2019-ncov-cases

[11] Singh R P, Javaid M, Haleem A and Suman R 2020 Internet of things (IoT) applications to fight against COVID-19 pandemic *Diabetes Metab. Syndr. Clin. Res. Rev.* **14** 521–24
[12] Bai L *et al* 2020 Chinese experts' consensus on the internet of things-aided diagnosis and treatment of coronavirus disease 2019 (COVID-19) *Clin. eHealth.* **3** 7–15
[13] Chamola V, Hassija V, Gupta V and Guizani M 2020 A comprehensive review of the COVID-19 pandemic and the role of IoT, drones, AI, Blockchain and 5G in managing its impact *IEEE Access.* **1** 1–41
[14] Chakraborty T and Ghosh I 2020 Real-time forecasts and risk assessment of novel coronavirus (COVID-19) cases: a data-driven analysis *Chaos, Solitons Fractals* **135** 109850
[15] Javaid M, Haleem A, Vaishya R, Bahl S, Suman R and Vaish A 2020 Industry 4.0 technologies and their applications in fighting COVID-19 pandemic *Diabetes Metab. Syndr. Clin. Res. Rev.* **14** 419–22
[16] Kummitha R K R 2020 Smart technologies for fighting pandemics: the techno- and human-driven approaches in controlling the virus transmission *Gov. Inf. Q.* **37** 101481
[17] Khan I M, Jabeur N, Khan M Z and Mokhtar H 2012 An overview of the impact of wireless sensor networks in medical health care *Conf. Paper*
[18] Sadiku M N O, Eze K G and Musa S M 2018 Wireless sensor networks for healthcare *J. Sci. Eng. Res.* **5** 210–13
[19] Stanković S 2009 Medical applications based on wireless sensor networks *IPSI.*
[20] OECD *The impact of the coronavirus (COVID-19) crisis on development finance* (http://oecd.org/coronavirus/policy-responses/the-impact-of-the-coronavirus-covid-19-crisis-on-development-finance-9de00b3b/)
[21] Naudé W 2020 *Artificial intelligence against COVID-19: an early review* (https://towardsdatascience.com/artificialintelligence-against-covid-19-an-early-review-92a8360edaba)
[22] Smolaks M 2020 *Deep learning systems can speed up diagnosis of COVID-19 patients* (https://aibusiness.com/deeplearning-systems-can-identify-covid-19-infections-on-x-rays/)
[23] Esteva A, Kuprel B, Novoa R A, Ko J, Swetter S M, Blau H M and Thrun S 2017 Dermatologist-level classi_cation of skin cancer with deep neural networks *Nature* **542** 115–8
[24] Han S S, Kim M S, Lim W, Park G H, Park I and Chang S E 2018 Classification of the clinical images for benign and malignant cutaneous tumors using a deep learning algorithm, *J. Investigative Dermatol.* **138** 1529–38
[25] Menegola A, Tavares J, Fornaciali M, Li L T, De Avila S E F and Valle E 2017 RECOD titans at ISIC challenge arXiv:1703.04819
[26] Fujisawa Y, Otomo Y, Ogata Y, Nakamura Y, Fujita R, Ishitsuka Y, Watanabe R, Okiyama N, Ohara K and Fujimoto M 2019 Deep-learning based, computer-aided classifier developed with a small dataset of clinical images surpasses board-certified dermatologists in skin tumour diagnosis, *Brit. J. Dermatol.* **180** 373–81
[27] Rezvantalab A, Sa_gholi H and Karimijeshni S 2017 Dermatologist level dermoscopy skin cancer classi_cation using different deep learning convolutional neural networks algorithms arXiv:1810.10348
[28] Toh A 2020 *Big data could undermine the COVID-19 response* https://wired.com/story/big-data-couldundermine-the-covid-19-response/
[29] Combalia M *et al* 2019 BCN20000: Dermoscopic lesions in the wild arXiv:1908.02288
[30] Tschandl P, Rosendahl C and Kittler H 2018 The HAM10000 dataset, a large collection of multi-source dermatoscopic images of common pigmented skin lesions, *Sci. Data* **5** 180161

[31] Vaishya R, Javaid M, Khan I H and Haleem A 2020 Artificial intelligence (AI) applications for COVID-19 pandemic, *Diabetes Metab. Syndr. Clin. Res. Rev.* **14** 337–9
[32] Ardakani A A, Kanafi A R, Acharya U R, Khadem N and Mohammadi A 2020 Application of deep learning technique to manage COVID-19 in routine clinical practice using CT images: results of 10 convolutional neural networks, *Comput. Biol. Med.* **121** 103795
[33] Ravì D, Wong C, Deligianni F, Berthelot M, Andreu-Perez J, Lo B and Yang G-Z 2017 Deep learning for health informatics, *IEEE J. Biomed. Health Informat.* **21** 4–21
[34] Chung M *et al* 2020 CT imaging features of 2019 novel coronavirus (2019-nCoV), *Radiology* **295** 200230
[35] Kantor P 1999 *Foundations of Statistical Natural Language Processing.* (Cambridge, MA: MIT Press) pp 91–2
[36] NyÍri T and Kiss A 2018 Novel ensembling methods for dermatological image classification, *Proc. Int. Conf. Theory Pract. Natural Comput* (Cham, Switzerland: Springer) pp 438–48
[37] Bi L, Kim J, Ahn E and Feng D Automatic skin lesion analysis using large-scale dermoscopy images and deep residual networks arXiv:1703.04197
[38] Mahbod A, Schaefer G, Ellinger I, Ecker R, Pitiot A and Wang C 2019 Fusing fine-tuned deep features for skin lesion classification, *Comput. Med. Imag. Graph.* **71** 19–29
[39] Hagerty J R, Stanley R J, Almubarak H A, Lama N, Kasmi R, Guo P, Drugge R J, Rabinovitz H S, Oliviero M and Stoecker W V 2019 Deep learning and handcrafted method fusion: Higher diagnostic accuracy for melanoma dermoscopy images, *IEEE J. Biomed. Health Informat.* **23** 1385–91
[40] Ardila D *et al* 2019 End-to-end lung cancer screening with three-dimensional deep learning on low-dose chest computed tomography, *Nature Med.* **25** 954–61
[41] Serte S and Demirel H 2020 Wavelet-based deep learning for skin lesion classification, *IET Image Process.* **14** 720–26
[42] Codella N C F *et al* 2018 Skin lesion analysis toward melanoma detection: a challenge at the 2017 international symposium on biomedical imaging (ISBI), hosted by the international skin imaging collaboration (ISIC), *Proc. IEEE 15th Int. Symp. Biomed. Imag. (ISBI)* p 168
[43] Li Q *et al* 2020 Early transmission dynamics in Wuhan, China, of novel Coronavirus-infected pneumonia, *New England J. Med.* **382** 1199–207
[44] Wu J T, Leung K and Leung G M 2020 Nowcasting and forecasting the potential domestic and international spread of the 2019-nCoV outbreak originating in Wuhan, China: a modelling study, *Lancet* **396** 689–97
[45] Lei J, Li J, Li X and Qi X 2020 CT imaging of the 2019 novel coronavirus (2019-nCoV) pneumonia, *Radiology* **298** 200236
[46] Guan W-J *et al* 2020 Clinical characteristics of 2019 novel coronavirus infection in China MedRxiv doi: 10.1101/2020.02.06.20020974
[47] Zheng C, Deng X, Fu Q, Zhou Q, Feng J, Ma H, Liu W and Wang X 2020 Deep learning-based detection for COVID-19 from chest CT using weak label medRxiv doi: 10.1101/2020.03.12.20027185
[48] Ullah Z, Al-Turjman F, Mostarda L and Gagliardi R 2020 Applications of artificial intelligence and machine learning in smart cities, *Comput. Commun.* **154** 313–23
[49] Oueida S, Aloqaily M and Ionescu S 2019 A smart healthcare reward model for resource allocation in smart city *Multimedia Tools Appl.* **78** 24573–94
[50] Oueida S, Kotb Y, Aloqaily M, Jararweh Y and Baker T 2018 An edge computing based smart healthcare framework for resource management *Sensors* **18** 4307

[51] Hussain A A and Al-Turjman F 2020 Resource Allocation in Volunteered Cloud Computing and Battling COVID-19 *AI-powered IoT for COVID-19* (Boca Raton, FL: CRC Press) ch 2
[52] Ibrahim U, Ozsos M and Al-Turjman F 2020 Futuristic CRISPR-based biosensing in the cloud and internet of things era: an overview, *Multi-media Tools Appl.* https://doi.org/10.1007/s11042-020-09010-5
[53] Al-Zinati M, Alrashdan R, Al-Duwairi B and Aloqaily M 2020 A reorganizing biosurveillance framework based on fog and mobile edge computing *Multimedia Tools Appl.* **1** 1–21
[54] Al-Khafajiy M *et al* 2020 Intelligent control and security of fog resources in healthcare systems via a cognitive fog model, *Int. J. Wireless Inf. Netw.* **27** 467–83
[55] Pludderman A, Hobbs R and Mahtani K R 2020 Rapid diagnosis of community-acquired pneumonia for clinicians rapid review oxford COVID-19 evidence series (University of Oxford) https://cebm.net/rapid-diagnosis-strategy-ofcommunity-acquired-pneumonia-for-clinician/
[56] Mitchell B 2019 Computer network storage explained https://lifewire.com/what-is-computer-networking-816249
[57] Lawrence C 2020 Is cloud computing the superhero of COVID-19? https://codemotion.com/magazine/devhub/cloud-manager/cloud-computing-covid-19/
[58] Morrison C and Archer H 2020 Coronavirus resilience planning:use of near me video consulting in gp practices scottish government technology enabled care programme. https://sehd.scot.nhs.uk/pca/PCA2020(M)03
[59] Kostoff R N, Heroux P, Aschner M and Tsatsakis A 2020 Adverse health effects of 5G mobile networking technology under real-life conditions *Toxicol. Lett.* **323** 35–40
[60] Vaishya R, Javaid M, Khan I H and Haleem A 2020 Artificial Intelligence (AI) applications for COVID-19 pandemic *Diabetes Metab. Syndr. Clin. Res. Rev.* **14** 337–39
[61] Hussain A A, Bouachir O, Al-Turjman F and Aloqaily M 2020 AI Techniques for COVID-19 *IEEE Access* **8** 128776–95
[62] Iyengar K, Upadhyaya G K, Vaishya R and Jain V 2020 COVID-19 and applications of smartphone technology in the current pandemic *Diabetes Metab. Syndr. Clin. Res. Rev.* **14** 733–37
[63] Mishra S S and Rasool A 2019 IoT health care monitoring and tracking: a survey *Proc. of Int. Conf. on Trends in Electronics and Informatics (ICOEI 2019)* pp 1052–057
[64] Zhu H *et al* 2020 IoT PCR for pandemic disease detection and its spread monitoring *Sens. Actuators B Chem.* **303** 127098
[65] Harvey L Battling COVID-19 with disinfecting robots https://blogs.mathworks.com/headlines/2020/04/23/battling-covid-19-with-disinfecting-robots/
[66] DeCaprio D, Gartner J, Burgess T, Kothari S and Sayed S 2020 Building a COVID-19 vulnerability index arXiv:2003.07347
[67] Akkaş M A, Sokullu R and Ertürk Çetin H 2020 Healthcare and patient monitoring using IoT *Internet Things.* **11** 100173
[68] Singh R P, Javaid M, Haleem A and Suman R 2020 Internet of things (IoT) applications to fight against COVID-19 pandemic *Diabetes Metab. Syndr. Clin. Res. Rev.* **14** 521–24
[69] Bai L *et al* 2020 Chinese experts' consensus on the internet of things-aided diagnosis and treatment of coronavirus disease 2019 (COVID-19) *Clin. eHealth.* **3** 7–15
[70] Chamola V, Hassija V, Gupta V and Guizani M 2020 A comprehensive review of the COVID-19 pandemic and the role of IoT, drones, AI, Blockchain and 5G in managing its impact *IEEE Access.* **1** 1–41

[71] Javaid M, Haleem A, Vaishya R, Bahl S, Suman R and Vaish A 2020 Industry 4.0 technologies and their applications in fighting COVID-19 pandemic *Diabetes Metab. Syndr. Clin. Res. Rev.* **14** 419–22
[72] Wang C J, Ng C Y and Brook R H 2020 Response to COVID-19 in Taiwan: big data analytics, new technology, and proactive testing *JAMA* **323** 1341–2
[73] Chen F M, Feng M C, Chen T C, Hsieh M H, Kuo S H and Chang H L *et al* 2020 Big data integration and analytics to prevent a potential hospital outbreak of COVID-19 in Taiwan *J. Microbiol. Immunol. Infect* **54** 129–30
[74] Watanabe Y, Allen J D, Wrapp D, McLellan J S and Crispin M 2020 Site-specific glycan analysis of the SARS-CoV-2 spike *Science.* **369** 330–3
[75] Garattini C, Raffle J, Aisyah D N, Sartain F and Kozlakidis Z 2019 Big data analytics, infectious diseases and associated ethical impacts, *Philos. Technol.* **32** 69–85
[76] Li C, Debruyne D N, Spencer J, Kapoor V, Liu L Y, Zhou B, Lee L, Feigelman R, Burdon G and Liu J *et al* 2020 High sensitivity detection of coronavirus SARS-CoV-2 using multiplex PCR and a multiplex-PCR-based metagenomic method bioRxiv. https://doi.org/10.1101/2020.03.12.988246
[77] Ortea I and Bock J-O 2020 Re-analysis of SARS-CoV-2 infected host cell proteomics time-course data by impact pathway analysis and network analysis. a potential link with inflammatory response bioRxiv. doi: 10.1101/2020.03.26.009605
[78] Lon J R, Bai Y, Zhong B, Cai F and Du H 2020 Prediction and evolution of B cell epitopes of surface protein in SARS-CoV-2 bioRxiv. doi: 10.1101/2020.04.03.022723
[79] Brann D, Tsukahara T, Weinreb C, Logan D W and Datta S R 2020 Non-neural expression of SARS-CoV-2 entry genes in the olfactory epithelium suggests mechanisms underlying anosmia in COVID-19 patients bioRxiv. doi: 10.1101/2020.03.25.009084
[80] Jin Y-H, Cai L, Cheng Z-S, Cheng H, Deng T, Fan Y-P, Fang C, Huang D, Huang L-Q and Huang Q *et al* 2020 A rapid advice guideline for the diagnosis and treatment of 2019 novel coronavirus (2019-ncov) infected pneumonia (standard version), *Mil. Med. Res.* **7** 4
[81] Brauer F, Castillo-Chavez C and Castillo-Chavez C 2012 *Mathematical models in population biology and epidemiology* vol 2 (Berlin: Springer)
[82] Giordano G, Blanchini F, Bruno R, Colaneri P, Di Filippo A, Di Matteo A and Colaneri M *et al* 2020 A SIDARTHE model of COVID-19 epidemic in Italy *Nat. Med.* **26** 855–60
[83] Chen B, Shi M, Ni X, Ruan L, Jiang H, Yao H, Wang M, Song Z, Zhou Q and Ge T 2020 Visual data analysis and simulation prediction for COVID-19 arXiv:2002.07096
[84] Peng L, Yang W, Zhang D, Zhuge C and Hong L 2020 Epidemic analysis of COVID-19 in China by dynamical modeling medRxiv:2002.06563
[85] Tátrai D and Várallyay Z 2020 COVID-19 epidemic outcome predictions based on logistic fitting and estimation of its reliability arXiv:2003.14160
[86] Strzelecki A 2020 The second worldwide wave of interest in coronavirus since the COVID-19 outbreaks in South Korea, Italy and Iran: a Google trends study *Brain Behav. Immun.* **88** 950–1
[87] Long Y-S, Zhai Z-M, Han L-L, Kang J, Li Y-L, Lin Z-H, Zeng L, Wu D-Y, Hao C-Q and Tang M *et al* 2020 Quantitative assessment of the role of undocumented infection in the 2019 novel coronavirus (COVID-19) pandemic arXiv:2003.12028
[88] Heroy S 2020 Metropolitan-scale COVID-19 outbreaks: how similar are they? arXiv:2004.01248

[89] Ahmed S F, Quadeer A A and McKay M R 2020 Preliminary identification of potential vaccine targets for the COVID-19 coronavirus (SARS-CoV-2) based on SARS-CoV immunological studies, *Viruses* **12** 254

[90] Banerjee A, Santra D and Maiti S 2020 Energetics based epitope screening in SARS CoV-2 (COVID 19) spike glycoprotein by immunoinformatic analysis aiming to a suitable vaccine development bioRxiv: doi: 10.1101/2020.04.02.021725

[91] Sarkar B, Ullah M A, Johora F T, Taniya M A and Araf Y 2020 The essential facts of Wuhan novel coronavirus outbreak in China and Epitope-based vaccine designing against 2019-nCoV bioRxiv:doi: 10.1101/2020.02.05.935072

[92] Abdelmageed M I, Abdelmoneim A H, Mustafa M I, Elfadol N M, Murshed N S, Shantier S W and Makhawi A M 2020 Design of multi epitope-based peptide vaccine against E protein of human COVID-2019: an immunoinformatics approach bioRxiv:doi: 10.1101/2020.02.04.934232

[93] Li Z, Li X, Huang Y-Y, Wu Y, Zhou L, Liu R, Wu D, Zhang L, Liu H and Xu X *et al* 2020 FEP-based screening prompts drug repositioning against COVID-19 bioRxiv doi: 10.1101/2020.03.23.004580

[94] Ge Y, Tian T, Huang S, Wan F, Li J, Li S, Yang H, Hong L, Wu N and Yuan E *et al* 2020 A data-driven drug repositioning framework discovered a potential therapeutic agent targeting COVID-19 bioRxiv doi: 10.1101/2020.03.11.986836

IOP Publishing

Artificial Intelligence Strategies for Analyzing COVID-19 Pneumonia Lung Imaging, Volume 1
Characterization approaches
Ayman El-Baz and Jasjit S Suri

Chapter 2

Detecting COVID-19 in chest radiographs using machine learning and convolutional neural networks

Andrew C Li, David T Lee, Kristoff K Misquitta, Kaiji Uno and Sasha Wald

The accurate and efficient diagnosis of potential COVID-19 patients is vital in the fight against the current pandemic. However, even the gold-standard COVID-19 test—the reverse transcription polymerase chain reaction (RT-PCR) test—suffers from a high false negative rate and a turnaround time of up to one week, preventing the infected from accessing the timely care they require, and impeding efforts to isolate positive cases. To address these shortcomings, our study has developed a machine learning model based on the DenseNet-201 deep convolutional neural network, which can classify COVID-19 using chest radiographs in less than one minute and far more accurately than conventional tests (F1 score: 0.96; precision: 0.95; recall: 0.98). It uses a significantly larger dataset and more control classes than previously published models, demonstrating the promise of the machine learning approach for accurate and efficient COVID-19 screening. A live web application of the trained model can be accessed at https://cov2d19-classifier.herokuapp.com/.

2.1 Introduction

COVID-19 is a highly infectious disease that has been declared to be both a public health emergency and a pandemic by the World Health Organization (WHO) [1]. As of August 2020, the virus had infected more than 25 million people, killed upwards of 840 000, and disrupted the lives of millions more through travel restrictions, mandated quarantine periods, and school and business closures [2].

However, these aggressive lockdowns can only be so successful, given that new research suggests that current screening methods are imperfect. Take, for example,

doi:10.1088/978-0-7503-3795-3ch2

the only molecular test available that can diagnose the current COVID-19 infection: the RT-PCR test [3, 4]. Turnaround times for test results range from one day to an entire week, depending on the patient's risk level [5]. Furthermore, within the first five days of exposure, the false negative rate for the test is 67%. Eight days after exposure, when the false negative rate is supposedly lowest, it remains as high as 20% [6]. Thus, from 20% to 67% of the individuals being screened by RT-PCR at a given time may be diagnosed as healthy when they actually have COVID-19, disrupting efforts to isolate positive cases and diverting healthcare resources from where they are most needed.

Chest radiographs (x-rays) represent another potential tool for COVID-19 diagnosis. However, some chest x-ray features of COVID-19 are only moderately characteristic to the human eye, and are sometimes undetectable [7]. Thus, the diagnosis of COVID-19 by radiologists can be difficult and confusing, especially when distinguishing COVID-19 from other lung conditions, such as bacterial pneumonia or non-COVID-19 viral pneumonia.

Thus, an automatic COVID-19 diagnosis tool based on chest x-ray images that uses artificial intelligence and deep learning can provide two key benefits, compared to current testing methods:

1. **Faster, cheaper, and more accurate testing**. Automated tests free up resources and streamline the healthcare process for COVID-19 patients. Machine learning has already been successfully used in the diagnosis of other medical conditions, especially cancers, and sometimes offers greater accuracy than human doctors [8, 9].
2. **Increased test accessibility for burdened healthcare systems and developing countries**. Many healthcare centers already have radiological imaging machines, eliminating the logistical difficulties and expenses associated with the distribution of conventional tests. In addition, under-resourced and developing countries, where tests and human radiologists are in extremely short supply, stand to benefit from automated models that can serve as alternative testing processes. In Nigeria, only 1% of the population has been tested as of August 7, due to severe test shortages, multi-week test turnaround times, and limited government laboratories. Private facilities charge $132 per test. By comparison, a chest x-ray costs less than 5 USD (1,650 Naira) in Nigeria [10].

Thus, a machine learning model based on chest radiographs has the potential to offer improvements in performance and accessibility, compared to current methods.

In particular, convolutional neural networks (CNNs) have proven useful for automatically extracting features that are not obviously characteristic in the original image, greatly improving imaging models [11]. CNNs can be further refined using transfer learning, a technique in which the convolutional layers of a network are pre-trained on a large, unrelated data set of images, such as ImageNet. This provides unique advantages, including faster training on the new dataset, a smaller data requirement, and overall better performance.

This chapter proposes a transfer-learning-based CNN to predict cases of COVID-19 using simple chest x-ray images. The model is implemented using TensorFlow and a DenseNet-201 pre-trained model trained to classify normal, bacterial pneumonia, viral pneumonia, tuberculosis, and COVID-19 pneumonia radiographs. This constitutes a total of four control classes in addition to COVID-19.

Numerous other studies have created machine learning models to classify COVID-19 using radiological images [12–19]. However, these models were limited by their use of either a small data set or only a few control classes. The data set sizes in the studies reviewed ranged from 50 to approximately 1000 images; only two used data sets larger than the one used in this study. Additionally, there were a maximum of only two control classes, which always consisted of healthy images and non-COVID-19 pneumonia images. Our multiclass model uses four control classes: healthy, tuberculosis, and non-COVID-19 pneumonia, further subdivided into two classes labelled as bacterial and viral. In addition to being trained on a larger dataset, this model has the advantage of being more generalized and robust in a real-world setting.

2.2 Methods

2.2.1 Data collection

We compiled 9868 chest x-ray images of healthy individuals and those with COVID-19 pneumonia, bacterial pneumonia, viral pneumonia, or tuberculosis using several publicly available and open-source datasets [20–27]. The numbers of x-ray images were distributed as follows: 34% healthy, 28% viral pneumonia, 27% bacterial pneumonia, 5% COVID-19, and 4% tuberculosis (figure 2.1).

2.2.2 Data preprocessing

To improve model generalization and processing speed, all x-ray scans were downsampled and resized to dimensions of 128×128×3 pixels. The images were then converted to the RGB scale and their labels one-hot encoded to be compatible with the most common transfer learning models.

To improve model generalization and reduce overfitting, the ImageDataGenerator function of Tensorflow Keras was used to randomly augment each image in real time before it was used to train the model. The augmentation parameters applied were horizontal flip, random rotation from 0 to 8 degrees, random width and height shift from 0% to 15%, and random zoom from 0% to 20%.

The data was then split into training, validation, and test sets. The same disease distribution was preserved across all split datasets. The training set consisted of 6324 images, the validation set of 1574 images, and the test set of 1970 images.

2.2.3 Model and architecture

DenseNet-201, trained on the ImageNet dataset, was used as the convolutional layer of the proposed model. Training was performed using the following algorithm and architecture:

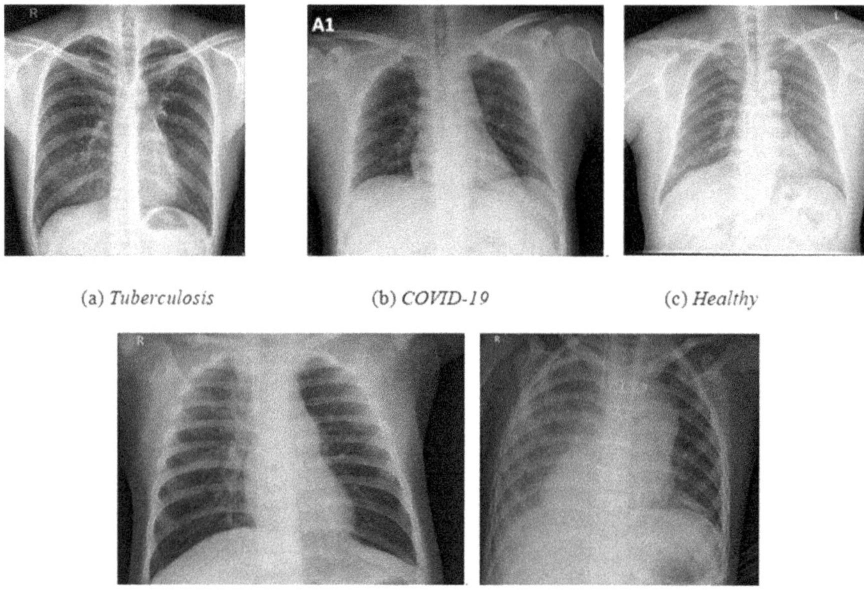

(a) *Tuberculosis* (b) *COVID-19* (c) *Healthy*

(d) *Viral Pneumonia* (e) *Bacterial Pneumonia*

Figure 2.1. Example chest x-ray images: (a) tuberculosis, (b) COVID-19, (c) healthy, (d) viral pneumonia, (e) bacterial pneumonia.

1. Apply convolutions to the training images using DenseNet-201, freezing the model weights.
2. Apply two-dimensional global average pooling.
3. Flatten data.
4. Feed data into a fully-connected dense layer consisting of 32 nodes, using the ReLU activation function.
5. Feed data into a fully-connected dense layer consisting of five nodes, using the softmax activation function for final disease classification (figure 2.2).

The default Adam optimizer and the categorical cross-entropy loss function were used due to the multiclass nature of the model. Training took place over 50 epochs using a batch size of five. Early stopping that monitored the validation accuracy was also implemented with a patience of five epochs. The model was stopped at epoch 22 after the validation accuracy dipped below a prior accuracy for five epochs in a row, indicating overfitting, and the weights of the best earlier epoch were restored for the final model (figure 2.3).

2.3 Results

The training accuracy steadily rose to 88.71% in the epoch which was selected for the final model. The validation accuracy stood at 82.97%, and the test set accuracy was 83.4%. More metrics are described in table 2.1. The average area under the receiver operating curve (AUROC) for the model was 0.8963 (figure 2.4). Figures 2.5 and 2.6

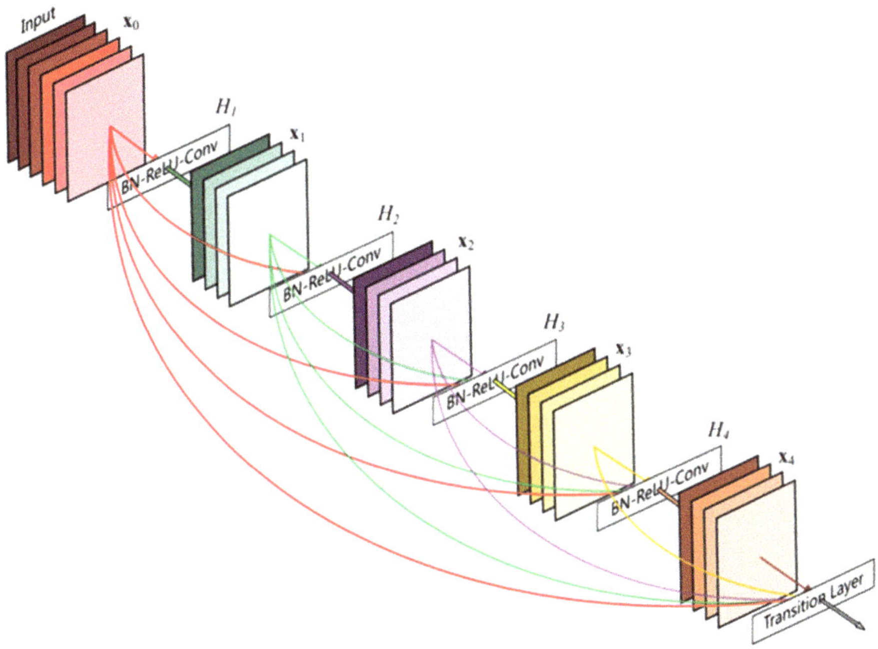

Figure 2.2. A visualization of the DenseNet-201 architecture. 'Each layer takes all preceding feature-maps as input' [28].

```
base_model = tf.keras.applications.DenseNet201(input_shape=(image_height, image_width, 3), include_top=False, weights='imagenet')
base_model.trainable = False

global_average_layer = tf.keras.layers.GlobalAveragePooling2D()
flatten_layer = Flatten()
dense_layer1 = tf.keras.layers.Dense(32, activation='relu')
dense_layer2 = tf.keras.layers.Dense(5, activation='softmax')

model = tf.keras.Sequential([
    base_model,
    global_average_layer,
    flatten_layer,
    dense_layer1,
    dense_layer2
])

model.compile(optimizer='adam', loss='categorical_crossentropy', metrics=['accuracy'], run_eagerly=True, loss_weights=[1, 6, 1, 1, 6])
```

Figure 2.3. Python code used to build the model with TensorFlow Keras.

Table 2.1. Precision, recall, F1 score, and support metrics for each class.

Class	Precision	Recall	F1 score	Support (number images in test set)
Normal	0.93	0.96	0.95	639
COVID-19	0.95	0.98	0.96	125
Bacterial pneumonia	0.76	0.77	0.76	556
Viral pneumonia	0.76	0.74	0.75	567
Tuberculosis	0.88	0.73	0.80	83

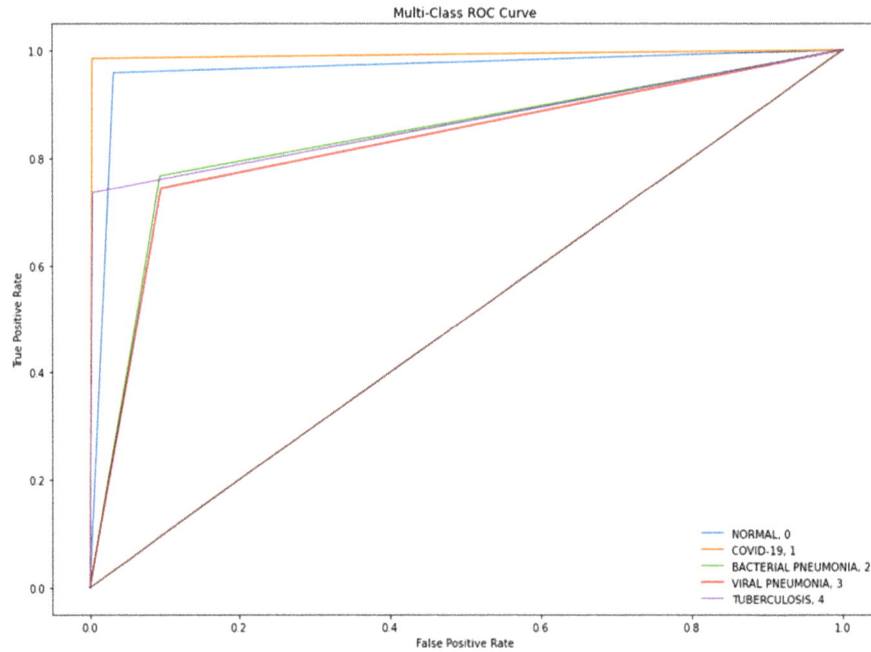

Figure 2.4. Receiver operating curve for the model's performance on each class.

```
Predicted Label
NOR [[612 2   2   15  8]
COV  [2   123 0   0   0]
BP   [9   1   426 120 0]
VP   [14  0   132 421 0]
TB   [18  4   0   0   61]]
      NOR COV BP  VP  TB
          True Label
```

Figure 2.5. Raw confusion matrix for the model test predictions. NOR: normal, COV: COVID-19, BP: bacterial pneumonia, VP: viral pneumonia, TB: tuberculosis.

represent a confusion matrix of the raw classification values and a heatmap of the normalized confusion matrix.

2.4 Discussion

While our overall model classification accuracy of 83.4% could be improved upon, the classification accuracy for COVID-19 chest x-rays was exceptional, with a precision of 0.95, a recall of 0.98, and an F1 score of 0.96 (figure 2.4). This represents an extremely accurate diagnosis of COVID-19: the false negative rate achieved of

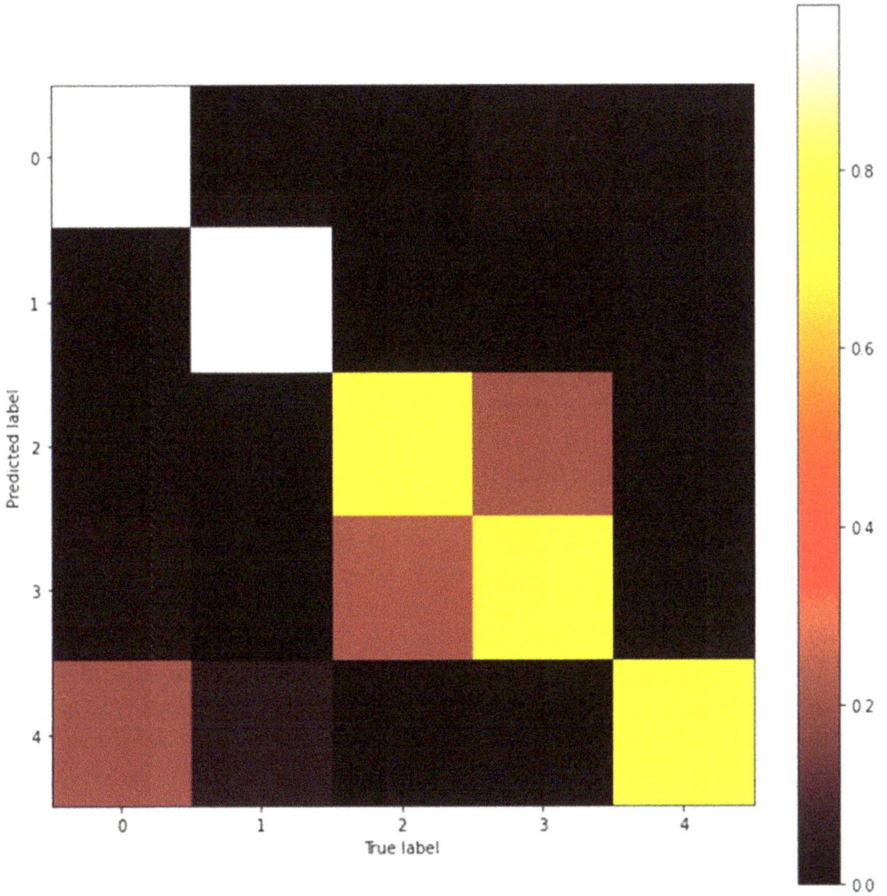

Figure 2.6. Normalized confusion matrix heatmap for the model test predictions. 0: normal, 1: COVID-19, 2: bacterial pneumonia, 3: viral pneumonia, 4: tuberculosis.

5.38% is far lower than the minimum false negative rate of 20% for RT-PCR tests, and false positives are minimized as well.

Most of the reduction in the model's accuracy can be traced to its difficulty in distinguishing between bacterial and viral pneumonia. While this limits the model's usability as a general-purpose diagnostic tool across all five lung classes, it does not interfere with its primary goal of identifying new COVID-19 infections. Ultimately, the model was able to classify COVID-19 chest x-rays more accurately than the common tests used today and also differentiate COVID-19 from numerous other lung conditions.

It should be noted that future studies should investigate the use of more common respiratory infections, such as the common cold or seasonal flu, as control classes to confirm the model's robustness. Furthermore, due to the contagious nature of COVID-19, the physical practicalities of using imaging equipment on COVID-19 patients are complex, as the equipment must be thoroughly cleaned between each screening, and patients are at risk of transmitting the virus whilst moving to and from the equipment [29].

A live web application of the trained model can be found at https://cov2d19-classifier.herokuapp.com/. Given an x-ray image, the app will return the probability that it belongs to each class along with a final prediction. This application is in a beta development stage and has not been tested in a professional environment; therefore, it is not recommended for official medical use.

2.5 Conclusions

In this chapter, we have described a convolutional neural network that uses the DenseNet-201 model to detect cases of COVID-19 pneumonia using chest radiographs. It is robust and reliable, as it uses a larger dataset and more control classes than most other models published. It is able to accurately distinguish COVID-19 from healthy, viral pneumonia, bacterial pneumonia, and tuberculosis x-ray images. It achieves an F1 score of 0.96 and a COVID-19 classification accuracy that far exceeds those of RT-PCR tests, which suffer from a high false negative rate.

Given the sheer volume of patients that must be screened, this automated tool can save valuable time, money, and resources that are scarce in healthcare systems around the world. It may especially impact developing countries and resource-starved regions where both molecular tests and trained radiologists are in short supply, as it is an automated diagnosis tool that provides a simple detection solution. We believe that this model, and machine learning as a whole, can significantly improve current COVID-19 diagnosis practices—vital in a pandemic in which accurate and efficient screening is a must.

Acknowledgements

This paper and model would not have been possible without the support of the MIT Lincoln Laboratory, the Beaver Works Summer Institute, and Medlytics course instructors. In particular, the instructors Jordan Montgomery (PhD), Jeffrey Arena, and Thomas Curtis helped immeasurably with their expertise and teaching.

References

[1] 2020 Listings of WHO's Response to COVID-19.World Health Organization

[2] Dong E, Du H and Gardner L 2020 An interactive web-based dashboard to track COVID-19 in real time *Lancet Infect. Dis.* **20** 533–4

[3] Wang W *et al* 2020 Detection of SARS-CoV-2 in different types of clinical specimens *JAMA* **323** 1843–4

[4] CDC 2020 'Testing for COVID-19.'

[5] Mukherjee S 2020 The average turnaround for COVID test results is now 7 days or more *Fortune*

[6] Kucirka L M *et al* 2020 Variation in false-negative rate of reverse transcriptase polymerase chain reaction–based SARS-CoV-2 tests by time since exposure *Annal. Int. Med.* **173** 262–67

[7] Ng M-Y *et al* 2020 Imaging profile of the COVID-19 infection: radiologic findings and literature review *Radiol.: Cardiothorac. Imaging* **2** e200034
[8] Kann B H *et al* 2019 Artificial intelligence in oncology: current applications and future directions *Oncology* **33** 46–53
[9] Walsh F 2020 AI 'outperforms' doctors diagnosing breast cancer
[10] Nigeria Healthcare Service Cost Comparison 2018 https://knoema.com/jlebqif/nigeria-healthcare-service-cost-comparison
[11] Krizhevsky A *et al* 2017 ImageNet classification with deep convolutional neural networks *Commun. ACM* **60** 84–90
[12] Apostolopoulos I D and Tzani A M 2020 Covid-19: automatic detection from x-ray images utilizing transfer learning with convolutional neural networks. *Phys. Eng. Sci. Med.* **43** 635–40
[13] Asif S *et al* 2020 Classification of COVID-19 from chest x-ray images using deep convolutional neural networks. medRxiv https://www.medrxiv.org/content/10.1101/2020.05.01.20088211v2
[14] Ozturk T *et al* 2020 Automated detection of COVID-19 cases using deep neural networks with x-ray images *Comput. Biol. Med.* **121** 103792
[15] Sethy P K and Behera S K 2020 Detection of coronavirus disease (COVID-19) based on deep features *Preprints* **2020** 2020030300
[16] Xu X *et al* 2020 A deep learning system to screen novel coronavirus disease 2019 pneumonia *Engineering* **6** 1122–9
[17] Yoo S H *et al* 2020 Deep learning-based decision-tree classifier for COVID-19 diagnosis from chest x-ray imaging *Front. Med.* **7** 427
[18] Hemdan E E-D, Shouman M A and Karar M E 2020 Covidx-net: A framework of deep learning classifiers to diagnose covid-19 in x-ray images arXiv:2003.11055
[19] Wang L, Mo J, Zhou G, Xu L and Liu Y 2020 An efficient mixture of deep and machine learning models for COVID-19 diagnosis in chest X-ray images *PLoS ONE* **15** e0242535
[20] Kermany D, Zhang K and Goldbaum M 2018 Labeled optical coherence tomography (OCT) and chest x-ray images for classification Mendeley Data https://data.mendeley.com/datasets/rscbjbr9sj/2
[21] Kermany D S *et al* 2018 Identifying medical diagnoses and treatable diseases by image-based deep learning *Cell* **172** 1122-31.e9
[22] Jaeger S *et al* 2014 Two public chest x-ray datasets for computer-aided screening of pulmonary diseases. *Quant. Imaging Med. Surg.* **4** 475-7
[23] Chowdhury M E H *et al* 2020 Can AI help in screening viral and COVID-19 pneumonia? *IEEE Access* **8** 132665–76
[24] Singh T 2020 COVID-19 & normal posteroanterior(PA) x-rays. *Kaggle* https://www.kaggle.com/tarandeep97/covid19-normal-posteroanteriorpa-xrays
[25] Patel P 2020 Chest x-ray (Covid-19 & pneumonia). *Kaggle* https://www.kaggle.com/prashant268/chest-xray-covid19-pneumonia
[26] Raddar 2020 Chest x-rays tuberculosis from India. *Kaggle* https://www.kaggle.com/raddar/chest-xrays-tuberculosis-from-india
[27] Larxel 2020 COVID-19 x rays. *Kaggle* https://www.kaggle.com/andrewmvd/convid19-x-rays
[28] Huang G *et al* 2016 Densely connected convolutional networks arXiv:1608.06993
[29] Uvaradweb and UVA | Physician Resource 2020 COVID-19 and imaging: why CT scans and x-rays are not recommended for diagnosing coronavirus (UVA Radiology and Medical Imaging Blog for Patients)

IOP Publishing

Artificial Intelligence Strategies for Analyzing COVID-19 Pneumonia Lung Imaging, Volume 1
Characterization approaches
Ayman El-Baz and Jasjit S Suri

Chapter 3

Inf-Net: an automatic lung infection segmentation network that uses CT images

Tao Zhou, Dengping Fan, Gepeng Ji, Geng Chen, Huazhu Fu and Ling Shao

Coronavirus disease 2019 (COVID-19) has spread aggressively since early 2020, causing the world to suffer from an existential health crisis. In practice, the identification of infected regions using chest CT images is of great significance for the diagnosis and treatment of COVID-19 patients. Although progress has been made, lung infection segmentation still faces various challenges, including low levels of contrast between normal tissues and infections as well as large variations in infection characteristics. Deep-learning-based techniques require huge volumes of labelled data to train an effective model; however, it is difficult to collect a large amount of data within a short period. To overcome these challenges, in this study, we propose a novel lung infection segmentation network, called Inf-Net, which can automatically segment infected regions of chest CT images. Specifically, a parallel partial decoder is adopted to aggregate the high-level features and then produce a global map. Next, Inf-Net jointly utilizes edge attention and reverse attention to obtain enhanced representations and model the boundaries, which can effectively boost the segmentation performance. Furthermore, a semi-supervised segmentation framework based on a randomly selected propagation strategy is proposed; this can make full use of unlabelled samples to improve the network's learning ability and its performance. Experimental results obtained using the COVID-SemiSeg data set and real CT images show that the proposed Inf-Net and Semi-Inf-Net outperform other cutting-edge segmentation methods.

3.1 Introduction

The novel coronavirus disease (COVID-19) that emerged in December 2019 has led to a worldwide crisis that has severely impacted healthcare systems, economies, and

doi:10.1088/978-0-7503-3795-3ch3

personal wellbeing all around the world [1]. The reverse-transcription polymerase chain reaction (RT-PCR) test has been regarded as the major means of detecting COVID-19 infection in screening programmes [2, 3]. However, the shortage of equipment and the restrictions of test settings limit the rapid and precise screening of suspected subjects. In addition, the RT-PCR test has been reported to produce high false negative rates [4]. Medical radiological imaging, e.g., x-rays and computed tomography (CT), have been used as supplements to the RT-PCR test and their efficiency has been validated for lung disease diagnosis and quantification [5, 6]. Furthermore, in comparison with the RT-PCR test, various studies have shown that chest CT analysis can result in higher performance (e.g. greater sensitivity) in COVID-19 diagnosis [7, 8]. In comparison with X-rays [9, 10], CT screening is widely preferred due to its ability to provide a three-dimensional view of the patient's lung [11]. The qualitative evaluation of infected lung regions and longitudinal changes using CT images can provide important and useful information in the diagnosis and treatment of COVID-19 [12–14]. However, the manual calibration of lung infections is a tedious and time-consuming task [15]. Moreover, infection calibration strongly depends on the expertise of radiologists, which could be influenced by clinical experience and individual bias. Thus, it is very important to develop accurate and automatic lung infection segmentation algorithms.

Recently, several deep-learning-based methods have been developed for the detection of COVID-19 and the segmentation of lung infections [5, 16, 17]. For example, Rajinikanth *et al* [16] proposed COVID-Net to detect COVID-19 cases using chest radiography images. Chen *et al* [17] proposed a modified U-Net model for accurate and rapid segmentation of COVID-19 infection regions from chest CT images. In addition, Xu *et al* [18] proposed a location–attention-oriented model to compute the infection probability of COVID-19. Wu *et al* [19] proposed a joint framework to perform classification and segmentation to achieve real-time diagnosis of COVID-19 patients. Wang *et al* [20] proposed a weakly supervised deep-learning-based framework to detect COVID-19 in 3D CT volumes. Although these methods have made progress in diagnosing COVID-19 in clinical practice, there are still several challenges to achieving accurate COVID-19 infection segmentation using CT images. Specifically, (1) there are large variations in the texture, size, and position of infections shown in CT images, which causes a significant challenge for infection segmentation. For example, consolidations are tiny and small; thus, it is easy to obtain false negative segmentation results from a whole CT image. (2) The inter-class variance is very small. For example, blurring and low contrast often appear at ground-glass opacity (GGO) boundaries, making it difficult to identify such boundaries. (3) Due to the COVID-19 crisis, it has been difficult to collect a large amount of labelled data within a short time, but sufficient labelled data is crucial to train deep learning models. Moreover, collecting high-quality pixel-level annotations of lung infections in CT images is still expensive and time-consuming.

To address these challenges, we developed an automatic COVID-19 lung infection segmentation network (Inf-Net) for CT Images. The motivation for our Inf-Net stems from the fact that, during lung infection segmentation, clinicians often utilize a coarse-to-fine strategy, i.e. they first roughly locate the infected regions and then accurately extract contours according to the local appearance information. In other words, the boundary and the area are two key characteristics that can be used to effectively distinguish between normal tissues and infections. Thus, the proposed Inf-Net first locates coarse areas and then implicitly models the boundaries via reverse attention and edge preservation constraints to explicitly enhance the boundary identification. Furthermore, we propose a semi-supervised segmentation framework which can leverage an amount of unlabelled data to improve the segmentation performance. The experimental results obtained for the collected COVID-SemiSeg data set demonstrate that the proposed Inf-Net and Semi-Inf-Net networks outperform most cutting-edge segmentation methods. The main contributions are threefold: (1) we propose a novel lung segmentation model, i.e. Inf-Net, for CT images. By aggregating features from high-level layers via a parallel partial decoder (PPD), the combined features can include much contextual information and produce a global map of initial guidance areas for the fine segmentation steps. Moreover, we leverage a set of recurrent reverse attention (RA) modules and an edge preservation module to exploit the relationship between areas and boundary cues. (2) To alleviate the shortage of labelled data, we propose a semi-supervised segmentation framework for COVID-19 infection segmentation. This framework offers a better learning ability via a randomly selected propagation strategy. (3) We build a novel COVID-SemiSeg data set, which includes 100 labelled CT slices from the COVID-19 CT Segmentation data set [21] and 1600 unlabelled images from the COVID-19 CT Collection data set [22]. The COVID-SemiSeg data set is publicly available at https://github.com/DengPingFan/Inf-Net

3.2 Method

We propose a novel COVID-19 lung infection segmentation deep network (Inf-Net) to automatically segment infected regions of CT images. In the following sections, we first introduce the details of the proposed Inf-Net and then introduce the semi-supervised Inf-Net. Finally, we introduce an extension of the proposed framework for the multiclass labelling of different types of lung infection.

3.2.1 Lung infection segmentation network

Figure 3.1 shows the overall architecture of our Inf-Net, which consists of three key components: the edge preservation module (EPM), the RA module, and the PPD. Specifically, CT images are first fed to two convolutional blocks to extract high-resolution (i.e. low-level) features. In addition, an EPM is proposed to improve the representation of objective region boundaries. Then, we adopt a PPD to aggregate high-level features (i.e., f_i, $i = 3, 4, 5$) and obtain a coarse global map S_g of lung infections. Furthermore, these high-level features combined with f_2 are fed to RA modules under multi-scale supervision. Finally, the output S_s is fed to a sigmoid activation function to obtain the final prediction of the infected lung regions. The details of each key component and our loss function will be given in the following sections.

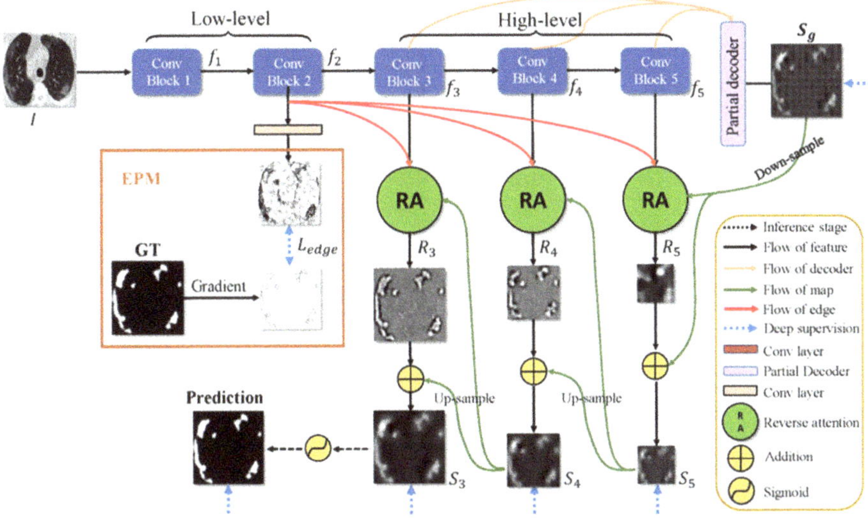

Figure 3.1. The architecture of the proposed Inf-Net model, which consists of three key components, i.e., the EPM, the RA module, and the PPD.

3.2.1.1 Edge preservation module

Recently, several related studies [22–24] have shown that edge information can provide useful fine-grained constraints to guide feature extraction during object segmentation, while low-level features often preserve sufficient edge information. Thus, we propose an EPM to capture edge information in order to boost the segmentation performance. Specifically, the low-level features (e.g., f_2) are fed into a convolutional layer with one filter to produce the edge map, which is supervised using the edge detection loss. The dissimilarity between the produced edge map and the edge map G_e derived from the ground truth (GT) is then measured using the standard binary cross-entropy (BCE) loss; thus, we can obtain:

$$L_{\text{edge}} = -\sum_{x=1}^{w}\sum_{y=1}^{h}[G_e \text{loglog}\,(S_e) + (1 - G_e)\log(1 - S_e)], \tag{3.1}$$

where G_e denotes the gradient of the ground-truth map G_s, and (x, y) are the coordinates of each pixel; w and h represent the width and height of the predicted edge map and the ground-truth map, respectively.

3.2.1.2 Parallel partial decoder

A recent study [25] has pointed out that low-level features provide fewer contributions to object segmentation than high-level ones, but they often require more computational resources due to their relatively large spatial resolutions. Thus, in the proposed model, we adopt a parallel partial decoder to aggregate the high-level features (as shown in figure 3.2). Specifically, we utilize Res2Net as a backbone to extract two sets of low-level features (f_1 and f_2) and three sets of high-level features (f_3, f_4, and f_5). The partial decoder is then adopted to aggregate the high-level

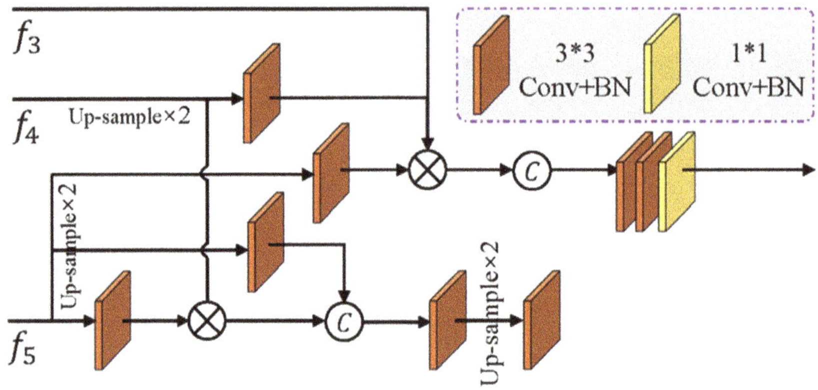

Figure 3.2. The structure of the parallel partial decoder.

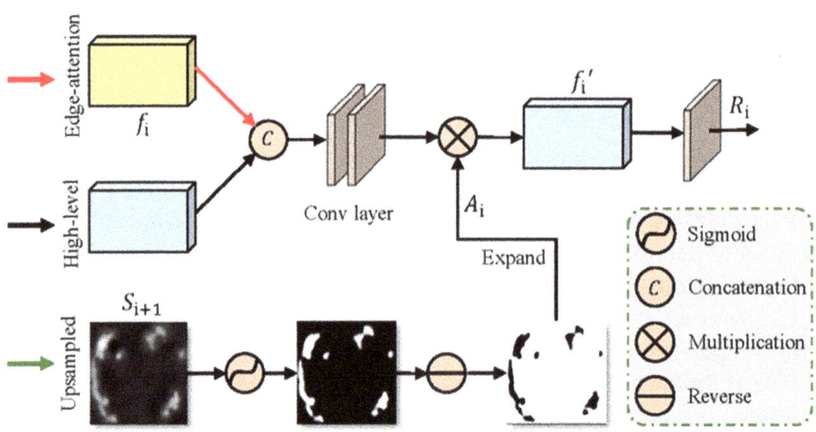

Figure 3.3. Illustration of the reverse attention module.

features using a parallel connection. We can also obtain a coarse global map using the high-level features, which is used to guide the RA modules.

3.2.1.3 Reverse attention module

To accurately determine infected lung regions, clinicians often utilize a two-step strategy. The first step is to roughly localize the infected regions, and the second step is to inspect some local tissue structures to accurately label the infected regions. Inspired by this two-step strategy, the proposed Inf-Net uses two key components in its design, i.e. a rough locator and a fine labeller. Specifically, the partial decoder is regarded as a rough locator, which is guided by a global map, S_g. A progressive framework is the proposed to segment the infection regions in an erasing manner, which is regarded as a fine labeller. Furthermore, to exploit complementary regions and details, we consider adaptively using reverse attention on the three parallel high-level features. As shown in figure 3.3, we can obtain the reverse attention features R_i by multiplying the fused high-level features and the edge attention features, i.e., $R_i = C(f_i, D(e_{att}))A_i$, where $C(\bullet)$ denotes a concatenation operation followed by a 2D convolutional layer with 64 filters, and $D(\bullet)$ denotes a downsampling operation. In addition, the weight A_i is defined by $A_i = E(\ominus(\sigma(U(S_{i+1}))))$, where $U(\bullet)$ denotes an upsampling operation, $\ominus(\bullet)$ is an inversion operation performed by subtracting the input from matrix E, and $\sigma(\bullet)$ denotes the sigmoid activation function. In addition, $E(\bullet)$ denotes the expansion of a single channel feature to 64 repeated tensors; and the detailed procedures are shown in figure 3.3.

3.2.1.4 Overall loss function

In the proposed model, the loss function includes two key components, i.e. the loss function L_{edge} for edge supervision, and the loss function L_{seg} for segmentation supervision. To achieve accurate segmentation, we define a combination of a weighted intersection over the union (IoU) loss (L_{IoU}^{w}) and a weighted BCE loss (L_{BCE}^{w}) for the segmentation supervision, as follows:

$$L_{seg} = L_{IoU}^{w} + L_{BCE}^{w}. \tag{3.2}$$

The two components effectively provide global and local supervision for accurate segmentation, as the standard IoU loss is widely adopted in segmentation tasks, while the weighted IoU loss can increase the weights of hard pixels to highlight their importance. Compared with the BCE loss, the weighted BCE loss pays more attention to hard pixels rather than treating all pixels equally. The definitions of the losses are the same as those used in [26, 27].

Finally, the overall loss is defined as follows:

$$L_{total} = L_{edge} + L_{seg}\left(G_s, S_g^{up}\right) + \sum_{i=3}^{5} L_{seg}(G_s, S_i^{up}), \tag{3.3}$$

where G_s denotes the object-level segmentation ground-truth map, S_g^{up} denotes the upsampled global map, and S_i^{up} denotes the ith upsampled side-output map.

3.2.2 Semi-supervised Inf-Net

Because it is difficult and time-consuming to manually label infected lung regions, we are only able to obtain a very limited number of annotated CT images. To overcome this problem, we present a novel framework for the semi-supervised Inf-net, which can leverage various unlabelled CT images to improve the generalization of the proposed model. The proposed semi-supervised infected lung region segmentation framework is shown in figure 3.4. The proposed framework is based on a random sampling strategy, which can progressively enlarge the training set using the unlabelled samples. Algorithm 1 shows the procedure used to assign pseudo labels to unlabelled CT images; these CT images with pseudo labels are then adopted to train the proposed infected lung region segmentation model.

3.2.3 Multiclass infection labelling task

In the clinical setting, it is often necessary to conduct a quantitative evaluation of different types of lung infection, e.g., GGO and consolidation. To achieve this task,

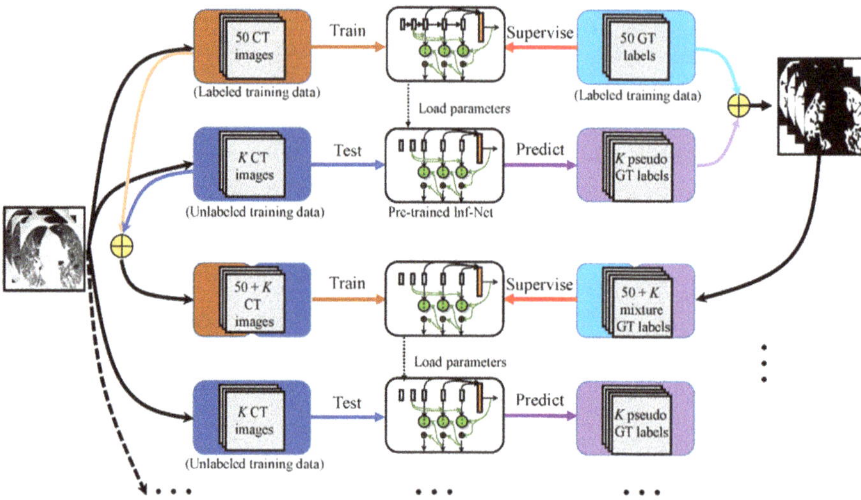

Figure 3.4. Illustration of the proposed semi-supervised Inf-Net framework.

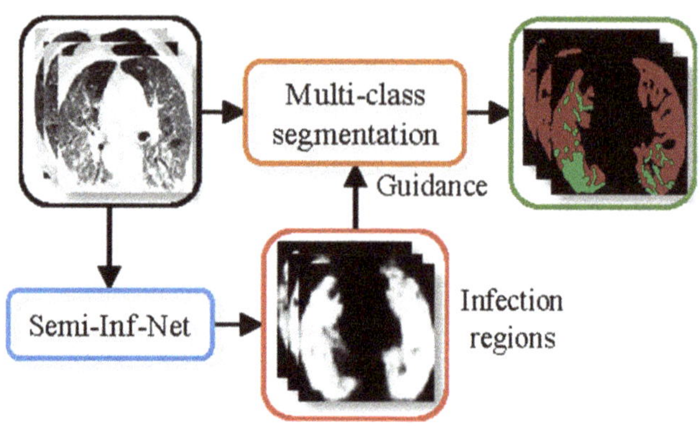

Figure 3.5. Illustration of the use of segmented infection regions to guide multiclass segmentation.

we extend the proposed Semi-Inf-Net to a multiclass lung infection labelling framework, in which the infected regions are utilized to guide the multiclass labelling task. Figure 3.5 shows the main structure of the multiclass lung infection labelling framework. Specifically, we first obtain the Semi-Inf-Net infection segmentation results and then utilize them to guide the multiclass labelling of different kinds of lung infection. To achieve this, both the segmentation results and their corresponding CT images are fed to a multiclass segmentation network (as shown in figure 3.5), e.g. FCN8s [28], or U-Net [29]. It is worth noting that the multiclass labelling framework can take full advantage of the infection segmentation results obtained by the proposed Semi-Inf-Net model, boosting the performance of the multiclass infection labelling task.

Algorithm 1 Semi-supervised Inf-Net
Input: Labelled training data D_{labeled} and unlabelled training data set $D_{\text{unlabeled}}$.
Output: Trained model M
1: Conduct the model M training on D_{labeled};
2: **Repeat**
4: Conduct testing using the trained model M and K randomly selected CT images from $D_{\text{unlabeled}}$, which forms a network-labelled data set $D_{\text{Net-labeled}}$, consisting of K CT images with pseudo labels;
5: Enlarge the training data set, i.e. $D_{\text{training}} = D_{\text{training}} \cup D_{\text{Net-labeled}}$;
6: Remove K CT images from the unlabelled data set $D_{\text{unlabeled}}$;
7: Fine-tune the model M using the training data set D_{training};
8: **Until**: $D_{\text{unlabeled}}$ is empty.
9: **Return**: Trained model M.

3.3 Experimental results and analysis

3.3.1 Data set

In this work, we form a semi-supervised COVID-19 infection segmentation data set (COVID-SemiSeg), which includes: (1) 100 labelled CT images [21], from which 45 CT images are randomly selected as training samples, five CT images are selected as validation samples, and the remaining 50 CT images are regarded as testing samples; (2) 1600 2D CT axial slices, which are extracted from 3D volumes in the COVID-19 CT Collection data set [22].

3.3.2 Experimental settings

Comparison methods: To evaluate the effectiveness of the proposed model, we compare the proposed Inf-Net and Semi-Inf-Net with the following five methods: U-Net3 [29], U-Net++3 [30], Attention-UNet4 [31], Gated-UNet4 [32], and Dense-UNet5 [33]. In addition, for the multiclass labelling experiments, we compare the proposed framework with three models: DeepLabV3+ [34], FCN8s [28], and multiclass U-Net [29].

Evaluation metrics: Six metrics are employed for performance evaluation, including the Dice similarity coefficient, sensitivity (Sen.), specificity (Spec.), precision (Prec.), structural measure [35], enhanced-alignment measure [36], and mean absolute error. The details of each evaluation metric can be found in [37].

3.3.3 Segmentation results

Quantitative comparison: The quantitative results are shown in table 3.1. From table 3.1, we can observe that our Inf-Net performs better than U-Net and U-Net++ in terms of Dice, S_α, E_φ^{mean}, and MAE. The main reason for the superior performance of Inf-Net is that the implicit reverse attention and explicit edge-attention modeling can provide robust feature representations. It is worth noting that our

Table 3.1. Quantitative results of infected lung region segmentation using different methods with the COVID-SemiSeg data set .

Method	Backbone	Param.	FLOPs	Dice	Sen.	Spec.	S_α	E_ϕ^{mean}	MAE
U-Net	VGG16	7.853 M	38.116G	0.439	0.534	0.858	0.622	0.625	0.186
Attention-U-Net	VGG16	8.727 M	31.730G	0.583	0.637	0.921	0.744	0.739	0.112
Gated-U-Net	VGG16	175.093M	714.419M	0.623	0.658	0.926	0.725	0.814	0.102
Dense-U-Net	DenseNet161	45.082M	43.785G	0.515	0.594	0.840	0.655	0.662	0.184
U-Net++	VGG16	9.163M	65.938G	0.581	0.672	0.902	0.722	0.720	0.120
Inf-Net	Res2Net	33.122M	13.922G	0.682	0.692	0.943	0.781	0.838	0.082
Semi-Inf-Net	Res2Net	33.122M	13.922G	0.739	0.725	0.960	0.800	0.894	0.064

Table 3.2. Quantitative results for ground-glass opacities in the COVID-SemiSeg data set.

Methods	Dice	Sen.	Spec.	S_α	E_ϕ^{mean}	MAE
DeepLabV3+(stride=8)	0.375	0.478	0.863	0.544	0.675	0.123
DeepLabV3+(stride=16)	0.443	0.713	0.823	0.548	0.655	0.156
FCN8s	0.471	0.537	0.905	0.582	0.774	0.101
Multiclass U-Net	0.441	0.343	0.984	0.588	0.714	0.082
Semi-Inf-Net & FCN8s	0.646	0.720	0.941	0.711	0.882	0.071
Semi-Inf-Net & MC	0.624	0.618	0.966	0.706	0.889	0.067

Table 3.3. Quantitative results for consolidation in the COVID-SemiSeg data set.

Methods	Dice	Sen.	Spec.	S_α	E_ϕ^{mean}	MAE
DeepLabV3+(stride=8)	0.148	0.152	0.738	0.500	0.523	0.064
DeepLabV3+(stride=16)	0.238	0.310	0.708	0.517	0.606	0.077
FCN8s	0.279	0.268	0.716	0.560	0.560	0.050
Multiclass U-Net	0.403	0.414	0.967	0.577	0.767	0.055
Semi-Inf-Net & FCN8s	0.301	0.235	0.808	0.571	0.571	0.045
Semi-Inf-Net & MC	0.458	0.509	0.967	0.603	0.767	0.047

model can obtain a further 5.7% improvement in the Dice metric when the semi-supervised learning strategy is introduced.

An assistant diagnostic model is often expected to provide additional relevant information regarding the infected areas. Thus, we applied the proposed model to a multiclass (i.e. GGO and consolidation segmentation) labelling task. Tables 3.2 and 3.3 show a comparison of the segmentation results for the COVID-SemiSeg data set, in which 'Semi-Inf-Net & FCN8s' and 'Semi-Inf-Net & MC' denote the combinations of our Semi-Inf-Net with FCN8s [28] and multiclass U-Net [29], respectively.

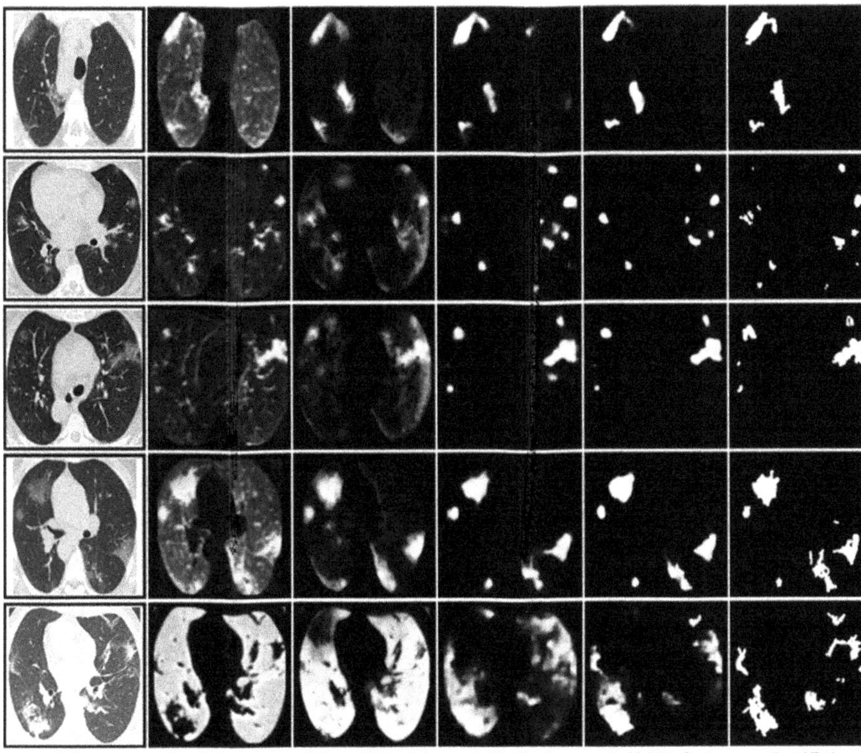

Figure 3.6. Visual comparison of infected lung segmentation results using different methods.

From table III, it can be observed that our 'Semi-Inf-Net & MC' obtains better performance for GGO segmentation, according to most of the evaluation metrics. The proposed model also achieves better performance for consolidation segmentation than the other compared methods. For instance, our method outperforms multiclass U-Net [29] by 12% according to the Dice metric for the average segmentation results.

Qualitative comparison: The qualitative results of the infected lung segmentation results are shown in figure 3.6. Based on the results, we offer the following observations: (1) our Semi-Inf-Net and Inf-Net outperform other comparison methods; (2) the U-Net model achieves unsatisfactory results, as various mis-segmented tissues are present; (3) the U-Net++ model improves the segmentation results, but the performance still needs to be improved. The performance of the proposed Inf-Net is mainly due to the advantage of the coarse-to-fine segmentation strategy, in which a parallel partial decoder is regarded as a rough labeller to first locate infected lung regions and then fine segmentation based on multiple edge attention modules is utilized to achieve the final results. It is also worth noting that our semi-supervised learning strategy can obtain better infected lung segmentation results. From figure 3.6, one can observe that Semi-Inf-Net obtains more accurate

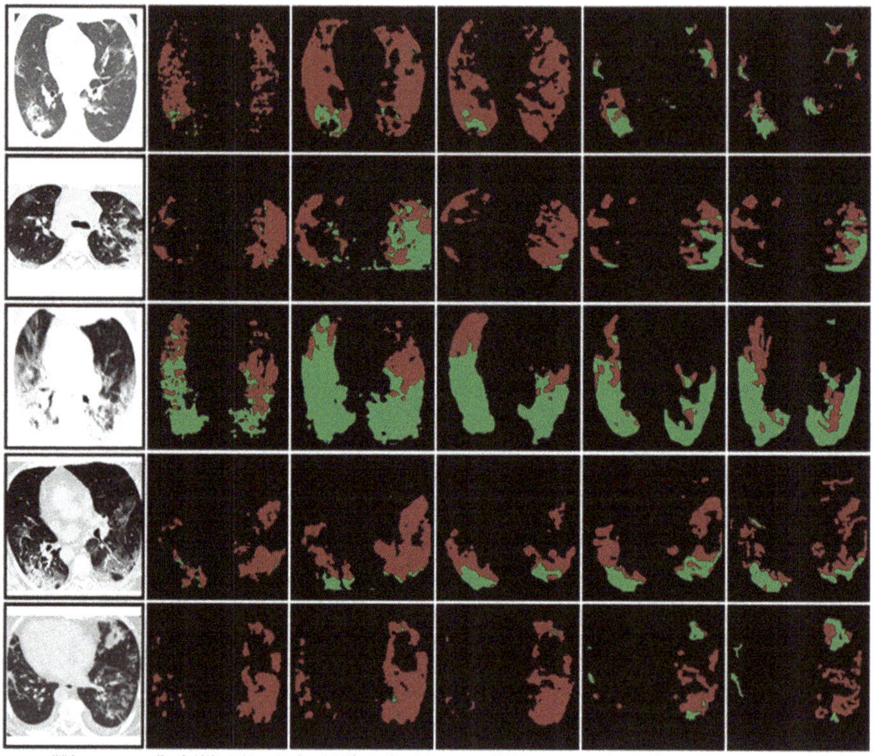

Figure 3.7. Visual comparison of multiclass infected lung segmentation results using different methods. Red and green labels denote GGO and consolidation, respectively.

boundaries than Inf-Net, while Inf-Net often obtains blurred boundaries, especially in subtle infection regions.

In addition, figure 3.7 shows the multiclass infection labelling results. From figure 3.7, it can be observed that our Semi-Inf-Net & MC consistently performs better than all the compared methods. Specifically, GGO and consolidation infections can be accurately segmented using the proposed Semi-Inf-Net & MC model, which further validates the advantage of the proposed model. The DeepLabV3+ method obtains unsatisfactory results with different strides and fully convolutional networks (FCNs), in which consolidation and GGO infections can be inaccurately segmented.

3.3.4 Ablation study

To validate the effectiveness of each key component of the proposed Semi-Inf-Net (i.e., PPD, RA, and EA modules), we conducted the following ablation studies.

(1) Effectiveness of PPD: to investigate the importance of the parallel partial decoder, we conducted a comparison between s1 (backbone only) and s3 (backbone + PPD) in table 3.4. The results clearly demonstrate that PPD can effectively boost the segmentation performance.

Table 3.4. Ablation study of the proposed Semi-Inf-Net.

Method	Dice	Sen.	Spec.	S_α	E_ϕ^{mean}	MAE
(s1) Backbone	0.442	0.570	0.825	0.651	0.569	0.207
(s2) Backbone+EPM	0.541	0.665	0.807	0.673	0.659	0.205
(s3) Backbone+PPD	0.669	0.744	0.880	0.720	0.810	0.125
(s4) Backbone+RA	0.625	0.826	0.809	0.725	0.814	0.102
(s5) Backbone+RA+EPM	0.515	0.594	0.840	0.655	0.662	0.184
(s6) Backbone+PPD+RA	0.581	0.672	0.902	0.722	0.720	0.120
(s7) Backbone+PPD+RA+EPM	0.739	0.725	0.960	0.800	0.894	0.064

Table 3.5. Quantitative results of infected lung region segmentation using different methods with the COVID-SemiSeg data set.

Method	Dice	Sen.	Spec.	Prec.	MAE
U-Net	0.308	0.678	0.836	0.265	0.214
Attention-U-Net	0.466	0.723	0.830	0.390	0.095
Grated-U-Net	0.447	0.674	0.956	0.375	0.066
Dense-U-Net	0.410	0.607	0.977	0.415	0.167
U-Net++	0.444	0.877	0.929	0.369	0.106
Inf-Net	0.579	0.870	0.974	0.500	0.047
Semi-Inf-Net	0.597	0.865	0.977	0.515	0.033

(2) Effectiveness of RA: from the results shown in table 3.4, we can see that s4 (backbone + RA) improves the segmentation performance (s1) in terms of metrics such as Dice, sensitivity, MAE, etc. This confirms that the RA module can help our model to accurately distinguish true infected areas.
(3) Effectiveness of PPD and RA: as shown in table 3.4, it can be observed that s4 performs better than the other models (i.e., s1–s4) in most metrics. Thus, the comparison results demonstrate that the RA together with the PDD contribute to improving the performance of our Inf-Net.
(4) Effectiveness of EPM: we also investigated the effectiveness of the EPM module. From table IV (i.e. s2 vs. s1, s5 vs. s4, s7 vs. s6), we can observe that the EPM module effectively boosts the segmentation performance.

3.3.5 Evaluation using real CT volumes

In clinical use, we may need to face the fact that some CT images show no infection. Thus, to validate the effectiveness of our model on real CT images, we tested the proposed model on the recently released COVID-19 infection segmentation data set [9]. This data set consists of 638 slices, in which 285 non-infected slices and 353 infected slices are extracted from nine CT volumes of real COVID-19 patients. Table 3.5 shows a comparison of the results obtained using different methods. It can be observed that our model still achieves the best segmentation when the data contains some non-infected slices. This is mainly because the unlabelled data used in our semi-supervised learning framework contains a lot of uninfected slices, which ensures that our model deals effectively with uninfected slices.

3.4 Conclusions

The accurate segmentation of infected lung regions in COVID-19 CT scans plays a critical role in the quantitative management of patients. In this study, we have presented a novel COVID-19 infected lung CT segmentation network (i.e., Inf-Net), which utilizes explicit edge attention and implicit reverse attention to improve the segmentation of infected regions. Moreover, to make use of various unlabelled samples, we built a semi-supervised segmentation framework named Semi-Inf-Net. Extensive experiments were conducted on the collected COVID-SemiSeg data set and real CT volumes. The experimental results demonstrate that the proposed Inf-Net and Semi-Inf-Net perform better than other state-of-the-art segmentation models. It is worth noting that the proposed framework can be used to assess a diagnosis of COVID-19, e.g. by quantifying infected lung regions and monitoring longitudinal changes. We hope that this work will accelerate related studies for the diagnosis of COVID-19 and provide a baseline semi-supervised model with limited data for future research.

References and further reading

[1] Wang C, Horby P W, Hayden F G and Gao G F 2020 A novel coronavirus outbreak of global health concern *The Lancet* **395** 470–3

[2] Tahamtan A and Ardebili A 2020 Real-time RT-PCR in COVID-19 detection: issues affecting the results. *Expert Rev. Mol. Diagn.* **20** 453–4

[3] Lan L, Xu D, Ye G, Xia C, Wang S, Li Y and Xu H 2020 Positive RT-PCR test results in patients recovered from COVID-19. *JAMA* **323** 1502–3

[4] Ai T, Yang Z, Hou H, Zhan C, Chen C, Lv W, Tao Q, Sun Z and Xia L 2020 Correlation of chest CT and RT-PCR testing for coronavirus disease 2019 (COVID-19) in China: a report of 1014 cases. *Radiology* **296** E32–40

[5] Shi F, Wang J, Shi J, Wu Z, Wang Q, Tang Z, He K, Shi Y and Shen D 2020 Review of artificial intelligence techniques in imaging data acquisition, segmentation, and diagnosis for COVID-19 *IEEE Rev. Biomed. Eng.* **14** 4–15

[6] Xiong Y, Sun D, Liu Y, Fan Y, Zhao L, Li X and Zhu W 2020 Clinical and high-resolution CT features of the COVID-19 infection: comparison of the initial and follow-up changes. *Invest. Radiol.* **55** 332–9

[7] Fang Y, Zhang H, Xie J, Lin M, Ying L, Pang P and Ji W 2020 Sensitivity of chest CT for COVID-19: comparison to RT-PCR. *Radiology* **296** E115–7

[8] Tahamtan A and Ardebili A 2020 Real-time RT-PCR in COVID-19 detection: issues affecting the results. *Expert Rev. Mol. Diagn.* **20** 453–4

[9] Ozturk T, Talo M, Yildirim E A, Baloglu U B, Yildirim O and Acharya U R 2020 Automated detection of COVID-19 cases using deep neural networks with X-ray images. *Comput. Biol. Med.* **121** 103792

[10] Wang L, Lin Z Q and Wong A 2020 Covid-net: a tailored deep convolutional neural network design for detection of covid-19 cases from chest x-ray images. *Sci. Rep.* **10** 19549

[11] Ye Z, Zhang Y, Wang Y, Huang Z and Song B 2020 Chest CT manifestations of new coronavirus disease 2019 (COVID-19): a pictorial review. *Eur. Radiol.* **30** 4381–9

[12] Lyu P, Liu X, Zhang R, Shi L and Gao J 2020 The performance of chest CT in evaluating the clinical severity of COVID-19 pneumonia: identifying critical cases based on CT characteristics *Invest. Radiol.* **55** 412–21

[13] Shan F, Gao Y, Wang J, Shi W, Shi N, Han M, Xue Z, Shen D and Shi Y 2020 Abnormal lung quantification in chest CT images of COVID-19 patients with deep learning and its application to severity prediction *Med. Phys.* **48** 1633–45

[14] Sun N, Wei L, Shi S, Jiao D, Song R, Ma L and Wang H *et al* 2020 A qualitative study on the psychological experience of caregivers of COVID-19 patients. *Am. J. Infect. Control* **48** 592–8

[15] Chen X, Yao L, Zhou T, Dong J and Zhang Y 2021 Momentum contrastive learning for few-shot COVID-19 diagnosis from chest CT images. *Pattern Recognit.* **113** 107826

[16] Rajinikanth V, Dey N, Noel Joseph Raj A, Ella Hassanien A, Santosh K C and Raja N 2020 Harmony-search and Otsu based system for coronavirus disease (COVID-19) detection using lung CT scan images arXiv:2004.03431

[17] Chen X, Yao L and Zhang Y 2020 Residual attention U-Net for automated multi-class segmentation of COVID-19 chest CT images arXiv:2004.05645

[18] Xu X, Jiang X, Ma C, Du P, Li X, Lv S and Yu L *et al* 2020 A deep learning system to screen novel coronavirus disease 2019 pneumonia. *Engineering* **6** 1122–9

[19] Wu Y-H, Gao S-H, Mei J, Xu J, Fan D-P, Zhang R-G and Cheng M-M 2021 JCS: an explainable covid-19 diagnosis system by joint classification and segmentation. *IEEE Trans. Image Process.* **30** 3113–26

[20] Wang X, Deng X, Fu Q, Zhou Q, Feng J, Ma H, Liu W and Zheng C 2020 A weakly-supervised framework for COVID-19 classification and lesion localization from chest CT. *IEEE Trans. Med. Imaging* **39** 2615–25

[21] COVID-19 CT segmentation dataset https://medicalsegmentation.com/covid19/

[22] Cohen J P, Morrison P and Dao L 2020 COVID-19 Image Data Collection arXiv:2003.11597

[23] Wu Z, Su L and Huang Q 2019 Stacked cross refinement network for edge-aware salient object detection *Proc. of the IEEE/CVF Int. Conf. on Computer Vision* 7264–73

[24] Zhang Z, Fu H, Dai H, Shen J, Pang Y and Shao L 2019 Et-net: a generic edge-attention guidance network for medical image segmentation. *Int. Conf. on Medical Image Computing and Computer-Assisted Intervention* (Cham: Springer) pp 442–50

[25] Wu Z, Su L and Huang Q 2019 Cascaded partial decoder for fast and accurate salient object detection *Proc. of the IEEE/CVF Conf. on Computer Vision and Pattern Recognition* 3907–16

[26] Qin X, Zhang Z, Huang C, Gao C, Dehghan M and Jagersand M 2019 Basnet: boundary-aware salient object detection *Proc. of the IEEE/CVF Conf. on Computer Vision and Pattern Recognition* 7479–89

[27] Wei J, Wang S and Huang Q 2020 F^3Net: fusion, feedback and focus for salient object detection *Proc. of the AAAI Conf. on Artificial Intelligence* **34** 12321–8

[28] Long J, Shelhamer E and Darrell T 2015 Fully convolutional networks for semantic segmentation *Proc. of the IEEE conf. on Computer Vision and Pattern Recognition* 3431–40

[29] Ronneberger O, Fischer P and Brox T 2015 U-net: convolutional networks for biomedical image segmentation *Int. Conf. on Medical image computing and Computer-assisted Intervention* (Cham: Springer) pp 234–41

[30] Zhou Z, Siddiquee M M R, Tajbakhsh N and Liang J 2018 Unet++: a nested u-net architecture for medical image segmentation *Deep learning in medical image analysis and multimodal learning for clinical decision support* (Cham: Springer) pp 3–11

[31] Oktay O, Schlemper J, Folgoc L L, Lee M, Heinrich M, Misawa K and Mori K *et al* 2018 Attention u-net: learning where to look for the pancreas *Conf. on Medical Imaging with Deep Learning (MIDL)*

[32] Schlemper J, Oktay O, Schaap M, Heinrich M, Kainz B, Glocker B and Rueckert D 2019 Attention gated networks: learning to leverage salient regions in medical images. *Med. Image Anal.* **53** 197–207

[33] Li X, Chen H, Qi X, Dou Q, Fu C-W and Heng P-A 2018 H-DenseUNet: hybrid densely connected UNet for liver and tumor segmentation from CT volumes *IEEE Trans. Med. Imaging* **37** 2663–74

[34] Chen L-C, Zhu Y, Papandreou G, Schroff F and Adam H 2018 Encoder-decoder with atrous separable convolution for semantic image segmentation *Proc. of the European conf. on computer vision (ECCV)* 801–18

[35] Fan D-P, Cheng M-M, Liu Y, Li T and Borji A 2017 Structure-measure: a new way to evaluate foreground maps *Proc. of the IEEE Int. Conf. on Computer Vision* 4548–57

[36] Fan D-P, Ji G-P, Qin X and Cheng M-M 2021 Cognitive vision inspired object segmentation metric and loss function *SCIENTIA SINICA Informationis* **51** 1475

[37] Fan D-P, Zhou T, Ji G-P, Zhou Y, Chen G, Fu H, Shen J and Shao L Inf-net: automatic covid-19 lung infection segmentation from CT images *IEEE Trans. Med. Imaging* **39** 2626–37

[38] Zhao J-X, Liu J-J, Fan D-P, Cao Y, Yang J and Cheng M-M 2019 EGNet: edge guidance network for salient object detection *Proc. of the IEEE/CVF Int. Conf. on Computer Vision* 8779–88

IOP Publishing

Artificial Intelligence Strategies for Analyzing COVID-19 Pneumonia Lung Imaging, Volume 1
Characterization approaches
Ayman El-Baz and Jasjit S Suri

Chapter 4

A comprehensive review of radiology smartphone applications

Mohammad (Behdad) Jamshidi, Mohammad Heydari[1], Jakub Talla, Zdeněk Peroutka, Maryam Ahmadi, Esmaeil Mehraeen, Hamid Abdollahi and Amirali Karimi

Background and purpose: Mobile applications (apps) are fast-growing tools that offer a wide range of services in the field of medical sciences, especially in the era of COVID-19, and can help medical systems efficiently. This study aims to present and introduce radiology apps (RadApps) to their sizeable potential target group and discuss the issues facing them.

Materials and methods: We conducted a systematic search on two major mobile platforms; Google Play for Android and the App Store for iOS for English-language apps. Researchers used four smartphones to install and analyze these apps, two for each of the operating systems. The following terms were applied for the search strategy: radiology, x-ray, ultrasound, MRI, medical imaging, CT, and radiography.

Results: The search results included a total of 153 apps, of which 46 (30%) were iOS apps, and the other 107 (70%) were for Android. Based on a careful review of these applications, we further divided them into four main categories, including 1. general, 2. educational, 3. guideline, and 4. tools apps. The largest numbers of apps were in the educational and tools categories. These applications seemed to offer an extensive range of services, fulfilling the needs of a diverse group of users.

Conclusion: Overall, RadApps seems to offer a feasible, user-friendly, and cost-effective approach to radiology. A large variety of radiology-related smartphone applications are available, with many potential benefits. They have opened a new horizon of education, research, and clinical decision-making. Nevertheless, in the

[1] Author to whom any correspondence should be addressed.

doi:10.1088/978-0-7503-3795-3ch4

era of technology and online communications, providers should comprehend and try to fix their shortcomings in newer versions, to achieve optimal efficiency.

4.1 Introduction

Our experience of the COVID-19 era has presented us with a number of uncertainties and nonlinearities related to the efficiency of conventional medical methodologies in coping with such epidemiological diseases [1–3]. One of the most important lessons that can be mentioned is the importance of new technologies and artificial intelligence in overcoming some of the problems associated with COVID-19 [4, 5]. In this respect, the use of emerging technologies, such as smartphone applications, telemedicine interfaces [6], and AI-based techniques empowering medical systems is the most important. Since the day the world first faced this pandemic disease, a great deal of research into AI-based methods and emerging technologies has been conducted [7]. In particular, a lot of effort has benefited applications such as radiology smartphone applications. For example, since mobile applications (apps) were first introduced in 2008, they have experienced an exponential growth in number [8, 9]. The use of apps in medicine is the subject of a wide and active area of research. Studies have indicated that these apps display enormous potential to change modern medicine based on their uses and audiences [10–13]. Several pieces of research had been done concerning the utilization of these apps in medicine. It has been demonstrated that medical apps (MedApps) are available for patients, researchers, clinicians, and medical students to help them undertake their daily tasks faster and more efficiently [14–16]. MedApps are released by many different providers, either on a commercial basis (with charges) or as open access software. Therefore, it seems essential to provide physicians and healthcare staff with training and education in how to use new technologies efficiently [17–19].

The RadApps are a wide range of MedApps, either developed or in progress [20], designed to assist a wide range of users in several areas [21, 22]. The current RadApps have opened new approaches to more advanced medical research, education [23, 24], diagnosis [25], and decision-making [26]. Nevertheless, they have many shortcomings, some of which are still unclear and which need to be discussed and clarified [27–30]. However, since these apps have high potential, there is an ever-increasing need to address and solve these issues so that they can reach the peak of their potential advantage. On the other hand, if they introduced quantitative imaging approaches into medicine, along with an increased need for radiation dose assessment, these apps would be more beneficial [31, 32].

In this chapter, we aim to introduce the advantages and features of RadApps, based on different categories and their target population. For this purpose, we carefully searched for, reviewed, and analyzed RadApps displayed in the Google Play store and the App Store for Android and iOS users, respectively. This chapter introduces, categorizes, and presents a scientific approach toward these apps, guiding users to choose the most suitable ones for their needs. We also discuss the numerous shortcomings they exhibit, paving the way for researchers and developers to solve these issues for the benefit of the users.

4.2 Material and methods

We conducted a systematic search on two major mobile platforms selected for this research, Google Play for Android and the App Store for iOS for English-language apps. Android apps were identified by a search of the Goggle Play store interface and iOS apps were identified via the iTunes/iOS search application interface. The keywords, including radiology, CT, MRI, x-ray, ultrasound, radiotherapy, medical imaging, medical image, DICOM, were searched. Available smartphones were used to install and analyze these apps. We recruited two smartphones running by iOS and two running the Android operating system for this purpose. Two reviewers independently screened the app store description of each app. Although studies on some parts of this paper are related to between December 2018 and January 2020, it had been completed to October 2020. Apps that were not English and not free were excluded. Free apps were downloaded and analyzed on two smartphones. We analyzed all the applications in terms of name, category of use, description, need to connect to the internet, and the number of installations.

4.3 Results

A total of 153 apps were found; based on the results obtained, these were further divided into four main categories, including general apps, educational apps, guideline apps, and tools apps; each category is defined and discussed in a separate section. Figure 4.1 and table 4.1 summarize our findings and present the total number and percentage of available applications for each category and indicate the number and percentage of applications that need an internet connection. A wide range of radiology apps are available in the educational category and this category is the most populous, followed by the tools apps. Also, the Android operating system provides more apps for its users, compared to iOS.

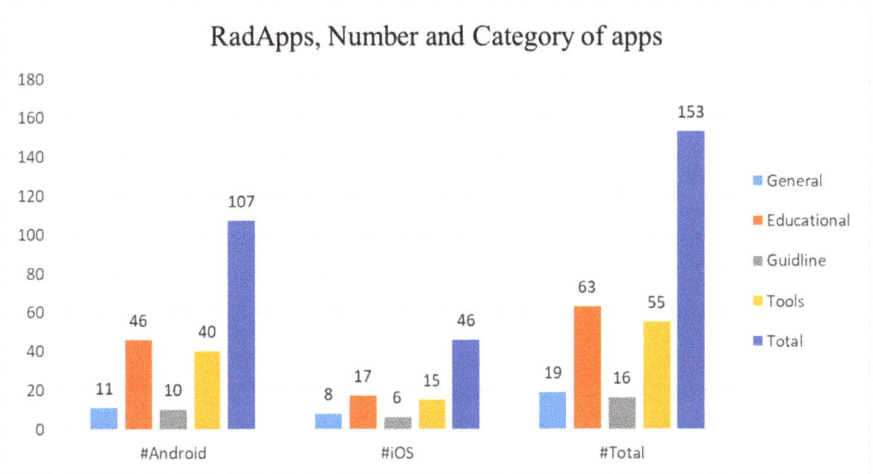

Figure 4.1. Chart of the number of RadApps per category.

Table 4.1. RadApps, categories, frequency, and percentage in each category.

App information		# Number (%) of android (n = 107)	#Number (%) of iOS (n = 46)	Total number (%) (n = 153)
General category				
Number		11 (10)	8 (17)	19 (12)
Internet connection required	Yes	6 (6)	4 (9)	10 (7)
	No	5 (5)	4 (9)	9 (6)
Educational category				
Number		46 (43)	17 (37)	63 (41)
Internet connection required	Yes	14 (13)	6 (13)	20 (13)
	No	32 (30)	11 (24)	43 (28)
Guideline category				
Number		10 (9)	6 (13)	16 (11)
Internet connection required	Yes	4 (4)	4 (9)	8 (5)
	No	6 (6)	2 (4)	8 (5)
Tools category				
Number		40 (38)	15 (33)	55 (36)
Internet connection required	Yes	12 (11)	8 (17)	20 (13)
	No	28 (26)	7 (15)	35 (23)
Total				
Number		107 (70)	46 (30)	153 (100)
Internet connection required	Yes	36 (33)	22 (48)	58 (38)
	No	71 (67)	24 (52)	95 (62)

Our comprehensive results for apps based on their name, description, category of use, need to connect to the internet, number of installations (for Android), and ratings (for IOS) are shown in tables 4.2 and 4.3, respectively. These carefully extracted findings for the 153 apps show the diversity of utilizations available.

4.3.1 General RadApps

General apps have a wide range of applications, from public information to advanced imaging techniques. This category includes different apps, such as atlas, flashcards, and games. As an intriguing discovery, social networks are found to be highly applicable frameworks for radiologists to share fascinating cases, improve radiological knowledge, and discuss and get the latest news related to their specialty [33].

Table 4.2. Categories of identified Android RadApps.

Category	Name	Description	Target community	App store	Internet connection required	Number of installations
General	Atlas of emergency radiology	Includes radiographic method and technique	Students	Google Play	No	+500
	Radiology manual	Manual of exposure positions	Students/radiology staff	Google Play	No	+10000
	Pocket atlas CT (abdomen)	Explains in detail the names of the organs in abdominal CT scans	Radiology students/ radiologists	Google Play	Yes	+1000
	Pocket atlas of CT (head)	Best way to reference anatomy and very easy to use for the field of radiology	Radiology students/ clinicians	Google Play	Yes	+10000
	Pocket atlas Ct (thorax)	Anatomical view of the thorax	Radiology students/ radiologists	Google Play	Yes	+1000
	Radiology ultrasound	Radiology ultrasound multiple-choice question review	Students	Google Play	No	+500
	CT scan cross sectional anatomy	A training atlas for viewing 3D images of the brain and other parts of the body	Students/junior doctors	Google Play	No	+10000
	Atlas of CT anatomy	Atlas of anatomy for CT scans, PET scans, and MRI scans of the abdomen, joints, chest, neck, cardiac area, and brain	Students/clinicians	Google Play	No	+1000
	Imaging Anatomy -Ct Mri Xr Us	An interactive atlas of normal imaging anatomy and a learning device	Radiologists/ clinicians	Google Play	Yes	+10000
	Jnl Amer Coll Radiology	Journal of the American College of Radiology	Researchers	Google Play	Yes	+1000
	Radiology management	The top professional journal for leaders in medical imaging management	Researchers	Google Play /App Store	Yes	+100

(*Continued*)

Table 4.2. (*Continued*)

Category	Name	Description	Target community	App store	Internet connection required	Number of installations
Educational	UBC radiology	To increase confidence in identifying normal anatomic structures, identify the most appropriate imaging test and common pathologies	Clinicians/students	Google Play	No	+10000
	Clinical chest radiology	Clinical teaching about the relevant aspects of the chest	Medical students/ radiology residents	Google Play	No	+500
	Chest Radiology	This app educates the user in how to review chest x-rays accurately.	Students/junior doctors	Google Play	No	+100
	Radiology quiz	This app discusses radiological images consisting of CT scans, x-rays, and MRI scans.	Radiographers/ radiology students	Google Play	Yes	+1000
	Clinical radiology	Clinical radiology is designed to help students, young doctors, and medical professionals.	Students/junior doctors	Google Play	No	+500
	Radiology mnemonics	Provides images of related topics and explanations of what the user is studying	Medical students	Google Play	Yes	+1000
	Chest radiology	This app promotes the understanding chest x-rays using images	Residents/clinicians	Google Play	No	+10000
	Normal findings in CT and MRI brain	For any beginning radiologist who wishes to recognize pathological conditions	Radiologists	Google Play	Yes	+500
	Radiology quiz for ultrasound	A game for sonographers and radiology doctors	Clinicians	Google Play	Yes	+1000

MSK Radiology 4 U	This educational application comprises over 3000 anonymized case studies in musculoskeletal imaging.	Clinicians/students	Google Play	Yes	+1000
Radiology tutor	Radiology tutor is intended for information only rather than diagnosis or treatment guidance	Students/junior doctors	Google Play	Yes	+100000
Radiology radio graphic imaging	Expand your knowledge and expertise in radiology, x-ray, and medical imaging using a quiz and self-learning	Students	Google Play	No	+1000
Medical radiology	Helps the user to understand the detailed interpretation and management of common emergency cases in radiology.	Students/ radiologists	Google Play	No	+100
Radiology & x-ray exam review	This app is a combination of practice questions, study cards, terms, and concepts for self-learning and exam preparation	Students	Google Play	Yes	+10000
Qevlar radiology	A special quiz tool designed for radiology residents	Residents/ physicians	Google Play	No	+1000
Plain films—radiology for medical students	Test yourself on basic x-ray interpretation, tracking your strengths and weaknesses as you go.	Students	Google Play	No	+1000
Radiology associates	Patient education and communication app for all patients of radiology associates	Patients	Google Play	No	+100
Radiologic signs	Identify different radiological signs in studies such as radiography, magnetic resonance, tomography, and ultrasound.	Students/Residents	Google Play	No	+100
Interactive CT & MRI Anat.Lite	Helps the user to understand the essential anatomical terms of the body	Medical students/ interns	Google Play	Yes	+100000
Basic RadiologyLite – SecondLook	Provides a series of radiographic images for students	Medical students	Google Play	No	+100

(*Continued*)

Table 4.2. (*Continued*)

Category	Name	Description	Target community	App store	Internet connection required	Number of installations
	Chest x-ray and pathology	A unique teaching and learning resource for understanding the principles of chest radiology.	Junior doctors/ students	Google Play	Yes	+100000
	ARRT® Radiography Q&A 2018 Ed	With this app you can pass the ARRT Radiography exam	Students	Google Play	No	+1000
	X-ray differential diagnosis	Provides a list of possible causes for each finding encountered in everyday medical practice	Students/junior doctors	Google Play	No	+1000
	Mani radiograph	Provides introductory information about x-ray equipment and accessories	Radiology staff	Google Play	No	+1000
	Radiographic anatomy x-ray	Allows the user to learn about the full extent of radiological projections used in daily patient care.	Clinicians	Google Play	Yes	+10000
	Radiodent	Learn and identify the normal anatomical landmarks, common radiographic errors, and pathological conditions.	Clinicians	Google Play	No	+10000
	Medical radiology	Helps the user to understand the detailed interpretation and management of common emergency cases in radiology	Students	Google Play	No	+50
	CT head basic interpretation	Helps the user to learn how to interpret head CT scans, how to understand hydrocephalus, brain abscesses, and brain edema.	Students/clinicians	Google Play	Yes	+500
	Radiological anatomy for FRCR1	To improve the anatomical knowledge of radiologists	Students/ radiologists	Google Play	No	+500

Radiology ultrasound	Multiple-choice question review	Students	Google Play	No	+500
Advanced radiology OnTheGo	Provides the user with interactive features and the ability to easily and constantly be in the know about the medical diagnostics and radiology industry.	Students	Google Play	No	+100
Radiology core: nuclear med	Free resource for radiology core exam preparation	Students	Google Play	No	+1000
Radiology by Dr Bipin Daga	A dynamic clinical radiologist famous for his excellent teaching techniques in radiology and imaging.	Students/ radiologists	Google Play	No	+1000
Radiology Toolbox	Designed by a practicing radiologist to help radiologists	Students/ health practitioners	Google Play	No	+1000
FRCR Physics for Radiology	True or false questions based on the format of the FRCR Physics exam	Students	Google Play	No	+100
Radiology Core: Physics	Free resource for radiology core exam preparation	Students	Google Play	No	+1000
Dental Radiography	Dental radiography quiz questions; free app for exam preparation for your dental radiography examination	Students	Google Play	No	+10000
RadioXtudy	Aims to assist graduate students in dentistry and dental surgeons in the study of radiographic interpretation.	Students	Google Play	No	+50000
Radiology Signs	A compilation of the most commonly signs seen in pre-postgraduate exams, in routine radiological investigations, such as x-rays, CT scans, MRI scans, ultrasonography, and nuclear imaging.	Students/ radiologists	Google Play	No	+10000
Radiology core: nuclear med	Free resource for radiology core exam preparation.	Students	Google Play	No	+1000

(*Continued*)

Table 4.2. (*Continued*)

Category	Name	Description	Target community	App store	Internet connection required	Number of installations
	Radiology measurements on finger tips	Useful for radiologists, radiology residents, medical students, and medical professionals	Radiologists/ students	Google Play	No	+1000
	Basic radiographic positioning	Provides guides for basic radiographic positioning	Radiologists	Google Play	Yes	+10000
	Radiodent	First smartphone application in the field of dental radiology that can be easily and effectively used	Students	Google Play	No	+10000
	Chest x-ray interpretation	CHEST x-rays (CXRs) are one of the oldest noninvasive methods for identifying abnormalities in the chest	Radiologists	Google Play	No	+10000
	Radiation oncology exam review	Board-style questions and rationales for over 200 boards	Students	Google Play	Yes	+10000
	MRI physics and imaging technology	This is a educational app for students and young doctors	Students	Google Play	Yes	+5000
Guideline	CT-guide & positioning	A teaching and learning resource for medical students	Students, junior doctors, trainee radiologists, CT radiographers	Google Play	Yes	+5000
	Radiology review manual—#1 for board review	A book application, which includes differential diagnoses for common clinical presentations and helps in making quick decisions	N/A	Google Play	No	+1000
	Navi radiography pro	Mobile guide for radiography with 3D images	Radiographers, radiologists, medical doctors,	Google Play	Yes	+500

	MRI positioning	This handbook on MRI is very useful for users	Radiology technicians, either studying or already working	Google Play	No	+10000
	CT positioning	Very useful handbook during work and study	Students	Google Play	No	+5000
	Placement coil MRI	This app explains how to install coils and how to position them correctly	N/A	Google Play	No	+1000
	Common imaging tests	Explains radiological medical categories; a guide that uses images	Patients	Google Play	No	+100
	Diagnologic for radiology	As a first social network in radiology, provides a social network for radiologists	Radiologists/ clinicians	Google Play	Yes	+5000
	Ultrasound guide	Contains ultrasound scan information with clear descriptions of some pathological ultrasound images	N/A	Google Play	No	+10000
	Radiotherapy & oncology	Provides published papers describing original research as well as review articles	N/A	Google Play	Yes	+10000
Tools	Contrast media in radiology	Guide for appropriate diagnosis and managing adverse reactions	Radiologists and technicians	Google Play	No	+500
	Chest x-ray made easy	Positioning techniques and chest x-ray interpretation	N/A	Google Play	No	+1000
	Port-ray: DICOM viewer for android	Viewer provides high-speed and quality access to any PACS (picture archiving and communication system)	Radiologists, surgeons	Google Play	Yes	+1000
	M Ray—DICOM viewer	Provides access your radiological images anywhere and anytime	N/A	Google Play	Yes	+10000
	Radiology key image archive	This app is intended solely for teaching purposes and is not intended for diagnosis purposes	N/A	Google Play	Yes	+1000

(*Continued*)

Table 4.2. (*Continued*)

Category	Name	Description	Target community	App store	Internet connection required	Number of installations
	Radiographic positioning and related anatomy	This is a tools app that is used to simulate positioning	N/A	Google Play	No	+10000
	Radiography safety distance	An app for calculating safe distances in radiography	Radiology staff	Google Play	No	+500
	NDT x-ray Toolbox	Provides geometric calculations, x-ray standards, image quality control, CT calculations	N/A	Google Play	No	+1000
	Radiography calculator	Provides radiographic inspection formulas	Radiology staff	Google Play	No	+5000
	X-ray interpretation	This app explains how to recognize basic radiological signs, pathology, and patterns	N/A	Google Play	No	+100000
	Radiography positioning of chest	An app for radiography positioning of the chest	Radiology staff/ radiologists	Google Play	No	+1000
	Exposure time calculator	This app is used to calculate exposure time for gamma rays (Ir-192) and x-rays	Radiology staff	Google Play	No	+1000
	DICOM medical image viewer	This orthogonal viewer supports overlays, atlases, GIFTI surface data, and DTI data	N/A	Google Play	No	+50
	iRadTech	This app places positioning information at the user's fingertips	Radiographers or students	Google Play	No	+500

Teleradio	This app helps radiologists to report on studies/scans with just the help of a browser	Radiologists	Google Play	No	+50
CT brain interpretation	Interpretation of CT scans of the brain	N/A	Google Play	Yes	+10000
Radiography Exposure Factors	This is a good tool for viewing an exposure chart radiography table	Radiologists	Google Play	No	+5000
Chest x-ray interpretation	Include anatomy and pathology of chest radiograph Chest x-ray	N/A	Google Play	No	+10000
MRI sequences	MRI signal production, MRI interpretation, MRI pulse sequences, gradient sequences	Radiology staff	Google Play	No	+5000
MRI Viewer	Provides a dynamic and interactive method of viewing cross-sections of human anatomy	Clinicians/ physicians	Google Play	No	+10000
MRI physics and imaging technology	Presents the the physics of imaging hardware magnetism, a pulse sequence overview, and diffusion weighted imaging	N/A	Google Play	No	+1000
CT Perfusion Imaging	Allows functional evaluation of tissue vascularity	N/A	Google Play	Yes	+100
Radiology acute abdomen	Explains radiology examinations for acute abdominal cases, handling of acute abdominal cases in radiology services	N/A	Google Play	No	+10000
Texas radiology associates	This app includes diagnostic image interpretation, interventional radiology procedures, pediatric procedures, and breast imaging	Students	Google Play	No	+1000

(*Continued*)

Table 4.2. (*Continued*)

Category	Name	Description	Target community	App store	Internet connection required	Number of installations
	pedsMRI	Provides pediatric MRI protocols at the user's fingertips	N/A	Google Play	Yes	+1000
	Mobile MIM	Used for the viewing, registration, fusion, and/or display for the diagnosis of medical images	Patients/clinicians	Google Play	No	+5000
	OsiriX HD	A full DICOM image viewer	N/A	Google Play	Yes	+1000
	Radiography exposure factors	Provides radiology articles, radiology journals	N/A	Google Play	Yes	+1000
	Radiology measurements	Gives the normal values of the anatomical measurements in radiology for adults and children	Radiologists, radiology residents	Google Play	No	+500
	Radiology acute abdomen	Handling of acute abdominal cases in radiology services	N/A	Google Play	No	+1000
	Radiology CT anatomy	Provides a dynamic and interactive method of viewing cross-sectional human anatomy in computed tomography (CT).	N/A	Google Play	Yes	+10000
	Radiology assistant	An invaluable imaging reference with over 90 articles written by expert radiologists.	Radiologists	Google Play	Yes	+50000
	Radiology rounds	Radiology rounds is an app that allows the user to share and learn from clinical cases.	Radiologists and residents	Google Play	No	+50000

Radiology CT viewer	Provides a dynamic and interactive method of viewing cross-sectional human anatomy in computed tomography (CT).	Radiologists and residents	Google Play	Yes	+10000
Interventional radiology	The interventional radiology app is a free resource for patients and professionals	Radiologists	Google Play	No	+100
X-ray timer	This app was modeled after the slide rules that industrial radiographers use to estimate their exposure times.	N/A	Google Play	No	+1000
Radiology Assistant	An invaluable imaging reference with over 90 articles written by expert radiologists!	Radiologists / Physicians	Google Play	Yes	+50000
Magnetic radiation detector-EMF Meter	Uses the magnetic sensor to detect radiation.	N/A	Google Play	No	+5000

Table 4.3. Categories of identified IOS RadApps

Category	Name	Description	Target community	App store	Internet connection required	Rating
General	Basic radiology	Provides a series of radiographic images for educating	Students	App Store	No	5
	Oral radiology lite	Provides a series of intraoral radiographs for students of dental sciences	Students	App Store	No	5
	Radiology Asia	Radiology Asia conference and exhibition	Researchers/ clinicians	App Store	No	+1
	Medications in radiology	Provides a quick and easy reference for commonly used medications in radiology	Students/ radiologists	App Store	Yes	+1
	Swiss Congress of Radiology	Displays the Congress program and also more detailed information about each session, speakers, exhibitors, and much more	Researchers	App Store	Yes	2
	Annual radiology meeting	Useful for exhibitors, visitors, speakers, and corporate partners	Researchers	App Store	Yes	+4
	Understanding Mri: MS	All patients with MS should have familiarity with this noninvasive test	Patients	App Store	No	5
Educational	UBC radiology	Learn anatomy and clinical reasoning using x-ray, CT, and MRI images	Students	App Store	No	+5
	Radiology core	Free resource for radiology core exam preparation.	Students	App Store	No	+ 3.5
	Holvan radiology	Office contacts, imaging locations, and patient education videos	Students/ radiologists	App Store	Yes	+1
	Radiology board reviewers	Multiple-choice questions with explanations for 20 different radiation board review topics	Students	App Store	Yes	+1
	Radiology & medical imaging	A combination of sets of practice questions, study cards, terms, and concepts for self-learning	Students	App Store	Yes	+1
	Oral radiology	For learners in the dental sciences to self-test their level of knowledge and their ability to recognize anatomical structures	Students	App Store	No	+5

	Pueblo radiology	Imaging locations and patient education videos	Radiologists	App Store	No	+1
	Qevlar radiology	The latest version of our special quiz tool designed for radiology residents and physicians	Radiology residents/ medical students	App Store	No	+1.2
	Diagnologic for radiology	Share interesting radiologic cases with worldwide radiologists—discuss or get second opinions from top subspecialists	Radiologists	App Store	Yes	+5
	Radiology associate app	Radiology associates office contacts, imaging locations, and patient education videos.	Radiology staff	App Store	No	+1
	Dental panoramic radiology	An interactive application designed to teach panoramic anatomy.	Students	App Store	Yes	+5
	KSTR weekly chest cases	High-quality education in thoracic radiology using a case-based approach	Students	App Store	No	+2
	Pediatric radiology	The most recent developments in all areas of pediatric imaging	Students	App Store	No	+1
	MRI contrast	Learn how scan parameters affect the MRI image.	Clinicians	App Store	No	+5
	MRI essentials	A comprehensive teaching tool for orthopedic MRI and a quick reference for picking up facts quickly in everyday practice.	Students/ clinicians	App Store	No	+4
	Interactive CT and MRI anatomy	Learn anatomy by learning the terms and answering step-by-step questions using a total of 241 CT and MRI images	Students	App Store	Yes	+2
Guideline	Real world radiology	Guide to the basics of thoracic imaging. Learn to read chest x-rays.	N/A	App Store	Yes	3.3
	Radiology toolkit	A collection of common references designed to help practicing radiologists	N/A	App Store	Yes	1
	Radiology management	Has been the top professional journal for leaders in medical imaging	N/A	App Store	Yes	+4
	Atlas of radiological image	A reference/learning tool for evaluating radiological images for diagnosis and therapy	Radiologists, surgeons, other physicians	App Store	No	4

(*Continued*)

Table 4.3. (*Continued*)

Category	Name	Description	Target community	App store	Internet connection required	Rating
	Images radiology	User-friendly App and is useful for guide patients check-up	N/A	App Store	No	1
	Rad once reference	This app provides fast access to cancer staging contouring atlases, DVH normal tissue constraints, and pertinent clinical calculators	N/A	App Store	Yes	1
Tools	Radiology rounds	Radiologists can share and learn from radiological images	Radiologists	App Store	Yes	4.9
	Anatomy on radiology CT	The app provides a dynamic and interactive method of viewing cross-sectional human anatomy in CT images	N/A	App Store	No	3
	Radiology toolbox pro	Designed to help users	Radiologists	App Store	Yes	3.3
	Radiology CT viewer	Provides a dynamic interactive method of viewing cross-sectional human anatomy in CT images	N/A	App Store	No	4.3
	Advance radiology on the GO	Provides the user with interactive features	N/A	App Store	No	1
	Radiology toolkit	A collection of common references designed to help practicing radiologists	Radiologists	App Store	Yes	1
	Applied radiology	Developed primarily for the radiology community.	Physicians	App Store	Yes	1
	Penn radiology meetings/Events	This application provides registered attendees with the essential tools to participate in live meetings and events	N/A	App Store	Yes	+4
	Elahiye radiology	Dentists can access the whole list of their patients who have been referred to Elahiye maxillofacial radiology for x-ray examinations	Dentists	App Store	Yes	1
	pedsMRI	This app provides pediatric MRI protocols at the user's fingertips.	Radiologists, MRI staff, residents	App Store	No	+4

Interventional radiology	Interventional radiology is a free resource with information on over 150 of the month's commonly performed interventional radiology procedures	Patients and professionals	App Store	No	5+
iRad MRI	Equipped with the most popular MRI protocols	N/A	App Store	Yes	3
Med film	Med film can query and retrieve DICOM images from any DICOM compatible software and PACS through some DICOM network protocols	N/A	App Store	Yes	4.7
Med ultra	N/A	Radiologists, radiology trainees	App Store	No	1
Mobile MIM	Mobile MIM can be used to review images, contours, DVH, and isodose curves from radiation treatment plans.	N/A	App Store	No	3

The top professional journals have introduced some applications for leaders in medical imaging. Self-learning apps are a group of general apps that are used to expand knowledge and expertise in Radiology imaging, learn the main concepts, and take quizzes. This group of apps is a combination of different app types, including practice questions and study cards, terms and concepts for self-learning, radiological exam preparation, and x-ray and medical imaging expertise.

Most atlas RadApps were used as a handy way to teach anatomy, a necessary concept for radiology specialists, students, and technicians. These apps are interactive tools, offering the normal body anatomy found in radiologic imaging for experts in the field, as well as assisting health students and professionals in learning general anatomy.

4.3.2 Educational RadApps

Most of the RadApps explored were classified as being in the educational category. We further divided this broad group into three subgroups: (1) User-based education apps; these apps aim to identify their audience, and provide them with suitable training based on their interests. Medical students, physicians, radiologists, residents, staff, or technicians are the primary users of these mobile apps. Twenty-one apps for Android and ten apps for iOS were designed for this type of audience. (2) Clinically based education apps, which provide their users with training in the concepts and terminology common in radiology, CT and MRI scanning, pathological diagnoses, interventions, and positioning. Instructing the users in how to correctly interpret images was the original clinical goal of the app designers. Nearly 18 educational apps for Android and seven for iOS were published online using a clinical approach. (3) Radiology quizzes and exam apps accounted for a minority of the educational apps, accounting for a total of about seven applications.

The target of educational apps is to help instruct young talented practitioners so that they can obtain the best clinical and academic qualifications. Some educational applications comprise many anonymized medical imaging case studies. Certain groups of educational applications target specific areas, to teach their users based on their needs. Comprehensive data on these applications are presented in tables 4.2 and 4.3, and we will discuss them in the following.

A variety of apps help users to identify normal anatomic structures and common pathologies. They guide learners towards learning about different aspects of radiology and medical imaging. Some apps offer specific types of education aimed at a particular body organ or region, such as dental radiology apps, which assist students in the field of dentistry. Applications providing differential diagnosis and those describing the full extent of radiological projections used in daily inpatient care also help healthcare workers and patients towards better management. The applications that centre their teachings on the detailed interpretation and management of common emergency cases in radiology also provide essential benefits. Another group provides learners with study notes and flashcards, explicitly targeting key unmissable points.

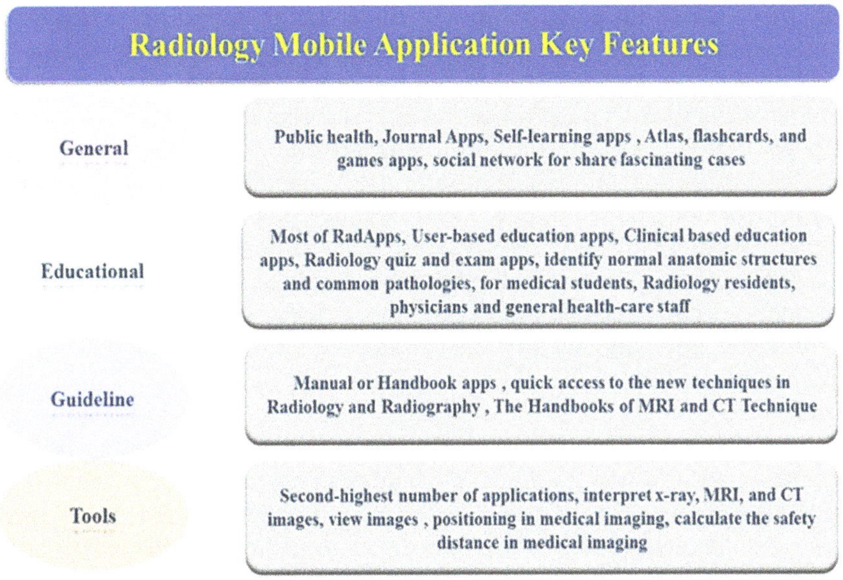

Figure 4.2. Radiology mobile application key features in each category.

Finally, quiz apps and practical radiology exams assist the students in evaluating their skills. These apps may also specifically target a specific exam, for example, the American Registry of Radiologic Technologists exam (ARRT). All these extensive materials can target specific audiences, such as medical students, radiology residents, physicians, general healthcare staff, and professionals in radiology.

4.3.3 Guideline RadApps

Guideline apps provide various imaging guides for radiologic technologists, residents, medical students, junior doctors, and professionals. The manual apps and handbook apps fall within this category. A few apps that introduce scientific radiology journals were placed in this group. Manual apps are used for quick access to new techniques in radiology and radiography. Chest radiology apps that provide comprehensive, concise, easily accessible radiological guide to the imaging of acute and chronic chest conditions are among the productive applications in this group, guiding their users to perform accurate reviews of chest x-rays. The Handbooks of MRI and CT Technique are guidelines for many practitioners, providing guides towards the best diagnoses and treatments for conditions of the brain, spine, abdomen, musculoskeletal system, and others.

4.3.4 Tools RadApps

This group accounts for the second-highest number of applications, which just fell short of the number of educational apps. We identified 40 Android apps and 15 iOS apps as belonging to this group. These apps can be used to interpret x-rays and MRI and CT images, view images in an interactive and dynamic environment, provide guidance about positioning in medical imaging, present tables for measurements, and calculate safety distances using medical imaging and radiology archives.

In some of the tools apps, professionals can upload and share clinical cases with their fellow radiologists. Some apps provide a dynamic and interactive method of viewing cross-sectional human anatomy in CT images. Most of the tools apps cover multiple imaging modalities: radiography, ultrasonography, and CT and MRI scans. Modules are split into six types, representing musculoskeletal, cervical, chest, cardiovascular, abdominal, and pelvic subspecialties. Some apps provide wireless and portable access to medical images. Some tools apps provide features assisting their users, mostly healthcare workers, with specific conditions. We will discuss this matter briefly. These features are thoroughly presented in tables 4.2 and 4.3.

The contrast media app describes the types of contrast media to be used for certain diagnoses and how to manage the adverse reactions. Interventional radiology apps are a group of tools apps designed for radiologists. Some viewer apps offer dynamic and interactive methods for viewing cross-sectional human anatomy in CT and MRI images. Medical DICOM image viewers provide the high-speed and -quality access needed for teleradiology. Various reviews of treatment plans can be achieved using specific applications. Some apps combine the power and mobility of modern mobile devices to access radiological images anywhere and anytime. These apps allow medical professionals to view and evaluate radiological images easily. Others help with CT calculations, positioning, and interpretation. Chest x-ray interpretations include not only healthy but also a large variety of pathological features. Exposure Time Calculator is an application used to calculate the exposure time for gamma- and x-rays, based on several factors. This app is recommended for use when processing films manually.

4.4 Discussion

Mobile apps have great potential to improve knowledge in a wide range of medical sciences. Several studies on the development of mobile apps for radiology applications have shown that these apps are useful and informative [34–36]. RadApps have several advantages, including their ease of use, portability, small size, and updatability. Furthermore, a large target group can benefit from these apps, including healthcare workers in different specialties, students, researchers, and even patients [37, 38]. In this chapter, we have provided an overview of the applications of RadApps for research, education, and clinical aims.

Based on the results of our careful review of the RadApps, we have further divided them into four main categories: general apps, educational apps, guideline apps, and tools. Educational apps, followed by tools apps, accounted for the majority of apps. Educational apps provide interested individuals with explicit knowledge and understanding of a topic, as well as providing access to portable and updatable data with which the user can learn scientific concepts. Some also contain quizzes that test the individuals' knowledge and help them to avoid errors and pitfalls. Tools apps, especially those with interesting designs and familiar and user-friendly interfaces, can potentially virtualize radiology in the best possible way.

A great benefit of online apps that is sometimes neglected is the rating of the applications and their numbers of downloads. This helps users in the process of choosing the application that is best suited for them. If users like the features of an application, they suggest them to others, resulting in a chain of downloads. This chain elevates the number of downloads, which in turn leads to recognition for the most useful apps and loss of viewers for the less useful ones.

Furthermore, RadApps can be specifically designed for a specific area of interest, providing detailed information on a specific subject. For instance, these applications have proved to be potentially useful in radiation oncology and pediatric radiology [35, 39]. Even in emergency situations, smartphones appear to be promising [40]. Specialized apps target not only different areas of interest but also a variety of specific body organs and areas, providing more expert information [41, 42].

Several studies have focused on RadApps. Székely *et al* reviewed smartphones, tablets, and mobile applications for radiological use. In their work, they listed 81 apps based on the five categories, including diagnostic reading, decision support applications, medical books, interactive encyclopedias, and journal reading programs [26]. The European Society of Radiology (ESR) published a report and clarified that mobile devices have three main applications, including the inspection or interpretation of radiological examinations, educational purposes, and social networking for clinical use [43]. A review article by Hirschorn *et al* provided several recommendations to minimize concerns about the ability of the existing mobile devices and networks to quickly and securely move medical images [44]. Kim *et al* explored the usability of mobile apps that support radiologists' training in diagnostic decision-making. In their study, they suggested that proficiency with mobile devices may not be equivalent to being an expert user who is proficient in using the apps [45]. Radiologic journals are also encouraged to design RadApps to help readers with their content [46].

Although they have numerous advantages, RadApps also have specific shortcomings. The use of these applications suffers from limitations imposed by the small sizes of mobile screens, the memory sizes of mobile phones, and the requirement for some apps to have an internet connection, irrespective of platform. Furthermore, some apps are expensive, have privacy policy limitations, or lack the image quality and tools available in routine clinical settings. On the other hand, radiologists, medical students, and researchers have to update their knowledge in the field of RadApps because they will imminently face more challenging radiological apps. Additionally, although apps have a high acceptability rate among patients and their families [47–49], the number of available online apps available for them is limited [39], since from a total of 153 RadApps, we could only locate five specifically introduced for patient use. These data suggest a possible need for more investment in introducing RadApps for patients and their families. Different applications can be used for control of the infectious disease [50].

Although it contains concurrent superior, detailed, and easy to interpret data and materials regarding different radiology applications, this study has limitations. First, we conducted this study based on Android and iOS devices, as they are the two leading platforms worldwide. There are other platforms, such as Windows or BlackBerry, which future studies will need to include. Second, our study was conducted using small phones and tablets and thus does not mention other, larger devices. Third, because many apps are not free of charge, our access was limited and we were not able to analyze all applications. Fourth, we report no analyses regarding various characteristics of the apps, including security, pricing, cost-effectiveness, protection, remote control, and app performance. Further work is required to assess these items.

4.5 Conclusions

One of the most powerful tools for helping physicians, healthcare systems, and medical centers in the era of COVID-19 is mobile applications. Not only can such applications efficiently mitigate the spread of the virus, but they can also speed up the processes of diagnosis and treatment. In this regard, this chapter provides a comprehensive review of radiology smartphone applications, which have been categorized into four groups, namely: (1) general, (2) educational, (3) guideline, and (4) tools apps. The results demonstrated that RadApps seem to offer a feasible, user-friendly, and cost-effective approach towards radiology, particularly for COVID-19 purposes. In addition, they have opened up new horizons of education, research, and clinical decision-making. The explosive growth in the number of these applications might help to address their problems and shortcomings in the ever-increasing newer versions. It seems logical to conceptualize these applications as the face of modern and technological future healthcare, although they need numerous improvements to reach their peak.

Ethical considerations

The Institutional Review Board of Iran University of Medical Sciences, Tehran, Iran, provided ethical approval for this study, No. 98-1-15/14945 (IR.IUMS.REC.1398.455).

Acknowledgment

This research was supported by the Ministry of Education, Youth, and Sports of the Czech Republic under the project OP VVV Electrical Engineering Technologies with High-Level of Embedded Intelligence CZ.02.1.01/0.0/0.0/18_069/0009855.

References

[1] Jamshidi M *et al* 2020 Artificial intelligence and COVID-19: deep learning approaches for diagnosis and treatment *IEEE Access* **8** 109581–95

[2] Vaishya R, Haleem A, Vaish A and Javaid M 2020 Emerging technologies to combat the COVID-19 pandemic *J. Clin. Exp. Hepatol.* **10** 409–11

[3] Ming L C *et al* 2020 Mobile health apps on COVID-19 launched in the early days of the pandemic: content analysis and review *JMIR mHealth uHealth* **8** e19796

[4] Jin C *et al* 2020 Development and evaluation of an artificial intelligence system for COVID-19 diagnosis *Nat Commun* **11** 1–14

[5] Portnoy J, Waller M and Elliott T 2020 Telemedicine in the era of COVID-19 *J. Allergy Clin. Immunol. Pract.* **8** 1489–91

[6] Saleem S M, Pasquale L R, Sidoti P A and Tsai J C 2020 Virtual ophthalmology: telemedicine in a COVID-19 era *Am. J. Ophthalmol.* **216** 237–42

[7] Abd-Alrazaq A *et al* 2020 Artificial intelligence in the fight against COVID-19: scoping review *J. Med. Internet Res.* **22** e20756

[8] Weinstein R S *et al* 2014 Telemedicine, telehealth, and mobile health applications that work: opportunities and barriers *Am. J. Med.* **127** 183–87

[9] Mehraeen E, Safdari R, Mohammadzadeh N, Seyedalinaghi S, Forootan S and Mohraz M 2018 Mobile-based applications and functionalities for self-management of people living with HIV *Health Informatics Meets EHealth: Biomedical Meets EHealth–From Sensors to Decisions. Proc. of the 12th EHealth Conf.* (Studies in Health Technology and Informatics vol 248) ed G Schreier and D Hayn (Amsterdam: IOS Press)

[10] Lewis T L and Wyatt J C 2014 mHealth and mobile medical apps: a framework to assess risk and promote safer use *J. Med. Internet Res.* **16** e210

[11] Mosa A S, Yoo I and Sheets L 2012 A systematic review of healthcare applications for smartphones *BMC Med. Inform. Decis. Mak.* **12** 67

[12] Niakan S, Mehraeen E, Noori T and Gozali E 2017 Web and mobile based HIV prevention and intervention programs pros and cons—a review *Health Informatics Meets eHealth* (Studies in Health Technology and Informatics vol 236) (Amsterdam: IOS Press) pp 319–27

[13] Mehraeen E, Safdari R, SeyedAlinaghi S and Mohammadzadeh N 2019 Exploring and prioritization of mobile-based self-management strategies for HIV care *Infect. Disord. Drug Targets* **19** 288–96

[14] Boulos M N K, Brewer A C, Karimkhani C, Buller D B and Dellavalle R P 2014 Mobile medical and health apps: state of the art, concerns regulatory control and certification *Online J. Public Health Inform.* **5** 229

[15] Ventola C L 2014 Mobile devices and apps for health care professionals: uses and benefits *Pharmacy and Therapeutics (PT)* **39** 356–64

[16] Free C, Phillips G, Felix L, Galli L, Patel V and Edwards P 2010 The effectiveness of M-health technologies for improving health and health services: a systematic review protocol *BMC Res. Notes* **3** 250

[17] Ratib O May 2011 From PACS to the clouds *Eur. J. Radiol.* **78** 161–2

[18] Mickan S, Tilson J K, Atherton H, Roberts N W and Heneghan C 2013 Evidence of effectiveness of health care professionals using handheld computers: a scoping review of systematic reviews *J. Med. Internet Res.* **15** e212

[19] Mehraeen E, Ghazisaeedi M, Farzi J and Mirshekari S 2017 Security challenges in healthcare cloud computing: a systematic *Glob J Health Sci.* **9** 3

[20] Kim M S, Aro M R, Lage K J, Ingalls K L, Sindhwani V and Markey M K 2016 Exploring the usability of mobile apps supporting radiologists' training in diagnostic decision making *J. Am. Coll. Radiol.* **13** 335–43

[21] Bolan C 2013 Cloud PACS and mobile apps reinvent radiology workflow *Appl. Radiol.* **42** 24–9

[22] Rodrigues M, Visvanathan A, Murchison J and Brady R 2013 Radiology smartphone applications; current provision and cautions *Insights Imaging* **4** 555–62
[23] Drnasin I and Grgic M 2010 The use of mobile phones in radiology *Proc. ELMAR-2010* (New York: IEEE) pp 17–21
[24] John S, Poh A C, Lim T C and Chan E H 2012 The iPad tablet computer for mobile on-call radiology diagnosis? Auditing discrepancy in CT and MRI reporting *J. Digit. Imaging* **25** 628–34
[25] Boonn W W and Flanders A E 2005 Survey of personal digital assistant use in radiology *RadioGraphics* **25** 537–41
[26] Székely A, Talanow R and Bágyi P 2013 Smartphones, tablets and mobile applications for radiology *Eur. J. Radiol.* **82** 829–36
[27] Ranschaert E R and Binkhuysen F H 2013 European Teleradiology now and in the future: results of an online survey *Insights Imaging* **4** 93–102
[28] Coppola F *et al* 2016 Results of an Italian survey on teleradiology *Radiol. Med.* **121** 652–9
[29] van Velsen L, Beaujean D J and van Gemert-Pijnen J E 2013 Why mobile health app overload drives us crazy, and how to restore the sanity *BMC Med. Inform. Decis. Mak.* **13** 23
[30] Misra S, Lewis T L and Aungst T D 2013 Medical application use and the need for further research and assessment for clinical practice: creation and integration of standards for best practice to alleviate poor application design *JAMA Dermatol.* **149** 661–2
[31] Abdollahi H, Shiri I and Heydari M 2019 Medical imaging technologists in radiomics era: an Alice in Wonderland problem *Iran J. Publ. Health* **48** 184
[32] Abdollahi H *et al* 2016 Radiation dose in cardiac SPECT/CT: an estimation of SSDE and effective dose *Eur. J. Radiol.* **85** 2257–61
[33] Ranschaert E R, van Ooijen P M, Lee S, Ratib O and Parizel P M 2015 Social media for radiologists: an introduction *Insights Imaging* **6** 741–52
[34] Rodrigues M A, Visvanathan A, Murchison J T and Brady R R 2013 Radiology smartphone applications; current provision and cautions *Insights Imaging* **4** 555–62
[35] Calero J J, Oton L F and Oton C A 2017 Apps for radiation oncology. A comprehensive review *Transl. Oncol.* **10** 108–14
[36] Szekely A, Talanow R and Bagyi P 2013 Smartphones, tablets and mobile applications for radiology *Eur. J. Radiol.* **82** 829–36
[37] Payne K B, Wharrad H and Watts K 2012 Smartphone and medical related App use among medical students and junior doctors in the United Kingdom (UK): a regional survey *BMC Med. Inform. Decis. Mak.* **12** 121
[38] Boulos M N, Wheeler S, Tavares C and Jones R 2011 How smartphones are changing the face of mobile and participatory healthcare: an overview, with example from eCAALYX *Biomed. Eng. Online* **10** 24
[39] Shelmerdine S C and Lynch J O 2015 Smartphone applications in paediatric radiology: availability and authority *Pediatr. Radiol.* **45** 1293–302
[40] Toomey R J *et al* 2010 Diagnostic efficacy of handheld devices for emergency radiologic consultation *AJR Am. J. Roentgenol.* **194** 469–74
[41] Yaghmai V, Kuppuswami S, Berlin J W and Salehi S A 2003 Evaluation of personal digital assistants as an interpretation medium for computed tomography of patients with intracranial injury *Emerg. Radiol.* **10** 87–9
[42] Johnston W K III, Patel B N, Low R K and Das S 2005 Wireless teleradiology for renal colic and renal trauma *J. Endourol.* **19** 32–6

[43] European Society of Radiology (ESR) 2018 ESR paper on the proper use of mobile devices in radiology *Insights Imaging* **9** 247–51
[44] Hirschorn D S, Choudhri A F, Shih G and Kim W 2014 Use of mobile devices for medical imaging *J. Am. Coll. Radiol.* **11** 1277–85
[45] Paul S *et al* 2016 An energy harvesting wireless sensor node for IoT systems featuring a near-threshold voltage IA-32 microcontroller in 14nm tri-gate CMOS 2016 IEEE Symp. on VLSI Circuits (VLSI-Circuits) (Piscataway, NJ: IEEE) pp 1–2
[46] Rahmani G and McCarthy P A 2017 The use of mobile apps by radiology journals *J. Digit. Imaging* **30** 529
[47] Singh A, Wilkinson S and Braganza S 2014 Smartphones and pediatric apps to mobilize the medical home *J. Pediatr.* **165** 606–10
[48] Glynn R W, O'Duffy F, O'Dwyer T P, Colreavy M P and Rowley H M 2013 Patterns of Internet and smartphone use by parents of children attending a pediatric otolaryngology service *Int. J. Pediatr. Otorhinolaryngol.* **77** 699–702
[49] Hand F, McDowell D T, Glynn R W, Rowley H and Mortell A 2013 Patterns of internet use by parents of children attending a pediatric surgical service *Pediatr. Surg. Int.* **29** 729–33
[50] Rodrigues M A, Murchison J T and Brady R R 2013 Radiology related applications: potential benefits and hazards *Eur. J. Radiol.* **82** 2406

IOP Publishing

Artificial Intelligence Strategies for Analyzing COVID-19 Pneumonia Lung Imaging, Volume 1
Characterization approaches
Ayman El-Baz and Jasjit S Suri

Chapter 5

A hybrid deep learning method with attention for COVID-19 spread forecasting

Abdelkader Dairi, Fouzi Harrou, Ying Sun and Sofiane Khadraoui

This chapter introduces a hybrid deep learning model for COVID-19 spread forecasting. Specifically, the proposed approach combines the desirable characteristics of bidirectional long short-term memory (BiLSTM), convolutional neural networks (CNN), and an attention mechanism. Importantly, this combination, called BiLSTM-A-CNN, is intended to amalgamate the ability of LSTMs to model time dependencies, the capability of the attention mechanism to highlight relevant features, and the noted ability of CNNs to extract features from complex data. The use of the BiLSTM-A-CNN model is expected to improve the forecasting accuracy of future COVID-19 trends. The performance of the proposed model is evaluated through comparisons with a recurrent neural network (RNN), a gated recurrent unit (GRU), long short-term memory (LSTM), and BiLSTM. The assessment is carried out using different statistical metrics, such as the coefficient of determination (R2), root mean square error (RMSE), mean absolute error (MAE), explained variance (EV), median absolute error (MdAE), mean absolute percentage error (MAPE), mean bias error (MBE), and relative mean bias error (rMBE). The daily records of confirmed and recovered cases from Austria, Brazil, Colombia, France, Germany, India, and Mexico are used to evaluate the investigated models. The results confirm the superior performance of the BiLSTM-A-CNN model for COVID-19 spread forecasting compared to those of the other models (i.e., RNN, GRU, LSTM, and BiLSTM).

5.1 Introduction

Today, artificial intelligence plays a prominent and growing role in the future development of science and technology. It has been introduced and applied in

doi:10.1088/978-0-7503-3795-3ch5

various areas of science, including computer science, finance, healthcare, robotics, and transportation. In the medical field, artificial intelligence-based medication is becoming an effective alternative to traditional medication approaches due to the availability of large-scale medical databases characterizing patient conditions, treatments, genetic information, and management decisions. Artificial intelligence has found a wide spectrum of application areas in the healthcare field, such as the early prediction of disease, the identification of mortality risk cases, the monitoring of disease trends, disease management, and the disease environment. In general, the use of artificial intelligence in healthcare greatly helps physicians to analyze complex data patterns, assists them in complex clinical decision-making and diagnosis, and enhances physicians' medical expertise. Early prediction is essential for the clinical diagnosis and treatment of many complex diseases, such as diabetes, cancer, heart disease, and the early stages of psychiatric disease. One of the most important applications of artificial medical intelligence, which has recently received much interest, is the forecasting and diagnosis of COVID-19 [1–4].

The current COVID-19 pandemic that was initially detected in Wuhan, China, in December 2019 is a critical problem confronting the modern world [5]. According to the World Health Organization, 213 countries and territories across the globe have been affected by COVID-19. Remarkably, several European countries, as well as North and South America, have been strongly affected by the COVID-19 outbreak. One major factor facilitating this virus's global propagation from its origin is the air traffic between Asia, North America, and Europe. Indeed, transmission from person to person has been recorded between close contacts of returned travelers. Besides, this virus can be propagated in different ways, including by direct body contact, contaminated cash, and air from infected persons who cough or sneeze [6]. It is worth pointing out that the incubation duration of COVID-19 is a minimum of fourteen days, which accelerates its propagation during the incubation period [7]. Accordingly, the forecasting of confirmed and recovered COVID-19 cases is essential for managing the outbreak and preparing efficient strategies to mitigate the spread of COVID-19.

AI has been utilized by expert epidemiologists for the real-time forecasting and monitoring of pandemic trends and public health threats. A group called HealthMap at Boston Children's Hospital, consisting of researchers, epidemiologists, and software developers, has recently implemented AI to monitor informal data sources for SARS-CoV-2 outbreaks and evaluate emerging public health threats in real time [8]. Another team of researchers at Carnegie Mellon University developed a forecasting model to accurately predict the spread of seasonal influenza based on Google's data and other social media data [9]. Google Flu Trends, which is a well-known model developed by Google.org, failed to track the flu epidemic mainly as a result of the poor design of the variables used in the prediction process [10]. A Canadian software company, called BlueDot, specializing in AI and infectious disease epidemiology, has successfully demonstrated a prediction of the spread of diseases such as the 2019-nCoV flu outbreak in China [11] and the international spread of the Zika virus from Brazil [12].

Over the last few months, COVID-19 has gained significant attention from among the research community, epidemiological experts, and local authorities.

Much work has been done to detect and diagnose COVID-19 disease using x-ray imagery, as described in the literature [13–16]. In [17], COVID-19 detection using x-ray imagery was addressed as a classification problem involving three classes: pneumonia, COVID-19 cases, and normal cases. To this end, a support vector machine (SVM) was applied to the extracted features using CNN models (MobileNetV2 and SqueezeNet). However, the detection was performed in a supervised way, which demands data labeling. In [18], deep learning models were applied for COVID-19 detection based on chest radiography images, in which different CNN architectures were initialized through transfer learning, exploiting other detection experience. However, the detection was performed using supervised binary classification (i.e., COVID-19 versus non-COVID-19). In [19], different CNN architectures were investigated for the classification of COVID-19 infection cases using computed tomography. First, the normal cases were eliminated, and then this approach focused on the abnormal cases by predicting COVID-19 infection or pneumonia. In [20], a COVID-19 detection system based on chest X-ray images was proposed that combined the CNN model and machine learning models, including SVM, decision tree, and nearest neighbors. In this system, Bayesian optimization was used for hyperparameter tuning.

In order to understand and manage this epidemic, numerous published studies have focused on the modeling, prediction, and forecasting of the spread of COVID-19 using recorded COVID-19 time series data. In [21], the capability and performance of four models, including autoregressive integrated moving average (ARIMA), a nonlinear auto-regression neural network, and LSTM, were evaluated for their ability to forecast confirmed COVID-19 cases. The results obtained demonstrated the superior performance of the LSTM model compared to those of the other models considered. Behnooda *et al* [22] investigated the impacts of weather conditions and the density of the population on the SARS-CoV-2 infection rate. To this end, they used a coupled adaptive network-based fuzzy inference system and virus optimization algorithms. The results reveal that the population density has the most crucial effect on the performance of the proposed models, which highlights the importance of social distancing to slow down the spread of COVID-19. Torrealba-Rodriguez *et al* [23] conducted a prediction of COVID-19 in Mexico based on daily confirmed cases up to 8 May 2020. They applied Gompertz, logistic, and artificial neural networks to model the number of cases of SARS-CoV-2 infection and showed that these models could describe the daily COVID-19 confirmed cases well. Ribeiro *et al* [24] considered regression models to forecast COVID-19 cases in Brazil. Specifically, they compared ARIMA, cubist regression, random forest, ridge regression, SVR, and stacking-ensemble learning for one, three, and six-step forecasts. They highlighted that SVM regression and stacking-ensemble learning achieved better forecasting than the other models. The method described in [25] used reduced-space Gaussian process regression to forecast and evaluate the spread of COVID-19 in the US from January 21 to April 12, 2020. Maleki *et al* [26] considered an AR time series model based on a two-piece scale mixture of normal distributions to forecast recovered and confirmed cases of COVID-19. Khan *et al* [6] applied a vector autoregressive (VAR) model to forecast new confirmed cases, deaths, and recovered cases of COVID-19 in Pakistan. They used data from March 8 to June 27, 2020, and demonstrated that the VAR model is effective in forecasting the spread of COVID-19. However, the major shortcoming of this study is the availability of a small amount of data, which makes model identification a difficult task.

A precise and convenient model for forecasting the spread of COVID-19 can be useful for improving resource allocation and strategic planning in hospitals and hence greatly help to slow or mitigate the propagation of COVID-19. Data-driven deep learning models have been shown to be very capable of modelling time series data in a wide range of applications [27]. Recently, deep learning methods have been applied to model and forecast the future trend of COVID-19 transmission [21, 28, 29]. For instance, in [28], the LSTM model was applied to forecast COVID-19 transmission. The model was trained using COVID-19 time series data up to March 31, 2020. In [29], five deep learning models were considered to forecast the recovered and confirmed COVID-19 cases in Italy, Spain, France, China, the US, and Australia with data up to June 17, 2020. The results showed that the best performance was obtained from the variational auto-encoder.

In this chapter, an innovative hybrid deep learning model is proposed to improve the forecasting accuracy of confirmed and recovered COVID-19 cases. The spread of this contagious disease is directly linked to existing confirmed counts, while its recovery is restricted by existing treatment capacity, which enables forecasting to be performed without the need for exogenous information. The proposed hybrid model amalgamates the desirable characteristics of BiLSTM, CNN, and the self-attention mechanism. The proposed flexible mode, the BiLSTM-A-CNN, exploits the capable performance of BiLSTM for time series modeling and flexible nonlinear approximation and the focus on the relevant features via the attention-based mechanism. Exploiting this sophisticated statistical tool is advantageous in the sense that it has the potential to improve the forecasting of COVID-19 confirmed and recovered time series data. COVID-19 datasets from seven countries (Austria, Brazil, Colombia, France, Germany, India, and Mexico) are used to evaluate BiLSTM-A-CNN and compare its forecasting performance with those of four deep learning models (i.e., the RNN, GRU, LSTM, and BiLSTM models). The adopted COVID-19 time series datasets cover the period from January 22, 2020, to April 7, 2021. The deep learning-driven models are constructed then assessed by several statistical metrics. The results demonstrate the effectiveness of the BiLSTM-A-CNN model.

The remainder of this article is organized as follows. In section 5.2, we first present the basic concepts of BiLSTM, CNN, and the attention mechanism. The proposed forecasting model is introduced in section 5.3. The results and discussions are given in section 5.4, which shows model performances and comparisons. The conclusions are drawn in section 5.5.

5.2 Materials

5.2.1 Preliminaries

Deep learning methods have been widely exploited in different areas because of their flexibility and extended ability to handle complex data [30–32]. They have demonstrated successful performance in different applications, including photovoltaic power forecasting [33], anomaly detection [34–37], and reinforcement learning [38, 39]. This section will describe the deep learning models used in our study (i.e., BiLSTM and CNN) and the attention mechanism.

5.2.1.1 Bidirectional long short-term memory

LSTM's key point is that its memory mechanism allows it to model time dependencies in data sequences [40]. This is due to the gating technique that acts as a filter that controls the amount of information that keeps or stops entering and updating the model states (weights). Indeed, LSTM consists of three nonlinear gates: (i) the forget gate (ii) the input gate (iii) and the output gate in the forward direction (past to future) for the time series data. The key idea of BiLSTM is to process data in the opposite direction of a given time series, i.e. backward (from the future to the past) [41]. This allows BiLSTM to profit from the advantage of using future information. Two LSTM instances are used to simultaneously learn and extract temporal features via double data processing [42]. Specifically, to this end, two hidden states are combined, enabling information to arrive from the backward layer and the forward layer. A schematic illustration of BiLSTM is given in figure 5.1.

The BiLSTM hidden layer can be written as:

$$\mathcal{H} = \vec{h}_{Forward} \otimes \vec{h}_{Backward} \tag{5.1}$$

where $\vec{h}_{Forward}$, $\vec{h}_{Backward}$ denote the hidden layer outputs for the LSTM instances that process data in the forward and backward directions, respectively. Indeed this duality of data processing enables BiLSTM to discover and learn more complex temporal features. BiLSTM has been widely employed in classification [43, 44], prediction [45], and forecasting [46].

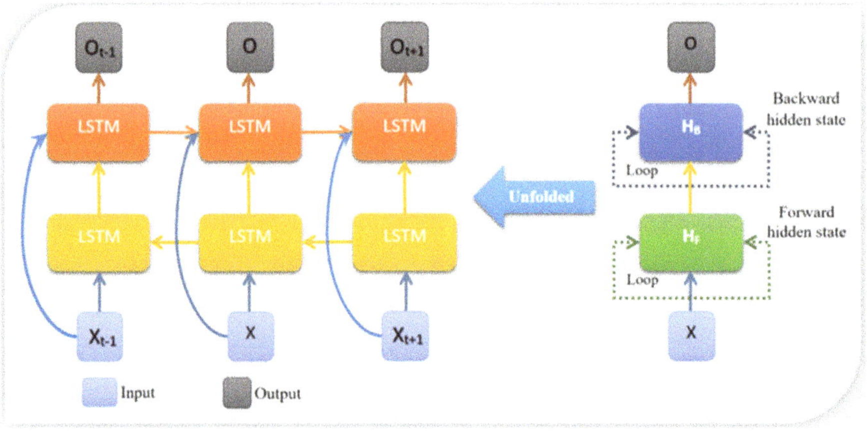

Figure 5.1. Schematic illustration of the BiLSTM structure.

5.2.1.2 Convolutional neural networks

CNNs are among the deep learning models mainly used to deal with computer vision classification problems via supervised learning [47–49]. The success of CNNs is due to their internal structure, which is composed of several nonlinear transformations that take place through convolutional operations, max-pooling features, map reduction, and a fully connected layer. This complex structure acts as a hierarchic feature extraction process (figure 5.2).

A CNN usually consists of stacked convolutional layers, including several filters that define the depth and aim to extract features through the nonlinear transformation of a given input. CNN proceeds to iteratively reveal and learn the features of the problem at hand using the convolution transformation and filtering operations, which are indeed dot products. The results of the hierarchical changes applied to the input are called a feature map. We briefly describe the main layers of a CNN, namely the convolution layer, the pooling layer, and the fully connected layer.

- *Convolution layer:* The input X is convolved by a set of learning kernels to construct new feature maps. The output of the convolution layer is computed as follows:

$$O_{Convolution\ Layer} = A\left(B + \sum_i K * X\right), \tag{5.2}$$

  where X denotes a given input, K is the convolution kernel, B represents the layer bias, and A denotes the nonlinear activation function.
- *Pooling layer:* The main objective of the pooling layer is to reduce the feature maps produced after a convolution operation. Moreover, the pooling operation decreases the computational complexity and serves to fuse features via operations such as max pooling, average pooling, and random pooling.

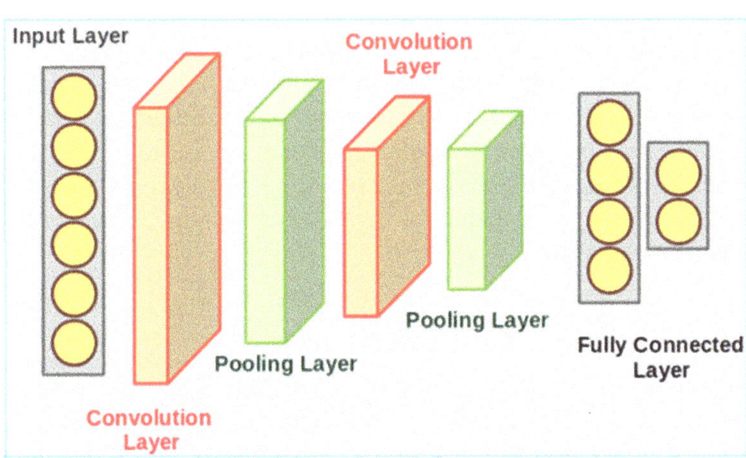

Figure 5.2. Schematic illustration of CNN structure.

Note that different window sizes can be used to create the pooling window that contains the features.

- *Fully connected layer:* The fully connected layer (FC) is like a traditional artificial neural network (ANN) or multilayer perceptron (MLP) and is composed of one or many layers that contain several neurons with an activation function A:

$$O_{FC} = A\left(B + \sum_{i} W * X\right), \tag{5.3}$$

where X denotes a given input, W and B denote the layer weight biases, and A denotes a nonlinear activation function such as a sigmoid function.

5.2.1.3 Attention mechanism

Human beings do not usually use all the available sensory information to perceive an evolving environment in order to perform specific tasks. Therefore, instead of scanning the full observed scene, human vision pays greater attention to the relevant parts of the image, which is called visual attention. This behavior acts as a filter or a mask by processing only valuable information and the pertinent features of the observed scene, optimizing the data processing time. Attention has been introduced [50, 51] to address natural language processing problems, image processing, machine translation, image recognition, and voice recognition. The attention approach highlights a valuable area in the feature space; this is achieved by computing a weighted sum called a context vector. Moreover, attention is employed as a special way to transport features between the encoder and the decoder; attention represented by the context vector highlights the most important features learned during the training process.

In contrast to attention, self-attention (SA) is flexible and can be applied to other models, not necessarily auto-encoders with recurrent neural networks. Furthermore, SA can be injected at any level of a neural network and deals with only one input, which improves the capture of the internal correlation of the input data [52]. Therefore, SA can be captured to improve the effectiveness of the learned representation and extract complementary information. Indeed, self-attention data processing starts by computing the weight vector (called the score) between the data points that belong to a given sequence X at positions i and j; the weight vector is computed as follows [52]:

$$\mathcal{X}_{scaled} = \frac{X - min(X)}{max(X) - min(X)} \tag{5.4}$$

where W_a denotes the self-attention model weight matrix, which is computed throughout the training, and d denotes the (W_a X_i) dimension; division by d speeds up convergence [52]. Furthermore, the weights S_{ij} are normalized using softmax, which gives a probability-like representation (the sum of all weight values is equal to one):

$$\mathscr{P}_{ij} = softmax(\mathscr{S}_{ij}) = \frac{\exp(\mathscr{S}_{ij})}{\sum_j \exp(\mathscr{S}_{ij})}. \tag{5.5}$$

The final self-attention model output is expressed as follows:

$$O_i = \sum_{j=1}^{n} \mathscr{P}_{ij} (W_a \mathscr{X}_i). \tag{5.6}$$

The obtained output improves the extracted features by highlighting the most relevant and describes the input elements' internal correlation. Moreover, the self-attention mechanism can derive global dependencies from the input itself, capturing item-to-item interactions across a given input sequence, regardless of their position or the distance between sequence elements.

5.3 The proposed hybrid deep model

The central idea is to build deep-stacked feature extractors of different kinds. In this study, a hybrid bidirectional recurrent model with an attention mechanism is proposed (see figure 5.3). The proposed approach consists of a robust deep recurrent feature extractor combined with a feature importance mechanism, a convolutional transformation that ends with a fully connected layer that plays the role of the real forecaster layer. Indeed, a novel effective deep architecture is designed to forecast COVID-19 confirmed and recovered cases over several locations. The recorded cases of COVID-19 are data sequences (time series) used as the inputs of the proposed model.

First of all, a feature scaling technique is used, in which data are normalized to the range [0, 1] using min-max normalization, where X is the input vector of the data sequence:

$$\mathscr{X}_{scaled} = \frac{X - min(X)}{max(X) - min(X)}. \tag{5.7}$$

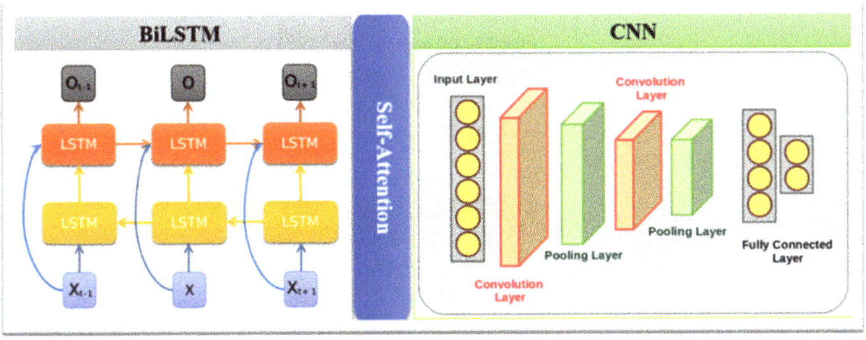

Figure 5.3. The proposed hybrid architecture.

Figure 5.4 illustrates an overview of the proposed approach steps used to provide a robust and effective COVID-19 deep forecasting framework. The normalization process aims to stabilize the model training. Furthermore, the normalized input serves to feed two LSTM recurrent neural network models, intended to model the time dependencies of the recorded COVID-19 cases (recovered and confirmed).

Indeed, one LSTM is trained using the time series data in the forward direction (past to future), while the second is trained using a reversed sense (future to past), which benefits from future context information to improve the modelling of the time series. The bidirectional data processing constitutes an enhanced feature space, which is used as an input for the self-attention mechanism. Moreover, the attention approach highlights relevant and particular features through a weighted vector. The obtained feature space is transformed through self-attention into a new feature map that helps the model to focus on a specific area containing more important features.

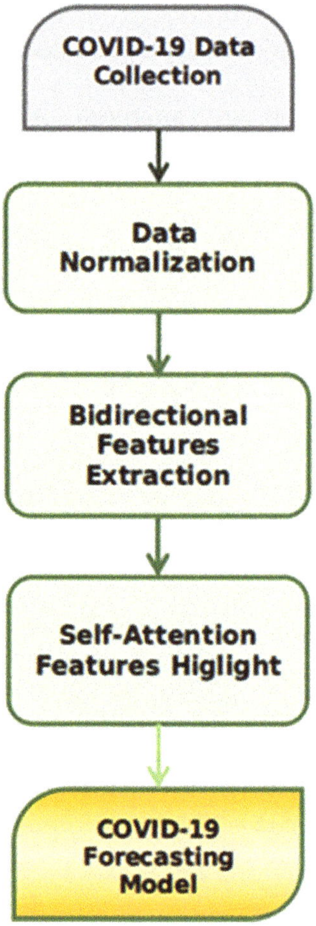

Figure 5.4. The proposed approach flowchart.

Attention acts like a feature importance approach. The self-attention mechanism uses a regularization approach to mitigate the bias (a bias-regularizer) and normalize the weights (a kernel-regularizer). This step of regularization improves of the attention mechanism's diversity and avoids overfitting.

The newly constructed features map represents the relevant features used to feed a CNN, a powerful feature extractor composed of convolutional operations and followed by a max-pooling transformation. Finally, a fully connected layer (the forecaster) is used to perform the forecasting. Moreover, to avoid overfitting situations, we use a regularization technique, namely 'dropout', which aims to randomly drop connections from the fully connected layer.

5.3.1 Evaluation metrics

For our performance comparisons, we adopted the following indexes to quantify the forecast values: the coefficient of determination (R^2), the RMSE, the MAE, the MAPE, the EV, the MdAE, the MBE, and the rMBE.

$$R^2 = \frac{\sum_{t=1}^{n}\left[(y_t - \bar{y}) \cdot (\hat{y}_t - \bar{y})\right]^2}{\sqrt{\sum_{t=1}^{n}(y_t - \bar{y})^2} \cdot \sqrt{\sum_{t=1}^{n}(\hat{y}_t - \bar{y})^2}}, \tag{5.8}$$

$$RMSE = \sqrt{\frac{1}{n}\sum_{t=1}^{n}(y_t - \hat{y}_t)^2}, \tag{5.9}$$

$$MAE = \frac{\sum_{t=1}^{n}\left|y_t - yt\right|}{n}, \tag{5.10}$$

$$MAPE = \frac{100}{n}\sum_{t=1}^{n}\left|\frac{y_t - \hat{y}_t}{y_t}\right|\%, \tag{5.11}$$

$$EV = 1 - \frac{\mathrm{Var}(\hat{y} - y)}{\mathrm{Var}(y)}, \tag{5.12}$$

$$MDAE = \mathrm{median}\left(\left|y_t - \hat{y}\right|\right), \tag{5.13}$$

$$rMBE = \frac{\sum_{t=1}^{n}(y_t - \hat{y})}{\sum_{t=1}^{n} y_t} \cdot 100, \tag{5.14}$$

where y_t represents the number of COVID cases, $\hat{y}_t$ is the corresponding forecast value, and n is the number of data points. Lower RMSE and MAE values imply better precision and forecasting quality.

In summary, this study aims to model and forecast the future trend (the upcoming ten days) of confirmed and recovered COVID-19 time series. Essentially, we investigate the performance of deep learning models when applied to a small amount of time series data and compare their forecasting accuracy with those of traditional time series models. Three deep learning models and five commonly used time series models are considered in this comparative study. The general procedure used in this study is depicted in figure 5.4. First, the daily recovered and confirmed time series data are divided into training and test subsets. All models are trained using the training set and evaluated using the test set. The best forecasting model is indicated by five statistical metrics, including R2, RMSE, MAE, EV, and MAPE.

5.4 Experiments and results

5.4.1 Data description

In this study, daily confirmed and recovered COVID-19 case time series data from seven different countries (Austria, Brazil, Colombia, France, Germany, India, and Mexico) are employed to assess the forecasting capacity of the investigated deep learning models. The data are offered to the public by the Center for Systems Science and Engineering (CSSE) at Johns Hopkins University (https://github.com/CSSEGISandData/COVID-19) and are shown in figure 5.5. We can see that India and Brazil have the largest numbers of confirmed cases. Considering the population in each country, India is experiencing the most significant impact of COVID-19. Both India and Brazil show a rapid increase in recovered cases, showing their quick and efficient response to this public health crisis. Table 5.1 provides the dates of the first case in the studied countries.

Table 5.2 summarizes the descriptive statistics of the COVID-19 datasets, indicating that the COVID-19 datasets have a non-Gaussian distribution with positive support and exhibit different intervals of variability.

5.4.2 Model performance assessment

We construct each deep learning model using the training datasets recorded from January 22, 2020, to March 8, 2021. We then use these constructed models to forecast the future trend of COVID-19 sequentially. The testing period is from March 9 to April 7, 2021.

In the training stage, we applied the grid search approach to set up the hyperparameters in the considered models. We adopted some common hyper-parameters for all the models used, such as the number of epochs (300), the learning rate (10–3), the batch size (5), the Rmsprop optimizer, and the lag (time steps) (12). Sixteen hidden units were used for all recurrent networks (RNNs), and an additional dense layer was used for the forecasting task; this layer was provided with a dropout technique for regularization to avoid overfitting.

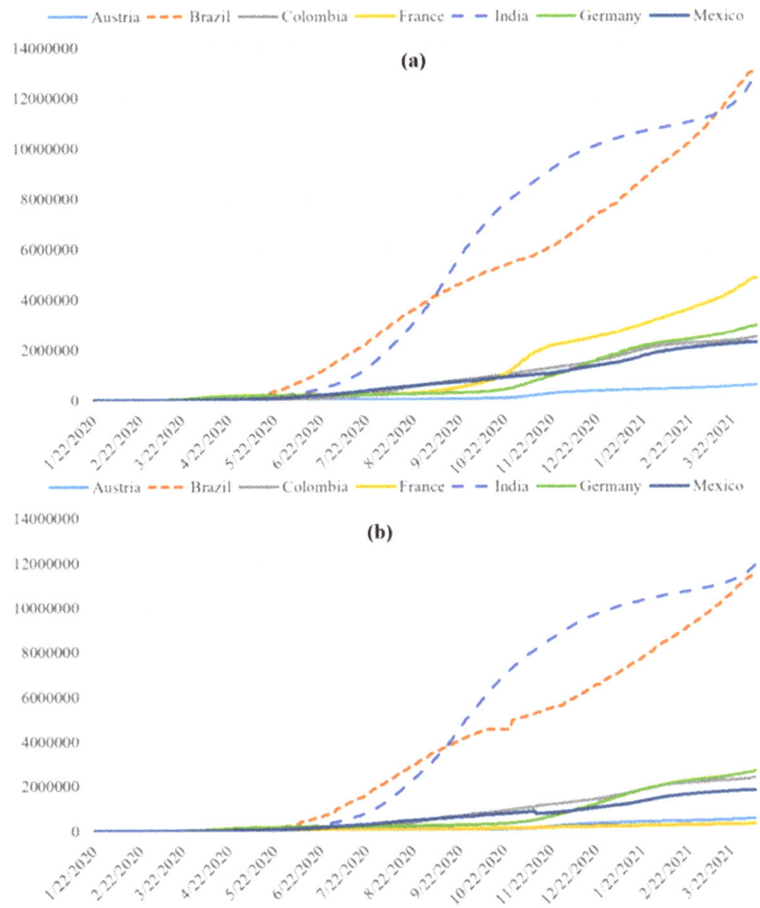

Figure 5.5. The number of (a) confirmed and (b) recovered COVID-19 cases from January 22, 2020 to April 7, 2021, in Austria, Brazil, Colombia, France, Germany, India, and Mexico.

Table 5.1. Date of the start of COVID-19 per country.

Country	Date
Austria	February 25, 2020
Brazil	February 26, 2020
Colombia	January 31, 2020
France	January 24, 2020
Germany	January 27, 2020
Mexico	February 28, 2020
India	January 30, 2020

Table 5.2. Statistical summary of the confirmed and recovered COVID-19 time series datasets.

Type, country	Min	Max	Std	Q-0.25	Q-0.5	Q-0.75	Skewness	Kurtosis
Confirmed, Austria	0	566008	184903.346	15882	27075.5	334913	0.904	2.149
Confirmed, Brazil	0	13193205	3942392.4	169594	3854232	7162978	0.541	2.108
Confirmed, Colombia	0	2479617	847526.044	11613	603894	1482072	0.595	1.886
Confirmed, France	0	4807123	1453137.49	176651	298909.5	2441737	0.917	2.383
Confirmed, India	0	12928574	4670878.9	70768	3581989	10004599	0.234	1.33
Confirmed, Germany	0	2940279	925587.265	172576	243070	1486839	1.046	2.485
Confirmed, Mexico	0	2261879	748126.294	36327	593776.5	1301546	0.66	2.105
Recovered, Austria	0	522774	171797.59	14061	22968	297424	0.988	2.276
Recovered, Brazil	0	11592159	3542770.71	67384	3219900	6322955	0.541	2.035
Recovered, Colombia	0	2345471	809042.588	2825	445585.5	1354021	0.668	1.964
Recovered, France	0	269989	76637.823	55569	73467	159138	0.62	2.37
Recovered, India	0	11851393	4509987.92	22549	2744367	9550712	0.315	1.358
Recovered, Germany	0	2638320	823940.251	145617	215036.5	1095982	1.195	2.841
Recovered, Mexico	0	1765244	580966.284	23100	487003.5	962397	0.653	2.164

The architecture of the proposed approach is composed of three parts:

- *The bidirectional LSTM layer*: the input of this layer is 3D with a *batch size* of, 12, 1, while its output has a *batch size* of 16, 1, and the activation function used at this level is *Relu.*
- *The self-attention layer*: this layer does not change the shape of the input; it just provides a weighted sum vector that highlights more relevant features computed using the input itself, so the input and output dimensions are the same (*batch size*, 12, 1). The activation function used at this level is *Tanh.*
- *The convolutional layer*: this layer performs convolution operations to extract more features and provides a feature map with a dimension of 16. The activation function used at this level is *Relu.*
- *The pooling layer*: in this layer, we use the max pool technique to reduce the dimensions of the feature map.
- *The fully connected layer*: This layer's dimension is 1; the forecasting is performed here. The activation function used at this level is a *sigmoid* function.

The five investigated deep learning models (BiLSTM-A-CNN, RNN, GRU, LSTM, and BiLSTM) are built for 412 days starting from January 22, 2020, and then applied to forecast COVID-19 confirmed and recovered cases for a 30 day forecast horizon from March 9, 2021. Figure 5.6 displays the observed model forecasts for the confirmed and recovered cases. Radar charts representing the rMBE computed for each model are displayed in figure 5.7. It can be seen from figure 5.6 that the five deep learning models provide reasonable forecasting of the confirmed and recovered cases. The proposed model provides good forecast quality, with relatively narrower bands around the actual observations. Radar graphs of the rMBE confirm the superior forecasting performance of the proposed approach, as it has the lowest rMBE values for all cases. The statistical metrics, including the RMSE, MAE, R2, EV, MDAE, and MAPE, are computed based on the confirmed and recovered test data, respectively, for the investigated countries, and are arranged in tables 5.3 and 5.4. The results in tables 5.3 and 5.4 shows that the five deep learning models provide a satisfactory forecasting performance for both confirmed and recovered time series data. Importantly, this is mainly due to the capacity of RNN-based models (i.e., RNN, GRU, LSTM, and BiLSTM) to model time dependencies in time series data. It is worth mentioning that deep learning models do not need *a priori* assumptions regarding the data, which makes them very attractive and easy to use. As expected, the proposed hybrid model exhibited better performance when compared to the RNN-based models. To facilitate comparison, the metrics for each series are further grouped and averaged either by model (table 5.5) or by series (table 5.6).

Table 5.5 presents the aggregated performance for each model. The EV values imply that all models provide a good fit. The proposed BiLSTM-A-CNN model showed the best forecasting compared with that of other deep learning models. Specifically, the BiLSTM-A-CNN model achieved outstanding performance with an R2 of 1, an EV of 1, and an MAPE of 0.790%. It was followed successively by LSTM, BiLSTM, GRU, and RNN. In terms of all the metrics calculated,

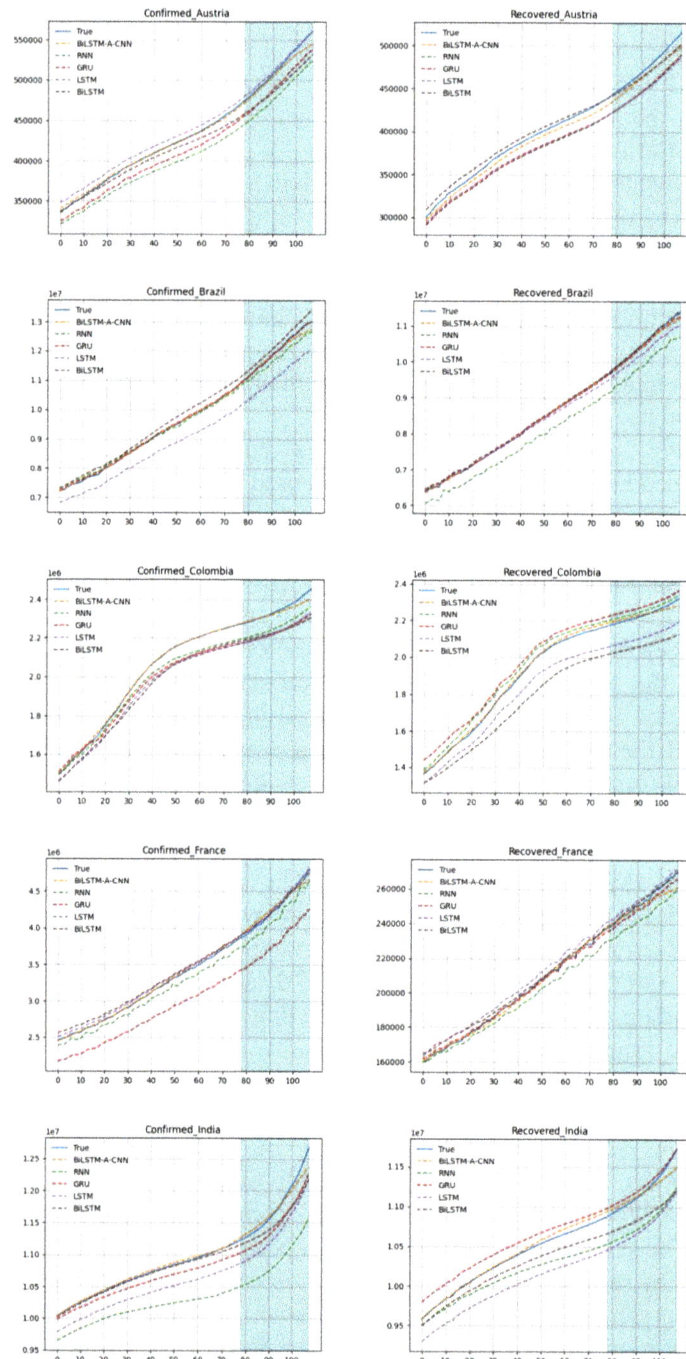

Figure 5.6. Forecast results of confirmed and recovered COVID-19 cases using five deep learning models for Austria, Brazil, Colombia, France, India, and Mexico. The green zone depicts the forecast range.

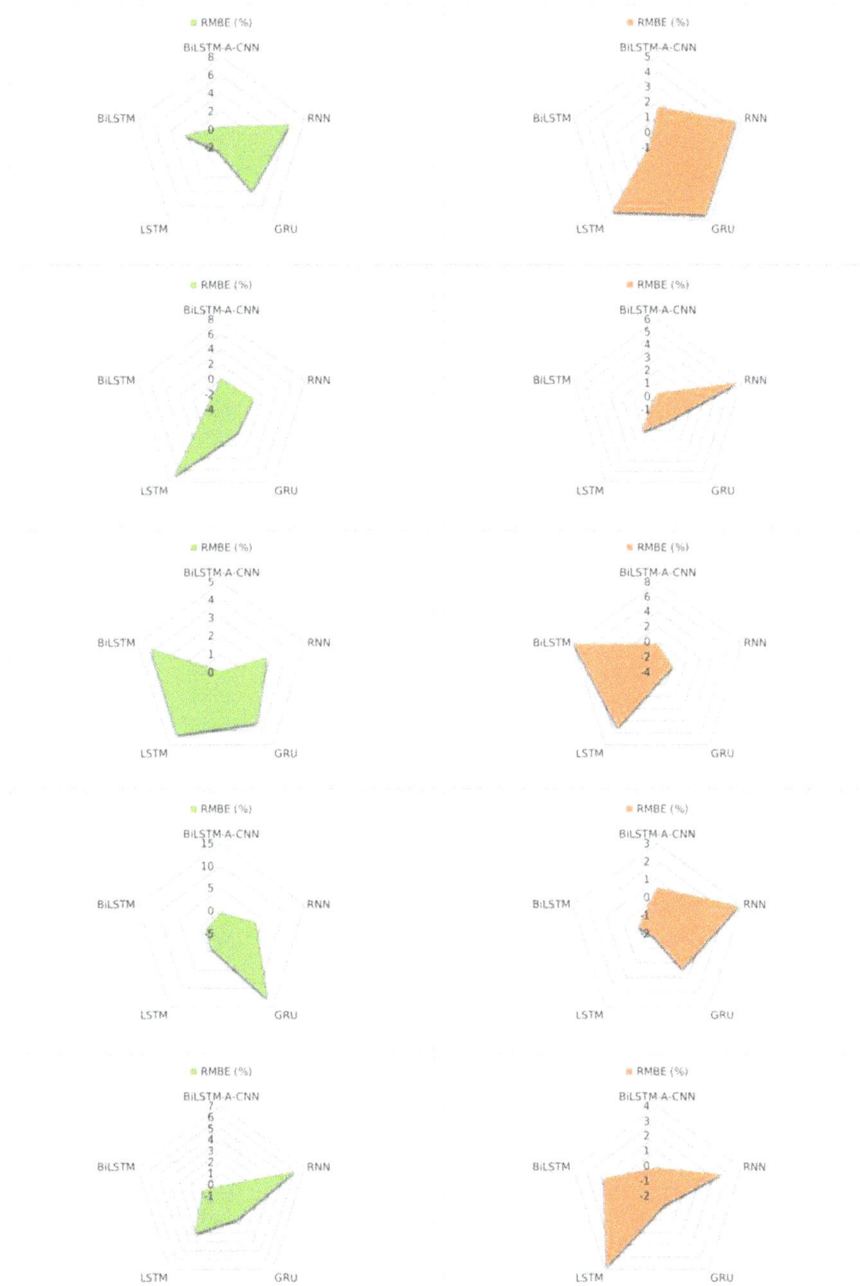

Figure 5.7. Radar charts of the rMBE (%) for each forecasting model for confirmed and recovered COVID-19 case data recorded in Austria, Brazil, Colombia, France, India, and Mexico.

Table 5.3. Performance of confirmed case forecasting performed by the proposed BiLSTM-A-CNN model, compared to the considered RNN models.

Model	Country	RMSE	MAE	R2	EV	MDAE	MAPE
RNN	Austria	18418	14147	0.989	0.995	14774	4.260
GRU	Austria	12906	10605	0.995	0.998	12585	4.099
LSTM	Austria	8113	7587	0.998	1.000	7262	6.647
BILSTM	Austria	9757	6174	0.997	0.998	3185	2.040
BILSTM-A-CNN	Austria	3514	2360	1.000	1.000	1693	1.148
RNN	Brazil	130428	108698	0.998	0.998	95033	1.550
GRU	Brazil	167652	97290	0.996	0.997	35937	2.111
LSTM	Brazil	499980	429853	0.964	0.991	361288	5.290
BILSTM	Brazil	170868	159907	0.996	0.999	140567	2.224
BILSTM-A-CNN	Brazil	58619	38100	1.000	1.000	24972	0.561
RNN	Colombia	45247	36265	0.994	0.996	25393	2.306
GRU	Colombia	63171	52270	0.989	0.990	47762	3.866
LSTM	Colombia	62560	48734	0.989	0.996	34510	2.649
BILSTM	Colombia	69055	62530	0.987	0.998	56224	4.281
BILSTM-A-CNN	Colombia	10003	6675	1.000	1.000	4963	0.580
RNN	France	81297	64211	0.996	0.999	66949	2.465
GRU	France	301198	252835	0.949	0.984	276918	9.790
LSTM	France	43010	40428	0.999	1.000	40212	3.186
BILSTM	France	63117	54073	0.998	0.999	53374	3.210
BILSTM-A-CNN	France	28318	17947	1.000	1.000	9506	0.931
RNN	Germany	171619	133766	0.965	0.986	139456	7.393
GRU	Germany	106756	80104	0.987	0.991	35946	5.564
LSTM	Germany	40737	29195	0.998	0.999	16146	2.632
BILSTM	Germany	70624	56020	0.994	0.994	49051	5.956
BILSTM-A-CNN	Germany	14506	10950	1.000	1.000	8468	1.109
RNN	India	489458	414024	0.961	0.978	385702	4.636
GRU	India	236339	192166	0.991	0.991	155245	3.008
LSTM	India	257545	228053	0.989	0.994	233846	2.565
BILSTM	India	205441	131955	0.993	0.993	52345	2.337
BILSTM-A-CNN	India	55946	38542	0.999	1.000	27693	0.598
RNN	Mexico	68506	57947	0.985	0.995	56747	3.957
GRU	Mexico	59666	55277	0.989	0.998	52084	4.109
LSTM	Mexico	68036	61466	0.985	0.997	56932	4.422
BILSTM	Mexico	49752	38766	0.992	0.995	24936	2.537
BILSTM-A-CNN	Mexico	8988	7452	1.000	1.000	6724	0.592

Table 5.4. Performance of recovered case forecasting performed by the proposed BiLSTM-A-CNN model, compared to the considered RNN models.

Model	Country	RMSE	MAE	R2	EV	MDAE	MAPE
RNN	Austria	12827	9496	0.994	0.997	7530	2.991
GRU	Austria	12671	9364	0.995	0.997	8080	3.092
LSTM	Austria	12300	8584	0.995	0.997	6162	2.319
BiLSTM	Austria	5945	5259	0.999	0.999	4711	4.939
BiLSTM-A-CNN	Austria	4961	3631	0.999	1.000	2819	1.402
RNN	Brazil	360551	318991	0.977	0.995	304549	4.551
GRU	Brazil	76170	64269	0.999	0.999	65109	1.290
LSTM	Brazil	147444	128353	0.996	0.996	131720	2.246
BiLSTM	Brazil	59698	47140	0.999	1.000	38340	0.942
BiLSTM-A-CNN	Brazil	54314	36100	0.999	0.999	23908	0.617
RNN	Colombia	54720	43851	0.992	0.997	32614	5.549
GRU	Colombia	59325	55246	0.990	0.999	56966	5.156
LSTM	Colombia	70391	56609	0.987	0.995	44616	3.429
BiLSTM	Colombia	106313	87247	0.969	0.979	65111	6.313
BiLSTM-A-CNN	Colombia	17777	10691	0.999	0.999	5929	0.829
RNN	France	4889	3901	0.994	0.995	3056	2.544
GRU	France	4110	3361	0.996	0.997	2557	3.406
LSTM	France	3355	2971	0.997	0.999	3270	1.941
BiLSTM	France	2258	1897	0.999	1.000	1567	1.454
BiLSTM-A-CNN	France	1842	1140	0.999	0.999	718	0.713
RNN	Germany	69084	47240	0.993	0.996	17077	3.338
GRU	Germany	109953	79797	0.983	0.992	55800	4.904
LSTM	Germany	62661	41308	0.995	0.996	8108	2.838
BiLSTM	Germany	46095	32286	0.997	0.998	12508	2.117
BiLSTM-A-CNN	Germany	12051	8567	1.000	1.000	5517	0.803
RNN	India	281548	230723	0.989	0.989	230263	3.896
GRU	India	210183	192556	0.994	0.999	178818	3.080
LSTM	India	288625	236394	0.988	0.996	264184	2.402
BiLSTM	India	175439	140865	0.996	0.996	112959	2.161
BiLSTM-A-CNN	India	45928	32997	1.000	1.000	24467	0.484
RNN	Mexico	48728	37418	0.987	0.992	24559	3.150
GRU	Mexico	126643	60871	0.911	0.926	14789	4.103
LSTM	Mexico	24182	18805	0.997	0.999	13626	1.478
BiLSTM	Mexico	60726	47858	0.980	0.990	41326	3.933
BiLSTM-A	Mexico	9591	6611	0.999	1.000	4961	0.699

Table 5.5. Averaged validation metrics per model.

MODEL	RMSE	MAE	R2	EV	MDAE	MAPE
RNN	131237.155	108619.871	0.987	0.993	100264.435	3.756
LSTM	113495.670	95595.676	0.991	0.997	87277.270	3.146
GRU	110481.687	86143.699	0.983	0.99	71328.255	4.113
BILSTM	78220.512	62283.971	0.993	0.996	46871.607	3.175
BILSTM-A-CNN	23311.250	15840.107	1	1	10881.188	0.79

Table 5.6. Averaged validation metrics per series.

Country	RMSE	MAE	R2	EV	MDAE	MAPE
Confirm Austria	10541.528	8174.704	0.996	0.998	7899.571	3.639
Confirm Brazil	205509.439	166769.608	0.991	0.997	131559.539	2.347
Confirm Colombia	50007.134	41294.682	0.992	0.996	33770.350	2.736
Confirm France	103387.985	85898.769	0.988	0.996	89391.804	3.916
Confirm Germany	80848.568	62006.843	0.989	0.994	49813.277	4.531
Confirm India	248945.774	200948.188	0.987	0.991	170966.076	2.629
Confirm Mexico	50989.411	44181.353	0.99	0.997	39484.591	3.123
Recover Austria	9740.877	7266.915	0.996	0.998	5860.493	2.949
Recover Brazil	139635.405	118970.365	0.994	0.998	112725.028	1.929
Recover Colombia	61705.078	50728.695	0.987	0.994	41047.141	4.255
Recover France	3290.915	2654.032	0.997	0.998	2233.512	2.012
Recover Germany	59968.537	41839.701	0.994	0.996	19802.257	2.8
Recover India	200344.818	166706.881	0.993	0.996	162137.941	2.405
Recover Mexico	53974.097	34312.570	0.975	0.981	19852.136	2.673

BiLSTM-A-CNN was the best forecasting model for solving this univariate time series forecasting problem with high efficiency and satisfying accuracy. This can be attributed to its capacity to extract relevant information and feature importance provided by the attention mechanism.

Table 5.6 shows the aggregated performance of each series. Overall, forecasts of confirmed cases outperform those for recovered cases. It is likely that the spread of the COVID-19 virus is linked to existing case counts and thus follows more predictable dynamics with memory, while treating and curing confirmed cases is more complicated.

5.5 Conclusions

Precise COVID-19 forecasts would support the control of medical resources and reinforce public policy formulation during this pandemic event. A hybrid deep learning model (called BiLSTM-A-CNN) that combines BiLSTM, CNN, and the attention mechanism, is proposed to enhance the accuracy of COVD-19 spread forecasting. The performance of the proposed hybrid model was assessed using the daily records of confirmed and recovered cases from Austria, Brazil, Colombia, France, Germany, India, and Mexico. Eight metrics of effectiveness were adopted to check the forecasting accuracy of the investigated deep learning models: R^2, RMSE, MAE, EV, MdAE MAPE, MBE, and rMBE. The results demonstrated that the proposed BiLSTM-A-CNN model provides better forecasting quality for the spread of COVID-19 than those of other deep learning models, namely RNN, GRU, LSTM, and BiLSTM. This could be attributed to the capacity and advantages of the BiLSTM-A-CNN due to its modeling of time dependencies by LSTM, the identification of relevant features using the attention mechanism, and the extraction of features from complex data via a CNN. Of course, this study demonstrated the promising performance of deep learning models in forecasting COVID-19 confirmed and recovered time series without exogenous information.

In a future work, we could update the dataset and incorporate additional input variables, such as weather data and lockdown indicators. We could also perform comparative studies to test the effects of measures installed during this pandemic event.

Acknowledgement

This chapter is based on work supported by the King Abdullah University of Science and Technology (KAUST), Office of Sponsored Research (OSR) under Award No: OSR-2019-CRG7–3800.

References

[1] Vaishya R, Javaid M, Khan I H and Haleem A 2020 Artificial Intelligence (AI) applications for COVID-19 pandemic *Diabetes Metab. Syndr.: Clin. Res. Rev.* **14** 337–9

[2] Naudé W 2020 Artificial intelligence vs COVID-19: limitations, constraints and pitfalls *AI Soc.* **35** 761–5

[3] Jamshidi M *et al* 2020 Artificial intelligence and COVID-19: deep learning approaches for diagnosis and treatment *IEEE Access* **8** 109581–95

[4] Dairi A, Harrou F, Zeroual A, Hittawe M M and Sun Y 2021 Comparative study of machine learning methods for COVID-19 transmission forecasting *J. Biomed. Inform.* 103791

[5] Toğaçar M, Ergen B and Cömert Z 2020 COVID-19 detection using deep learning models to exploit social mimic optimization and structured chest x-ray images using fuzzy color and stacking approaches *Comput. Biol. Med.* **121** 103805

[6] Khan F, Saeed A and Ali S 2020 Modelling and forecasting of new cases, deaths and recover cases of COVID-19 by using vector autoregressive model in Pakistan *Chaos, Solitons Fractals* **140** 110189

[7] Cheng Z J and Shan J 2020 2019 Novel coronavirus: where we are and what we know *Infection* **48** 155–63

[8] About Healthmap (accessed on January 12, 2022) https://healthmap.org/about/

[9] Brooks L C, Farrow D C, Hyun S, Tibshirani R J and Rosenfeld R 2018 Nonmechanistic forecasts of seasonal influenza with iterative one-week-ahead distributions *PLoS Comput. Biol.* **14** e1006134

[10] Lazer D and Kennedy R 2015 What we can learn from the epic failure of google flu trends Wired (Accessed January 12, 2022) https://www.wired.com/2015/10/can-learn-epic-failure-google-flu-trends/

[11] Long J B and Ehrenfeld J M 2020 The role of augmented intelligence (AI) in detecting and preventing the spread of novel coronavirus *J. Med. Syst.* **44** 1–2

[12] Bogoch I I *et al* 2016 Anticipating the int. spread of Zika virus from Brazil *Lancet* **387** 335–6

[13] Brunese L, Mercaldo F, Reginelli A and Santone A 2020 Explainable deep learning for pulmonary disease and coronavirus COVID-19 detection from x-rays *Comput. Methods Programs Biomed.* **196** 105608

[14] Khan A I, Shah J L and Bhat M M 2020 CoroNet: a deep neural network for detection and diagnosis of COVID-19 from chest x-ray images *Comput. Methods Programs Biomed.* **196** 105581

[15] Ucar F and Korkmaz D 2020 COVIDiagnosis-Net: deep bayes-squeezenet based diagnosis of the coronavirus disease 2019 (COVID-19) from x-ray images *Med. Hypotheses* **140** 109761

[16] Albahri O S *et al* 2020 Systematic review of artificial intelligence techniques in the detection and classification of COVID-19 medical images in terms of evaluation and benchmarking: taxonomy analysis, challenges, future solutions and methodological aspects *J. Infect. Public Health.* **13** 1381–96

[17] Toğaçar M, Ergen B and Cömert Z 2020 COVID-19 detection using deep learning models to exploit social mimic optimization and structured chest x-ray images using fuzzy color and stacking approaches *Comput. Biol. Med.* **121** 103805

[18] Minaee S, Kafieh R, Sonka M, Yazdani S and Soufi G J 2020 Deep-covid: predicting covid-19 from chest x-ray images using deep transfer learning *Med. Image Anal.* **65** 101794

[19] Ardakani A A, Kanafi A R, Acharya U R, Khadem N and Mohammadi A 2020 Application of deep learning technique to manage COVID-19 in routine clinical practice using CT images: results of 10 convolutional neural networks *Comput. Biol. Med.* **121** 103795

[20] Nour M, Cömert Z and Polat K 2020 A novel medical diagnosis model for COVID-19 infection detection based on deep features and Bayesian optimization *Appl. Soft Comput.* **97** 106580

[21] Kırbaş İ, Sözen A, Tuncer A D and Kazancıoğlu F Ş 2020 Comparative analysis and forecasting of COVID-19 cases in various European countries with ARIMA, NARNN and LSTM approaches *Chaos, Solitons Fractals* **138** 110015

[22] Behnood A, Golafshani E M and Hosseini S M 2020 Determinants of the infection rate of the COVID-19 in the US using ANFIS and virus optimization algorithm (VOA) *Chaos, Solitons Fractals* **139** 110051

[23] Torrealba-Rodriguez O, Conde-Gutiérrez R A and Hernández-Javier A L 2020 Modeling and prediction of COVID-19 in Mexico applying mathematical and computational models *Chaos, Solitons Fractals* **138** 109946

[24] Ribeiro M H D M, da Silva R G, Mariani V C and dos Santos Coelho L 2020 Short-term forecasting COVID-19 cumulative confirmed cases: perspectives for Brazil *Chaos, Solitons Fractals* **135** 109853

[25] Velásquez R M A and Lara J V M 2020 Forecast and evaluation of COVID-19 spreading in USA with reduced-space Gaussian process regression *Chaos, Solitons Fractals* **136** 109924
[26] Maleki M, Mahmoudi M R, Wraith D and Pho K H 2020 Time series modelling to forecast the confirmed and recovered cases of COVID-19 *Travel Med. Infect. Disease* **37** 101742
[27] Harrou F, Sun Y, Hering A S and Madakyaru M 2020 *Statistical Process Monitoring Using Advanced Data-Driven and Deep Learning Approaches: Theory and Practical Applications* (Amsterdam: Elsevier)
[28] Chimmula V K R and Zhang L 2020 Time series forecasting of COVID-19 transmission in Canada using LSTM networks *Chaos, Solitons Fractals* **135** 109864
[29] Zeroual A, Harrou F, Dairi A and Sun Y 2020 Deep learning methods for forecasting COVID-19 time-Series data: A Comparative study *Chaos, Solitons Fractals* **140** 110121
[30] Krizhevsky A, Sutskever I and Hinton G E 2012 Imagenet classification with deep convolutional neural networks *Adv. Neural Inform. Process. Syst.* **25** 1097–105
[31] Graves A, Mohamed A R and Hinton G 2013, May Speech recognition with deep recurrent neural networks *2013 IEEE International Conf. on Acoustics, Speech and Signal Processing* 6645–9
[32] Hochreiter S and Schmidhuber J 1997 Long short-term memory *Neural Comput.* **9** 1735–80
[33] Harrou F, Kadri F and Sun Y 2020 Forecasting of photovoltaic solar power production using LSTM approach *Advanced Statistical Modeling, Forecasting, and Fault Detection in Renewable Energy Systems* (Rijeka, Croatia: Intech Open)
[34] Harrou F, Hittawe M M, Sun Y and Beya O 2020 Malicious attacks detection in crowded areas using deep learning-based approach *IEEE Instrum. Meas. Mag.* **23** 57–62
[35] Wang W, Lee J, Harrou F and Sun Y 2020 Early detection of Parkinson's disease using deep learning and machine learning *IEEE Access* **8** 147635–46
[36] Dairi A, Cheng T, Harrou F, Sun Y and Leiknes T 2019 Deep learning approach for sustainable WWTP operation: a case study on data-driven influent conditions monitoring *Sustain. Cities Soc.* **50** 101670
[37] Harrou F, Dairi A, Sun Y and Kadri F 2018 Detecting abnormal ozone measurements with a deep learning-based strategy *IEEE Sens. J.* **18** 7222–32
[38] Silver D *et al* 2016 Mastering the game of Go with deep neural networks and tree search *Nature* **529** 484–9
[39] Mnih V *et al* 2015 Human-level control through deep reinforcement learning *Nature* **518** 529–33
[40] Hochreiter S and Schmidhuber J 1997 Long short-term memory *Neural Comput.* **9** 1735–80
[41] Schuster M and Paliwal K K 1997 Bidirectional recurrent neural networks *IEEE Trans. Signal Process.* **45** 2673–81
[42] Graves A and Schmidhuber J 2005 Framewise phoneme classification with bidirectional LSTM and other neural network architectures *Neural Netw.* **18** 602–10
[43] Sharfuddin A A, Tihami M N and Islam M S 2018 A deep recurrent neural network with bilstm model for sentiment classification *2018 Int. Conf. on Bangla Speech and Language Processing (ICBSLP)* (New York: IEEE) 1–4

[44] Graves A, Jaitly N and Mohamed A R 2013, December Hybrid speech recognition with deep bidirectional LSTM *2013 IEEE Workshop on Automatic Speech Recognition and Understanding* (Piscataway, NJ: IEEE) pp 273–8
[45] Zhang B, Zhang H, Zhao G and Lian J 2020 Constructing a PM2. 5 concentration prediction model by combining auto-encoder with Bi-LSTM neural networks *Environ. Modell. Softw.* **124** 104600
[46] Wang S, Wang X, Wang S and Wang D 2019 Bi-directional long short-term memory method based on attention mechanism and rolling update for short-term load forecasting *Int. J. Electr. Power Energy Syst.* **109** 470–9
[47] Kattenborn T, Leitloff J, Schiefer F and Hinz S 2021 Review on convolutional neural networks (CNN) in vegetation remote sensing *ISPRS J. Photogramm. Remote Sens.* **173** 24–49
[48] Khan A, Sohail A, Zahoora U and Qureshi A S 2020 A survey of the recent architectures of deep convolutional neural networks *Artif. Intell. Rev.* **53** 5455–516
[49] Krizhevsky A, Sutskever I and Hinton G E 2012 Imagenet classification with deep convolutional neural networks *Adv. Neural Inform. Process. Syst.* **25** 1097–105
[50] Bahdanau D, Cho K and Bengio Y 2014 Neural machine translation by jointly learning to align and translate arXiv:1409.0473
[51] Xu K, Ba J, Kiros R, Cho K, Courville A, Salakhudinov R, Zemel R and Bengio Y 2015 Show, attend and tell: neural image caption generation with visual attention *Int. Conf. on Machine Learning* arXiv:1502.03044
[52] Vaswani A, Shazeer N, Parmar N, Uszkoreit J, Jones L, Gomez A N, Kaiser L and Polosukhin I 2017 Attention is all you need arXiv:1706.03762

IOP Publishing

Artificial Intelligence Strategies for Analyzing COVID-19 Pneumonia Lung Imaging, Volume 1
Characterization approaches
Ayman El-Baz and Jasjit S Suri

Chapter 6

A residual network-based deep learning model for the detection of COVID-19 using cough sounds

Annesya Banerjee and Achal Nilhani

6.1 Introduction

The sudden outbreak of the COVID-19 virus in December 2019 imposed an unprecedented and tremendous load on healthcare systems worldwide. The strength, scalability, and preparedness of the healthcare industry have become key factors in deciding a nation's ability to combat the pandemic. Extensive efforts are being made by researchers across the globe to apply technological solutions to combat the extreme pressure being experienced by medical care systems. Emerging technologies, including artificial intelligence (AI), robotics, and automation, are being used to produce affordable, agile testing solutions, to implement contact tracing and social distancing, and to develop lung CT diagnostic tools [1, 2]. Different wearable technologies have shown promising applications in the domains of telehealth, patient monitoring, and disease detection [3] during the pandemic. The different acoustic signals produced by the human body, which provide valuable information that can be used to detect diseases, have also been analyzed. References [4, 5] offer detailed discussions of the use cases for acoustic signals (e.g. audio, speech, or language) in combination with computer audition amidst the COVID-19 crisis.

One such effort is the early diagnosis of the COVID-19 disease in the human body through cough symptom identification. As per the guidelines provided by the World Health Organization (WHO) [6], coughs, particularly dry and persistent ones, are among the most common symptoms of COVID-19 .patients. Almost 67.7% of patients have been reported to develop cough symptoms, according to an early report [7] by the WHO. Considering the fact that different diseases affect the respiratory system differently and thus produce cough signals with distinct acoustic

doi:10.1088/978-0-7503-3795-3ch6

patterns [8], several efforts have been made over the last few years to devise affordable diagnosis tools to identify a variety of respiratory diseases using analyses of cough sounds [9], [11–16]. Since the outbreak of the COVID-19, such cough-based diagnosis efforts have primarily been focused on the identification of COVID-19 symptoms. The authors of [17] developed an AI-engine implemented in a smartphone app named AI4COVID-19 to analyze the cough sounds recorded by the user and identify whether they are caused by COVID-19. A similar approach is adopted in [18] to develop a respiratory sound (cough and breath) -based automatic diagnosis tool for COVID-19 detection. This study used large-scale crowdsourced data collected through Android and web applications to perform the analysis. The studies described in [19–21] also pivoted on the deployment of a mobile-phone-based COVID-19 cough assessment system. The DiCOVA Challenge [10] organized by the Project Coswara group is a similar approach that aims to accelerate research into the diagnosis of COVID-19 using acoustics (mainly cough sounds, as given in Track 1, available at https://dicova2021.github.io/#challenges). The method proposed in this chapter addresses the task of Track 1, i.e. the discrimination of COVID-19 coughs from non-COVID-19 coughs by using a deep learning model fed with the log-Mel spectrum features of the audio signal. Our main contribution to this ongoing research into the audio-based detection of COVID-19 disease is that we have developed a classification mechanism which yields satisfactory results and is of sufficiently low complexity to be suitable for implementation in low-resource devices.

The rest of this chapter is arranged as follows: section 6.2 discusses the proposed algorithmic approach; section 6.3 describes the datasets used; section 6.4 reports the experimental results; and finally, section 6.5 concludes the work.

6.2 Algorithmic approach

Figure 6.1 represents the overall workflow of the proposed method. Details of each of the blocks are provided in the following subsections.

6.2.1 Audio preprocessing

To avoid any mechanical noise (e.g. audio recording device ON/OFF sounds, clicking sounds), the input audio data is first preprocessed. This preprocessing step consists of two main tasks: (1) identifying the portion of the audio that contains cough sounds and (2) centre-cropping the 'coughing' segment of the audio to address variable-length audio data present in the training/validation dataset. To accomplish

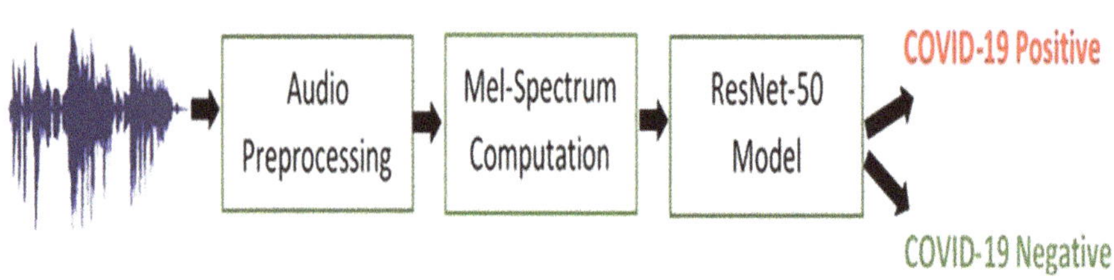

Figure 6.1. Overall workflow diagram of the proposed method.

task 1 of this step, we utilized a voice activity detector (VAD) [25, 26], considering the fact that all non-cough sounds in the audio data are noises or undesired artifacts. The VAD calculates the probability P_r of the presence of the desired (cough) sound in each 100 millisecond non-overlapping window of the audio data. The earliest window for which P_r is greater than a predefined threshold probability P_{TH} is considered to be the starting point of the preprocessed audio data. Audio segments that precede that window are completely discarded. In this case, setting P_{TH} equal to 0.6 yielded satisfactory results. Furthermore, since the provided data mainly contained cough sounds and no overlapping speech data, the current work has not focused on separating coughs from interfering speech sounds in real scenarios.

6.2.2 Mel spectrum computation

Mel scale features have been widely used in audio analysis tasks [22], from speech recognition and speaker recognition to musical genre classification, due to their perceptually motivated scales that resemble human auditory perception. The Mel scale frequency (f_{Mel}) is related to the normal frequency (f_{Hz}) using the relation given in (6.1):

$$f_{\mathrm{Mel}} = 2595\log_{10}\left(1 + \frac{f_{\mathrm{Hz}}}{700}\right) \tag{6.1}$$

so that the low frequencies (below 1 kHz) are linearly spaced, whereas the high frequencies (above 1 kHz) are logarithmically spaced. To obtain the Mel spectrum, the Fourier transformed acoustic signal (X(k)) is generally passed through a Mel filter bank that has filters with evenly spaced central frequencies and a triangular filter shaper. The Mel spectrum $S_{\mathrm{Mel}}(m)$ corresponding to the frequency domain signal X(k) is given by:

$$S_{\mathrm{Mel}}(m) = \sum_{k=0}^{N-1}[| X(k) |^2 H_m(k)],\ 0 \leqslant m \leqslant M - 1 \tag{6.2}$$

where M is the total number of Mel filters and $H_m(k)$ denotes the weight given to the kth energy bin for the output of the mth band. Figure 6.2 displays the Mel spectrums

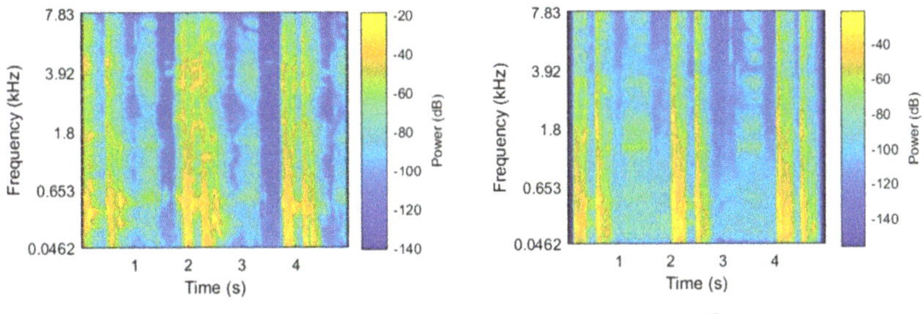

Figure 6.2. The Mel spectrums of (a) COVID-19-positive and (b) non-COVID-19 coughs.

of COVID-19-positive and non-COVID-19 cough samples, in which the spectrum was computed using M = 128 frequency bands over the frequency range of 32 Hz to 8 kHz with a sampling frequency of 16 kHz. As can be observed, there is a significant difference in the Mel spectrums of the two different coughs, and therefore, using this feature, it is possible for a machine learning model to discriminate between these two inputs.

6.2.3 Deep learning model

Motivated by the success of residual learning frameworks [23] in image recognition and computer vision tasks, we have used this residual learning based deep convolutional neural network (CNN) architecture for our audio classification. Analogously to an image identification task in which the input to the model is an image, the input for this audio classification task is an image equivalent of the audio data. In other words, the Mel spectrum itself works as a visual representation, similar to an image, of the time–frequency components of the input audio. Here, it should be noted that instead of directly feeding the Mel spectrum to the CNN, we use the log-Mel spectrum, which successfully tackles the general wide variation in audio spectrums. Figure 6.3 represents the detailed architecture of the residual network, which is 50 layers deep (ResNet-50) along with the expected sizes of the input and output data. For input in the form of an audio Mel spectrum or a log-Mel spectrum, the input size should be $M \times K \times 1$, where M is the number of frequency bands (e.g., 128) and K is the total number of time-frames used for analysis (here, 155 frames are required for a five-second audio segment; a 1024 point window and a 512 point overlap are considered). The network outputs the probabilities that the unknown audio segment represents COVID-19 or non-COVID-19.

6.3 Data set

For the training and validation of the proposed model, we have primarily used the Track 1 dataset provided by the DiCOVA Challenge 2021 organizers. This dataset contains 1040 audio samples that are divided into five-fold overlapping training–validation sets as per the challenge rule. Each audio sample is accompanied by data

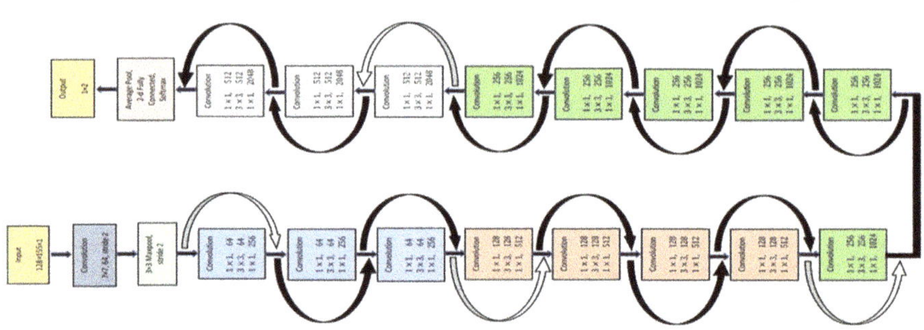

Figure 6.3. The residual network-50 architecture with a log-Mel spectrum as the input. Solid filled arrows (↷) denote direct addition (when the input and output have the same dimensions). Outlined arrows (↷) denote a convolution followed by an addition operation (when the input and output have different dimensions).

representing the patient's gender (Male - m/Female—f), nationality (India—I/Other—O), and COVID status (positive/negative). However, the number of COVID-19 positive samples is extremely low, compared to the non-COVID samples in this dataset. To address this class imbalance problem, our approach initially relied on data augmentation techniques, including pitch shifting, speeding up, time shifting, variation of the volume, the addition of noise, etc., which help to train the model with a variety of data representations. But since the class imbalance is very large (only 75 COVID samples compared to 965 non-COVID samples), data augmentation was not sufficient to achieve a satisfactory performance from the deep learning model. Therefore, to train our system, we also utilized the open-source dataset collected and released by the EPFL CoughVid team [19]. This additional dataset from EPFL consists of a total of 20,072 audio samples, out of which, 1010 samples were obtained from patients who had been diagnosed as COVID-19 positive. Also, each audio sample in this dataset is accompanied by the probability that the audio sample is a cough. For our purposes, we only considered those audio samples whose probability of being a cough was more than 0.6. Furthermore, from this subset of audio samples, we only used the confirmed COVID-positive samples. Using these selection rules, we finally obtained 640 additional COVID samples from this EPFL dataset. These data, along with the Track 1 Challenge dataset, were used to train the proposed log-Mel spectrum and ResNet-50 model. To test the model, the DiCOVA Blind Test Set of 233 audio samples was used.

6.4 Experimental results

6.4.1 Evaluation metrics

To evaluate the proposed model performance, we used the following metrics:

$$Accuracy\ (ACC) = \frac{TP + TN}{TP + TN + FP + FN}$$

$$Sensitivity\ (SE) = \frac{TP}{TP + FN}$$

$$Specificity\ (SP) = \frac{TN}{TN + FP}$$

$$Precision\ (PR) = \frac{TP}{TP + FP}$$

$$F1 - Score\ (F1) = 2 \times \left(\frac{PR \times SE}{PR + SE}\right)$$

where TP, TN, FP, and FN denote true positives, true negatives, false positives, and false negatives, respectively. Also, the receiver operating characteristics (ROC) curve was plotted to evaluate the area under the ROC curve (AUC) parameter. To adhere to the rules of the DiCOVA competition, the evaluation parameters were calculated using the mean confusion charts from the five-fold cross-validation.

6.4.2 Network training

The composite system shown in figure 6.1 was trained using the combined dataset with a 90%–10% non-overlapping training–validation data split. Although pretrained versions of ResNet-50 model are publicly available, we preferred training from scratch to adapt to the uniqueness of this problem. The Adam stochastic optimizer [24] was used to train the network because of its advantages, including a reduced memory requirement, computational efficiency, and small requirement for hyperparameter tuning. An initial learning rate of 0.0001, a mini-batch size of 20, and a total of 25 epochs were used for training. To improve the training, the order of the training samples was shuffled randomly after every epoch. All the model training and evaluation tasks in this work were executed by a system with an Intel® Core ™ i7–10510U CPU, 16 GB of RAM, and an NVIDIA GeForce MX250 GPU.

6.4.3 Baseline models

6.4.3.1 DiCOVA baseline [10]

The DiCOVA baseline systems provided by the challenge organizers extract the Mel frequency cepstral coefficients (MFCC) and their derivatives, as well as their double derivatives—a total of 39 dimensional features. This feature set was used to train three different machine learning classifiers: logistic regression (LR), a multi-layer perceptron (MLP), and random forest (RF). To train both the LR and the MLP, l_2 penalty regularization was used. Additionally, the MLP contained 25 hidden units followed by a tanh (.) activation layer. In the training of the RF classifier, the *gini* impurity criteria were used to measure the split quality. The best performance (an average validation AUC of 68.54% and a test AUC of 69.85%, as reported by the organizers) was obtained using the RF classifier and therefore, only this classifier was used for further comparisons.

6.4.3.2 Brown et al *[18]*

The authors propose a logistic regression model (LRM) to discriminate between the cough symptoms from people who tested COVID-19 positive and people with no COVID-19 positive result. The model takes as its input temporal features, such as duration, tempo, onset, root mean square energy; spectral features; and MFCC features along with their derivatives. In the case of spectral features, the statistical parameters (such as the mean, standard deviation, etc.) of the feature distribution are used in place of the exact feature values. The proposed model has been trained by a large-scale crowdsourced dataset collected by the authors. This work reports that the LRM achieved an ROC-AUC of 0.75 (0.19) with a precision of 0.82 (0.20) and a recall of 0.54 (0.23); the values in brackets denote the standard deviations.

6.4.4 Results

Here, we present the evaluation results obtained from our proposed model and also compare these results with the baseline model performance. It should be noted that the ground-truth labels for the blind test set have not yet been publicly made available. Thus, most of the evaluation performances presented in this section are calculated based on the five-fold cross-validation dataset. In the first experiment, we identify the relation between the number of frequency bands (M) used for the analysis of the audio and the deep learning model performance. The M values were varied from 32 to 512 in powers of 2.

Figure 6.4 represents the confusion matrices obtained from the ResNet-50 model for five different values of M. As can be observed, the highest classification accuracy of 96% is obtained for M = 32 and the accuracy value continuously decreases as M is increased. The five different ROC curves shown in figure 6.5 also depict that M = 32 yields the best performance, whereas M = 512 produces the worst performance. The AUC values for M = 32, 64, 128, 256 and 512 are 98.88%, 98.21%, 94.36%, 93.59%, and 86.24%, respectively.

A possible explanation for this deterioration of model performance with increasing M is as follows: while keeping the overall frequency range of the input audio constant, if M is increased then the dimension of each time–frequency bin is reduced; therefore, the audio feature information carried by each bin is also reduced. This ultimately results in poor classification performance of the deep learning model. However, making M very small (in the range from 4 to 16) is also unhelpful, because the sizes of the analysis bins become so large that extracting important information becomes complicated. Thus, the optimum value of M lies in the range from 32 to 64. We take M = 32 as the best case and proceed further.

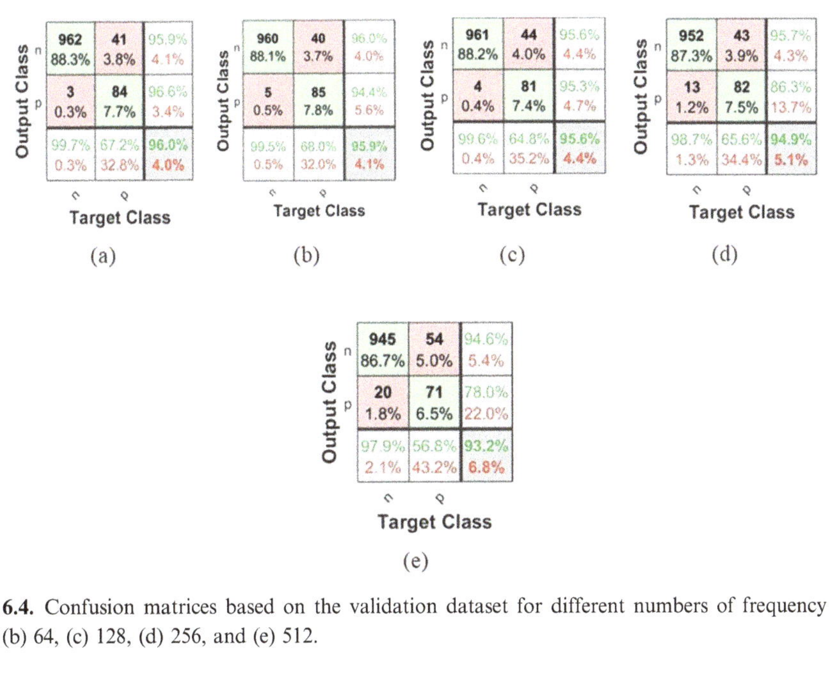

Figure 6.4. Confusion matrices based on the validation dataset for different numbers of frequency bands: (a) 32, (b) 64, (c) 128, (d) 256, and (e) 512.

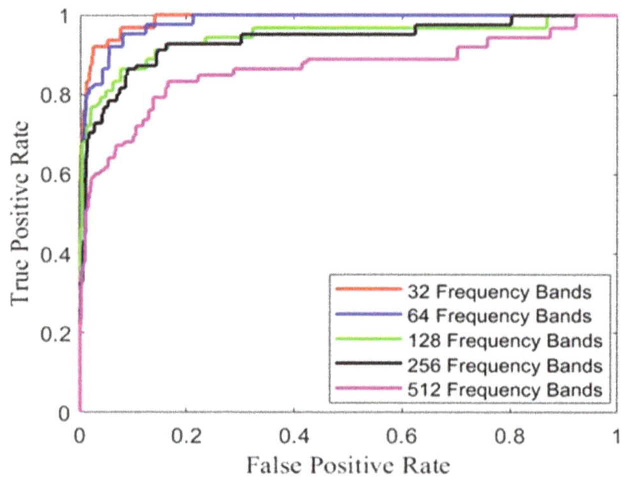

Figure 6.5. ROC curves for ResNet-50 models using five different numbers of frequency bands.

Table 6.1. Comparison of different model performances.

	Evaluation metrics				
Ref #	ACC	SE	SP	PR	F1
10	88.6	**77.5**	91.6	71.7	74.5
18	95.1	57.6	**100**	**100**	73.1
Our Work	**96.0**	67.2	99.7	96.6	**79.3**

In the next experiment, we compare the performance of the proposed model with the baseline systems. For this purpose, the baseline models mentioned in section 6.4.3 were trained and validated using the same data as that of the proposed model. Whenever possible, the model parameters were kept the same as those mentioned in the original papers [10, 18]. In other cases, standard values were assumed. Table 6.1 depicts the performance evaluation metrics yielded by these models; all values are in percentages (%) unless mentioned otherwise. As can be seen, the highest accuracy of 96% and an F1 score of 79.3% are obtained for the proposed model; however, the model described in [18] outperforms it in terms of specificity and precision. However, none of the three systems achieves a very satisfactory performance in terms of sensitivity. This can be a drawback for practical implementations and thus needs to be improved in future studies.

Also, from the submission results (using the blind test set) obtained from the organizer, it is observed that our proposed system achieves a test AUC of 75.91%, a test specificity of 62.50%, and a test sensitivity of 80.49%. Consequently, our submitted model has secured 16th position in the DiCOVA Challenge 2021 leader board.

6.5 Conclusions

To conclude, this chapter proposes a deep learning model based on the ResNet-50 architecture to discriminate between COVID-19 and non-COVID-19 coughs. The model accepts 32 frequency band-based log-Mel spectrums of the audio data as 'image-like' inputs and executes the two-class classification task. The developed model achieved an average validation AUC of 98.88%. Also, when this model was given the blind test set released by the DiCOVA challenge, the system achieved a test AUC of 75.91%, a test specificity of 62.50%, and a test sensitivity of 80.49%. Further improvements in the system will lead to better sensitivity of the classification model and enable the possibility of real-world implementation.

Acknowledgements

The authors would like to thank the DiCOVA Challenge 2021 organizers for making the crowdsourced dataset of COVID-19 coughs available for use by the scientific community and letting the authors contribute to this research progress for early detection of COVID-19-affected people.

References

[1] Ozturk T, Talo M, Yildirim E A, Baloglu U B, Yildirim O and Acharya U R 2020 Automated detection of COVID-19 cases using deep neural networks with x-ray images *Comput. Biol. Med.* **121** 103792

[2] Maghded H S, Ghafoor K Z, Sadiq A S, Curran K, Rawat D B and Rabie K 2020 A novel AI-enabled framework to diagnose coronavirus COVID-19 using smartphone embedded sensors: Design study *2020 IEEE 21st Int. Conf. on Information Reuse and Integration for Data Science (IRI)* 180–7

[3] Ding X *et al* 2020 Wearable sensing and telehealth technology with potential applications in the coronavirus pandemic *IEEE Rev. Biomed. Eng.* **14** 48–70

[4] Schuller B W, Schuller D M, Qian K, Liu J, Zheng H and Li X 2021 COVID-19 and computer audition: an overview on what speech & sound analysis could contribute in the SARS-CoV-2 corona crisis *Front. Digit. Health* **3** 564906

[5] Deshpande G and Schuller B W 2020 An overview on audio, signal, speech, & language processing for COVID-19 arXiv:2005.08579

[6] Sohrabi C, Alsafi Z, O'Neill N, Khan M, Kerwan A, Al-Jabir A, Iosifidis C and Agha R 2020 World Health Organization declares global emergency: a review of the 2019 novel coronavirus (COVID-19) *Int. J. Surg.* **76** 71–6

[7] World Health Organization 2020 Coronavirus disease 2019 (COVID-19): situation report, 82

[8] Thorpe W, Kurver M, King G and Salome C 2001 Acoustic analysis of cough *The Seventh Australian and New Zealand Intelligent Information Systems Conf.* **2001** 391–4

[9] Hee H I, Balamurali B T, Karunakaran A, Herremans D, Teoh O H, Lee K P, Teng S S, Lui S and Chen J M 2019 Development of machine learning for asthmatic and healthy voluntary cough sounds: a proof of concept study *Appl. Sci.* **9** 2833

[10] Muguli A *et al* 2021 DiCOVA challenge: dataset, task, and baseline system for COVID-19 diagnosis using acoustics *Proc. Interspeech 2021* 901–5

[11] Pramono R X A, Imtiaz S A and Rodriguez-Villegas E 2016 A cough-based algorithm for automatic diagnosis of pertussis *PLoS One* **11** e0162128
[12] Sharan R V, Abeyratne U R, Swarnkar V R and Porter P 2018 Automatic croup diagnosis using cough sound recognition *IEEE Trans. Biomed. Eng.* **66** 485–95
[13] Windmon A, Minakshi M, Bharti P, Chellappan S, Johansson M, Jenkins B A and Athilingam P R 2018 TussisWatch: a smart-phone system to identify cough episodes as early symptoms of chronic obstructive pulmonary disease and congestive heart failure *IEEE J. Biomed. Health Inform.* **23** 1566–73
[14] Bales C, Nabeel M, John C N, Masood U, Qureshi H N, Farooq H, Posokhova I and Imran A 2020 Can machine learning be used to recognize and diagnose coughs? *2020 Int. Conf. on e-Health and Bioengineering (EHB)* 1–4
[15] Amrulloh Y, Abeyratne U, Swarnkar V and Triasih R 2015 Cough sound analysis for pneumonia and asthma classification in pediatric population *2015 6th Int. Conf. on Intelligent Systems, Modelling and Simulation* 127–31
[16] Kosasih K, Abeyratne U R, Swarnkar V and Triasih R 2014 Wavelet augmented cough analysis for rapid childhood pneumonia diagnosis *IEEE Trans. Biomed. Eng.* **62** 1185–94
[17] Imran A, Posokhova I, Qureshi H N, Masood U, Riaz M S, Ali K, John C N, Hussain M I and Nabeel M 2020 AI4COVID-19: AI enabled preliminary diagnosis for COVID-19 from cough samples via an app *Inform. Med. Unlocked* **20** 100378
[18] Brown C, Chauhan J, Grammenos A, Han J, Hasthanasombat A, Spathis D, Xia T, Cicuta P and Mascolo C 2020 Exploring automatic diagnosis of covid-19 from crowdsourced respiratory sound data *Proc. of the 26th ACM SIGKDD Int. Conf. on Knowledge Discovery & Data Mining* 3474–84
[19] CoughVid 2021 https://coughvid.epfl.ch/about/
[20] COVID Voice Detector 2021 https://cvd.lti.cmu.edu/
[21] Sharma N, Krishnan P, Kumar R, Ramoji S, Chetupalli S R, R. N, Ghosh P K and Ganapathy S 2020 Coswara —a database of breathing, cough, and voice sounds for COVID-19 diagnosis *Proc. Interspeech 2020* 4811–5
[22] Rabiner L and Schafer R 2010 *Theory and Applications of Digital Speech Processing.* (Englewood Cliffs, NJ: Prentice-Hall)
[23] He K, Zhang X, Ren S and Sun J 2016 Deep residual learning for image recognition *Proc. of the IEEE Conference on Computer Vision and Pattern Recognition* 770–8
[24] Kingma D P and Ba J 2014 Adam: A method for stochastic optimization arXiv:1412.6980
[25] Sohn J, Kim N S and Sung W 1999 A statistical model-based voice activity detection *IEEE Signal Process Lett.* **6** 1–3
[26] Martin R 2001 Noise power spectral density estimation based on optimal smoothing and minimum statistics *IEEE Trans. Speech Audio Process.* **9** 504–12

IOP Publishing

Artificial Intelligence Strategies for Analyzing COVID-19 Pneumonia Lung Imaging, Volume 1
Characterization approaches
Ayman El-Baz and Jasjit S Suri

Chapter 7

Rapid and accurate AI-based diagnosis to distinguish COVID-19 from eight other lung respiratory diseases

Mugahed A Al-Antari, Cam-Hao Hua and Sungyoung Lee

7.1 Introduction

The recent spread of the COVID-19 pandemic throughout the world has caused a severe public health crisis for humanity [1]. In the early stages of this pandemic, more and more patients suffered from unknown respiratory complications in Wuhan, Hubei Province, China, at the end of December 2019 [2]. Between December 12, 2019, when the first case was confirmed, and January 25, 2020, at least 1975 more patients were diagnosed with COVID-19. This pandemic is notably caused by a new variant of coronavirus, known as severe acute respiratory syndrome coronavirus 2 (SARS-CoV-2) [2, 3]. Those who are exposed to this family of viruses experience symptoms such as fever, cough, dizziness, sore throat, fatigue, shortness of breath, loss of taste, to name a few [2–4]. Due to the unprecedented speed of person-to-person transmission in early stages of infection, more than 200 countries have been adversely affected globally [1]. This serious situation has prompted a series of responses in terms of healthcare infrastructure, public health systems, and economic activities to combat the impacts of the COVID-19 pandemic [5]. Obviously, the rapid daily growth of virus cases has led to a significant shortage of healthcare facilities, such as ventilators, beds, caregivers, masks, etc. As a result, millions of people are infected by this novel virus, while a much larger number of individuals are self-quarantined and/or unemployed [1, 2, 5]. It is worth noting that COVID-19 patients who have been affected by comorbidity face a much larger probability of mortality [6]. According to the World Health Organization (WHO), on June 30, 2021 [6] the numbers of confirmed and deceased COVID-19 patients were 182 and 3.94 M, respectively. Furthermore, this pandemic has caused

doi:10.1088/978-0-7503-3795-3ch7

tremendous difficulties for the educational system in many countries as well as in other fields, such as transport services, sports, logistics, etc. To address this challenging situation, the real-time reverse-transcription polymerase chain reaction (RT-PCR) toolkit [7] has been widely adopted for the diagnosis of COVID-19 infections. In addition, radiological imaging techniques, such as digital chest x-rays (CXR) and computed tomography (CT) scans have been used for the detection of pulmonary vulnerability, which is typically caused by COVID-19 [1, 8]. Despite the effectiveness of CT, digital chest x-ray systems are still widely used due to their benefits of cost-effectiveness, lower radiation dose, and speed of capture [4, 8]. In fact, the combination of a screening x-ray image or CT scan and an RT-PCR result is highly recommended to ensure the accuracy of a COVID-19 diagnosis [8]. Nevertheless, the necessity to regularly screen a huge number of patients exposed to SARS-CoV-2 causes considerable difficulties for radiologists. Therefore, the administration of the United States promoted the adoption of artificial intelligence (AI) algorithms to combat COVID-19 on March 16, 2020 [1]. To this end, research scientists and developers have constructed computer-aided design (CAD) systems using machine learning techniques to enhance physicians' efficiency in diagnosing and following up COVID-19 cases [1, 8]. Remarkably, over the past few years, the emergence of deep-learning (DL) techniques (a well-known branch of machine learning), has improved the effectiveness of screening-assisted schemes for physicians. Since then, deep-learning-based CAD systems have been capable of performing highly-qualified and trustworthy diagnosis with limited, or even no, requirements for manual intervention [9, 10]. It should be noted that deep-learning-based CAD systems have achieved remarkable outcomes in numerous medical applications, such as skin cancer [11, 12] and breast cancer [9, 10]. Clearly, their potential to efficiently combat the COVID-19 pandemic will be imminently realized [1]. Hence, these observations motivate the development of a deep-learning-based CAD system to diagnose COVID-19 using digital x-ray images in real time.

In this chapter, the contributions of the proposed methodology for COVID-19 diagnosis are summarized as follows. First, we describe a DL CAD system which employs the YOLO predictor to simultaneously detect and diagnose COVID-19 using chest x-ray images. Second, the proposed system can classify COVID-19 along with eight other respiratory diseases, which can be considered a multiclass recognition problem. Third, an exhaustive regularization mechanism that combines data augmentation and balancing with transfer learning is introduced to boost the performance of COVID-19 diagnosis in terms of both accuracy and processing time. Finally, the proposed methodology is evaluated using two digital x-ray data sets, i.e., the *COVID-19 data set* [13, 14] and the *Chestx-ray8 data set* [15], using a fivefold cross-validation strategy. Consequently, the outcomes of this work can be utilized to efficiently screen for the presence of COVID-19 and to construct the end-to-end pipeline of a DL CAD system for a given clinical task.

As the ultimate objective, this study aims to deliver an effective CAD framework using novel AI techniques to practically assist physicians and conventional systems in hospitals to diagnose COVID-19 and other respiratory diseases in an effective and convenient manner.

The remainder of this chapter is organized as follows. Section 7.2 presents a literature survey of research into COVID-19. Section 7.3 describes the relevant materials and technical details of the proposed DL CAD-based YOLO system. Section 7.4 presents the experimental results and corresponding analyses as well as a discussion. Section 7.5 draws conclusions from all the findings of this work.

7.2 Literature review

After the announcement of the new COVID-19 pandemic in early 2020, some studies based on artificial intelligence (AI) approaches were proposed for the detection of COVID-19 using digital CXRs or CT scans. In [16], Oh *et al* presented a patch-based DL CAD system consisting of segmentation and classification stages to detect COVID-19 using CXR images. For segmentation, FC-DenseNet103 was used to segment or extract complete lung regions from whole CXR images. For classification, several random regions (i.e., regions of interest) were extracted from the segmented lung regions, which served as inputs to the classification model's DL. They used CXR images from different classes, which were normal, bacterial pneumonia, tuberculosis, and viral pneumonia due to COVID-19. Ultimately, overall diagnostic performances of 84.40% and 88.9% were achieved for the F1 score and the overall accuracy, respectively. Ozturk *et al* [8] presented a DarkCovidNet DL model for COVID-19 detection using whole CXR images. Using seventeen convolutional layers, their model was developed for both binary classification (normal vs. COVID-19) and multiclass classification (normal vs. pneumonia vs. COVID-19). For the binary and multiclass classification tasks, the DL model proposed achieved overall diagnostic accuracies of 98.08% and 87.02%, respectively. In [17], Wang *et al* proposed a DL COVID network to distinguish COVID-19-infected lungs from normal lungs and diseased pneumonic lungs using CXR images. Their presented model outperformed ResNet-50 and VGG-16 and achieved positive predictive values (PPV) of 98.9%, 90.50%, and 91.30% for COVID-19, normal, and pneumonic cases, respectively. In [18], Hamdan *et al* proposed DL applications using seven well-established networks to diagnose COVID-19 in fifty CXR images. They reported that DensNet201 and VGG-19 achieved the best diagnostic performance of 90% accuracy. In [19], Ardakani *et al* presented an evaluation study of ten different well-established DL models used to diagnose COVID-19 in routine clinical practice using CT images. They diagnosed COVID-19 versus non-COVID-19 in a binary classification task and obtained the best diagnostic result with ResNet-101 and Xception DL networks, which had an overall accuracy of 99.40% each. In [20], Apostolopoulos *et al* used five established DL networks to detect COVID-19 in CXR images. They tested all five DL models using binary (i.e. COVID-19 vs. normal) and multiclass (i.e. pneumonia, COVID-19, and normal) recognition tasks. They concluded that the highest overall diagnostic accuracies of 93.48% and 98.75% were achieved using VGG-19 for binary and multiclass detection tasks, respectively. In [21], Khan *et al* presented a DL model called CORONET which was used to classify the lung disease COVID-19 in a multiclass task using whole CXR images. Their proposed model was able to distinguish COVID-19 from other respiratory diseases, including viral and bacterial pneumonia and negative cases, with an accuracy of 89.60%. Pereira *et al* [7] proposed a diagnostic scheme that used known texture descriptors in addition to a CNN. They used a resampling algorithm to balance the training set for a multiclass recognition task. They ultimately achieved a diagnostic F1 score of 65% for the classification of COVID-19 versus other lung diseases. In addition, comprehensive review studies of DL applications used to combat COVID-19 are presented in [22, 23]. However, the presented DL models were tested for the diagnosis of COVID-19 using whole CXR images. The whole CXR image always includes irrelevant or mixed-texture structural details, with the result that the derived deep features cannot represent a specific class. In fact, the diagnosis of knowledge extracted using the whole CXR image may not provide a superior practical solution for improving the diagnostic performance of any CAD system. Thus, the extraction of specific regions or patches representing lung disease (i.e. COVID-19 or another lung disease) from the whole CXR image to train DL models is key to improving the overall diagnostic performance. In this way, the DL model can derive more representative deep feature maps for just the exact abnormal patch regions, rather than using the whole CXR image. To the best of our knowledge, this is the first region-of-interest (ROI)-based DL CAD system that has been proposed that can automatically reveal and distinguish COVID-19 infections from all other respiratory diseases using whole input CXR images.

7.3 Methodology

The proposed AI-based CAD system has the ability to extract suspicious COVID-19 regions of interest (ROIs) from whole input CXR images and simultaneously distinguish them from eight other respiratory lung diseases. In this study, we diagnose the extracted regions for COVID-19 versus pneumonia, pneumothorax, atelectasis, effusion, masses, infiltration, nodules, and cardiomegaly. It is very important for physicians dealing with emergency cases, such as those of the COVID-19 pandemic, to easily and rapidly determine the nature of a lung disease when the patient arrives in the emergency room (ER). For this purpose, an AI-based CAD system in a unique pipeline framework is proposed. Figure 7.1 shows a general overview of the proposed AI-based CAD system in the patient triage workflow.

Recently, CAD systems based on DL have achieved impressive diagnostic performance for different diseases without user intervention. The rapid spread of COVID-19 has made it necessary to adopt and deploy such CAD systems to assist and support physicians and also patients. This issue has increased our determination to develop a rapid CAD system based on DL to diagnose COVID-19 lung disease using whole CXR images as the input. This will assist medical staff in hospitals by providing a smart patient triage workflow using the capability of DL based on CNNs. The smart patient triage workflow consists of three consecutive stages: support in contacting medical support, suspicious patient transportation, and an AI-based CAD system for COVID-19 diagnosis. During the COVID-19 pandemic, Korean government health centers have established strong healthcare systems

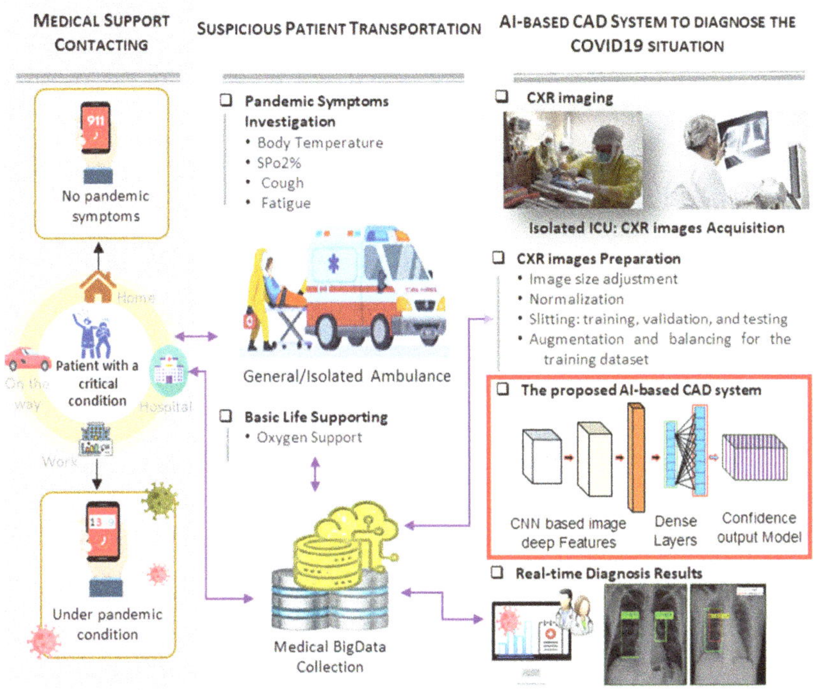

Figure 7.1. General overview of the proposed AI-based CAD system with the patient triage workflow for COVID-19 diagnosis.

especially for the COVID-19 situation. First, once a patient feels some possible symptoms of COVID-19, he/she has to call one of the emergency hotlines (i.e. 911 for a general emergency situation and 1339 for the pandemic). The patient may experience the pandemic symptoms at home, at work, in transit, at hospital, or in any other place. Second, once the healthcare center receives the suspicious patient call, it arranges a special isolated ambulance to transport the patient from the location of the call. In the ambulance, the professional medical team will investigate the pandemic symptoms (i.e. body temperature, SpO2%, cough, fatigue, etc.) and give the patient basic life-support such as oxygen. The patient information should be registered in the smart healthcare system and automatically synchronized with the private medical database of that healthcare center. Meanwhile, the medical staff in the emergency department can track the patient's status step-by-step and be ready to receive the patient. Third, once the patient reaches the emergency department, the physician and medical staff assign him/her directly to a special isolated intensive care unit (ICU). The first action of the ICU is to screen the patient using a standard x-ray machine and get an CXR image to support the diagnosis of COVID lung disease. The proposed AI-based CAD system could be used to rapidly and accurately complete the diagnosis process, especially for a vast number of patients. From a technical perspective, the proposed CAD system is first trained and validated using a large number of CXR images representing all lung diseases: COVID-19, pneumonia, pneumothorax, atelectasis, effusion, masses, infiltration, nodules, and cardiomegaly. In real time, the trained AI-based CAD system could provide the diagnosis results for the ROI around the suspicious lung region and provide a disease label for that region (either for COVID-19 or another disease). In this way, the physician could receive strong evidence for potential COVID-19 in a less than second. Such a practical solution is our objective, which can support physicians, medical staff, hospitals, or healthcare centers.

7.3.1 CXR image data set

To train and validate the proposed AI-based CAD system, two different CXR data sets are used: the *COVID-19 data set* [13, 14] and the *Chestx-ray8 data set* [15]. The total numbers of CXR images from each class used for training, validation, and testing are listed in table 7.1.

7.3.1.1 COVID-19 data set

Two publicly available sources related to COVID-19 are combined to form into the COVID-19 data set used in this work. The first source is digital chest x-ray images of patients suffering from COVID-19, which were collected by Cohen *et al* [13]. This image set is open access to enable research scientists and experts to flexibly develop AI algorithms to tackle the COVID-19 problem. It is noteworthy that researchers can easily increase the sample pool by including additional x-ray images. This work employs the x-ray images of 125 patients exposed to COVID-19, of which 82 are of males and 43 are of females. However, the metadata of this data set is incomplete. For instance, only 26 patients have age information; the average age is 55. The second x-ray image source is provided by Qatar University [14]. All the samples are encoded in portable network graphic (png) format with a fixed resolution of 1024 × 1024. Like the abovementioned data set, this image source is publicly available to facilitate COVID-19-oriented research, and its metadata is also unavailable for all patients. All the x-ray images, amounting to 201 patients, were used in our study. Accordingly, a total of 326 digital chest x-ray images were used to train and finalize the proposed DL CAD system. Although image-level labels of these images were known in advance, the details of the coordinates of ground-truth (GT) bounding boxes were unavailable. Therefore, in order to localize the abnormalities related to COVID-19, we requested two radiologists to annotate the lesions and/or nodules corresponding to COVID-19 disease. As illustrated in figure 7.2(a)–(c), it can be seen that some of the original images have small white or black arrows indicating the location damaged by SARS-CoV-2. Subsequently, the annotations of the two experts were compared with those signs and marked by rectangular symbols. Notably, each GT bounding box surrounding an abnormal lesion is defined by a width (w) value, a height (h) value, and a central (x, y) point. Typical views of COVID-19 regions and their corresponding GT information are added to the original CXR images, as shown in figure 7.2.

Table 7.1. CXR image distribution for each class of lung respiratory disease. The CXR images in each class are randomly split into 70% for training, 10% for validation, and 20% for testing.

#	COVID-19	Atelectasis	Infiltration	Pneumothorax	Lung mass	Effusion	Pneumonia	Cardiomegaly	Nodule
Training (70%)	228	126	86	69	90	107	84	102	228
Validation (10%)	33	18	12	10	9	15	12	15	33
Testing (20%)	65	36	25	20	17	31	24	29	65
Total	**326**	**180**	**123**	**99**	**116**	**153**	**120**	**146**	**326**

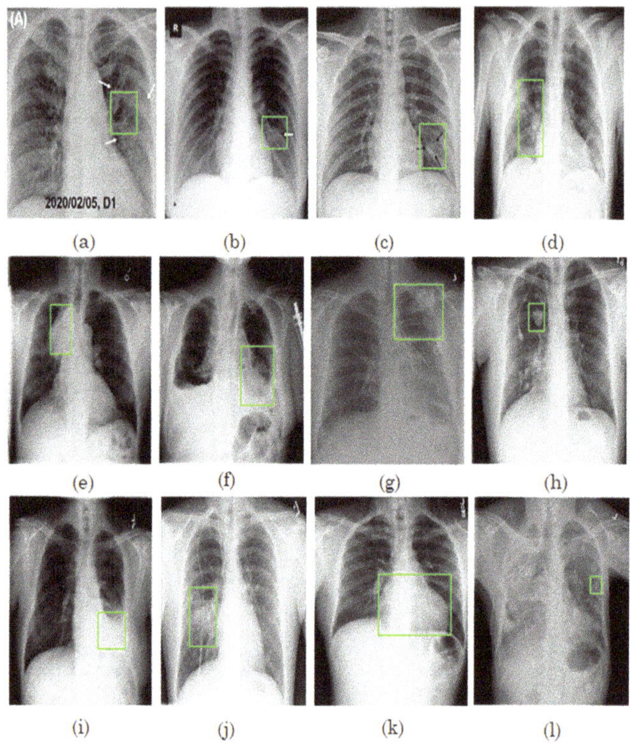

Figure 7.2. Representative CXR images for all lung respiratory diseases: (a)–(d) CXR images from COVID-19 data set. From the Chestx-ray8 data set, the CXR images are for (e) atelectasis, (f) infiltration, (g) pneumothorax, (h) lung mass, (i) effusion, (j) pneumonia, (k) cardiomegaly, and (l) nodule. The GT information is enclosed by a green box added to the original image.

7.3.1.2 Chestx-ray8 data set

The *Chestx-ray8* [15] data set is a popular data set for studies of eight different respiratory diseases, comprising atelectasis, infiltration, pneumothorax, masses, effusion, pneumonia, cardiomegaly, and nodules. All the chest x-ray images and corresponding GT details (consisting of the bounding box coordinates and the associated labels) are taken into account. It is notable that the parameters of the GT bounding box (which are the box's left-top coordinate (x, y), width (w), and height (h)) are predefined in XML format [15]. As shown in table 7.1, a total of 984 x-ray images, corresponding to eight respiratory diseases as mentioned above, are used for our training and validation process. They are all converted from DICOM into png format and then resized to 1024 × 1024. We show example CXR images with the corresponding GT information (disease labels and the coordinates of the bounding boxes) in figure 7.2.

7.3.2 CXR data preparation

Both the *COVID-19* [13, 14] and *Chestx-ray8* [15] data sets are employed to fine-tune and benchmark the proposed DL CAD system. In [9, 10], the images in these data sets are randomly split into 70% for training, 10% for validation, and 20% for testing at ratios of 70%, 10%, and 20%, respectively, as shown in table 7.1. Optimal hyperparameters are then investigated during the training phase based on the validation performance. Afterwards, the built model is benchmarked using the testing set. Meanwhile, the proposed methodology is evaluated by a fivefold cross-validation strategy. Specifically, all of the images are iteratively partitioned into either the training or the testing set. This allows an equal evaluation of each image and avoids unexpected error-prone bias. Notably, for the evaluation of small medical data sets, the k-fold cross-validation procedure offers a more reliable benchmark approach [9–11]. During the model learning process, mini-batches in the training set are shuffled automatically. In addition, a weighted cross-entropy loss function is adopted to maximize the optimization process [24]. Additionally, since the data set is small-scale and imbalanced class-wise, which certainly harms the modeling efficiency, balancing and augmentation strategies are applied, as discussed in the following subsection.

7.3.2.1 Deep-learning balancing and augmentation strategies

Data learning strategies, namely data balancing and augmentation, are used to improve the performance of the proposed AI-based CAD system [25, 26]. This kind of solution is proven to be effective in tackling the difficulties of learning from small-sized medical data sets [9, 10]. Another important point is that an equal number of classes in each mini-batch should be maintained throughout the training procedure [27, 28]. Such activity can prevent the trained DL architecture from learning about dominant classes (e.g. images with COVID-19 labels) in an adversely biased manner. For this purpose, the training images from the *Chestx-ray8* data set are doubled by simultaneous up–down and left–right flipping operations, which consequently results in 1378 images. Hence, the total number of training images increases to 2295, consisting of 1378 augmented versions of the *Chestx-ray8* data set and 917 images from the *COVID-19* data set.

Subsequently, we apply an augmentation procedure to the combined CXR image data set of eight plus one pulmonary disease labels, as follows. First, the raw CXR images are randomly scaled followed by a tenfold translation. Second, the scaled and translated versions are each rotated by 45 °. Finally, variants with rotations of 0° and 270° are flipped vertically and horizontally. In general, each input image is guaranteed to be augmented 22 times. As a result, a total of 50,490 digital chest x-ray images are finalized to train the proposed DL CAD system. Note that the same data balancing and augmentation scheme is applied for every fold in the k-fold cross-validation procedure. The initial parameters of the proposed model are those pre-trained with the ImageNet data set [9, 10], which are then fine-tuned using the training set of 50,490 images described above [29].

7.3.3 The proposed AI-based CAD system

To rapidly and accurately distinguish COVID-19 from the other eight lung diseases, an AI-based CAD system with the YOLO predictor is adopted and developed. The proposed CAD system has ability to extract the suspicious regions from whole CXR images and then classify them using different nine class labels. Previous research studies have used traditional image processing techniques or even complex machine learning or DL models [9, 10]. However, the proposed AI-based CAD system is developed as a compact model to simultaneously define and extract the suspicious lung ROIs and then classify them using nine class labels. The proposed CAD system has a unique CNN structure that extracts prominent 2D deep features from the input CXR images. It has ability to optimize the hypertrainable parameters end-to-end and fine-tune them simultaneously for the tasks of both ROI extraction and classification. This CAD system can extract the suspicious ROIs directly using the input CXR images. It does not have to divide the input CXR image into multiple subimages and feed each one separately into feature extraction (as in Faster R-CNN [30]) or use a sliding window [31] to define the localization of the lung ROIs. The YOLO DL model can divide the input CXR image into equal-sized $N \times N$ grid cells, as depicted in figure 7.3. If the extracted lung ROI center belongs to a specific grid cell, then this cell should be responsible for predicting the lung disease in the cell. For each grid cell, five boxes are used to represent the predicted disease class in terms of box location (x,y), height (h), width (w), and confidence score ($Pr_{conf.}$). Indeed, $Pr_{conf.}$ represents the confidence that the AI model will predict lung disease and denotes whether the extracted box has a real disease or or is part of the background. To calculate the confidence score for each cell during the training process, the probability of the existence of a respiratory disease (e.g. COVID-19) is the multiplied by the intersection over the union (IoU) value of that box, as follows:

$$Pr_{confidence} = Prob(ROI) \times IoU_{\text{Extracted box}}^{\text{Ground truth(GT)}}, \tag{7.1}$$

where the ROI represents the extracted objects in the CXR images and the IoU is the intersection over the union between the real GT and its extracted box. The confidence score equals zero when the grid cell contains background and not disease. If there is an object (e.g. COVID-19) in the detected ROI, the Prob(ROI) has a value between 0 and 1, which represents the probability that disease is present in that ROI. Each grid cell can predict the conditional probabilities $Prob(class_i|ROI)$ for the nine different disease classes. Thus, the confidence score for each box is calculated as follows:

$$Pr_{conf.} = Prob(Class_i) \times IoU_{\text{Extracted box}}^{\text{Ground truth}};\ i = 1, 2, 3, \ldots, \text{and } 9 \tag{7.2}$$

To calculate $Pr_{conf.}$ at the time of testing, the conditional probability should be multiplied by the specific box confidence value. Finally, the $Pr_{conf.}$ for each extracted box is calculated as follows:

$$Pr_{conf.Box_i} = \text{argmax}\{(Pr_{conf._i} \times Pr(class_i|ROI)), \ldots, (Pr_{conf._9} \times Pr(class_9|ROI))\}. \tag{7.3}$$

The extracted box with the maximum confidence score represents the final ROI that interprets the disease localization and its diagnostic label. Other boxes that have small values of $Pr_{conf.}$ are suppressed and excluded.

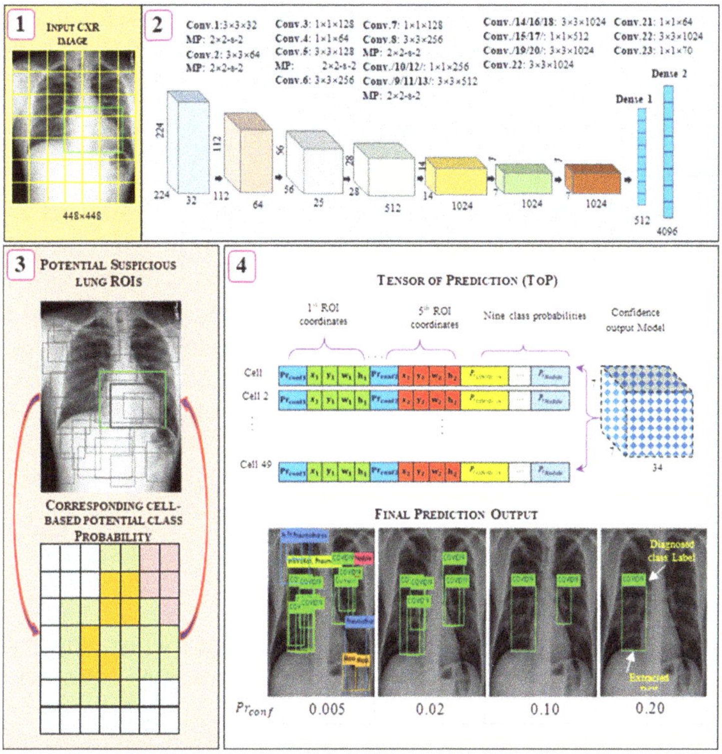

Figure 7.3. Detailed structure of the proposed AI-based CAD for distinguishing between COVID-19 and eight other eight lung respiratory diseases.

The proposed AI-based CAD system has a unique DL structure with 23 convolutional layers, two dense layers, and a tensor of prediction, as presented in figure 7.3. The convolution and dense layers use the leaky rectified linear activation function, except for the final dense layer, which uses the ReLU activation function, as in [32]. In addition, we use reduction convolution layers with a window of 1×1 pixel to compress the size of the deep features and make the training process faster [9, 10]. We then use a convolution layer with a window size of 3×3 followed by batch normalization layers to avoid overfitting and speed up the training [9, 10]. In addition, we use the max pooling (MP) strategy with a window size of 2×2 to shrink the deep features and estimate the powerful ones. In the final convolution layer, the deep feature maps are flattened using global average pooling (GAP) into a 1D vector shape that is suitable for the dense layers. The final output of the presented AI-based CAD system is called ToP; it contains all the predicted parameters for each box: the box coordinates (x, y, w, and h), $Pr_{conf.}$, and the nine probabilities for each lung disease class (e.g. $Pr_{COVID-19}$). In fact, the ToP is a 3D array with a size of $N \times N \times (5 \times B + C)$, where $N = 7$ represents the number of grid cells, $B = 5$ is the number of boxes, and $C = 9$ is the number of classes [5, 25, 26, 32]. Thus, the size of the final ToP is represented by $7 \times 7 \times 34 = 1666$ nodes. This means each 34 neurons in the last dense layer present all the predictors for all boxes in a specific cell in the actual CXR image. Thus, our presented CAD system is faster than other current predictors.

7.3.4 Experimental setting

Before they are fed into the DL model, the original input x-ray images are resized to a size of 448 × 448 using bilinear interpolation [9, 10]. Moreover, the pixel intensity in those images is normalized to range from 0 to 1, as in [9, 10]. Notably, we utilize a multi-scale strategy (i.e., applying input images of various resolutions) to train the teachable predictor [33]. It is obvious that the DL architecture reduces the spatial dimensions of the feature maps by five times; hence, we configure the model to preset a new spatial resolution for the input images in multiples of 32 for every ten batches. As a consequence, the smallest resolution should be 320 × 320, while the largest is 608 × 608. Notably, the mini-batch size is set to 24 and the total number of training epochs used to train the proposed architecture is set to 120.

7.3.5 Implementation environment

The whole data set loading pipeline and model training followed by evaluation are executed using an Intel® Core(TM) i7–6850K processor at 3.36GHz, 16 GB of RAM, and four NVIDIA GeForce GTX1080 GPUs.

7.3.6 Evaluation strategy

For evaluation, the predicted bounding box is considered to be a true positive if it fulfils the following two conditions: first, the IoU ratio between the extracted box and the corresponding GT representation should be equal to or greater than a predefined threshold value. Second, the confidence score (i.e., Pr_{conf}) of the predicted bounding box should be equal to or greater than another predefined threshold value [32, 34]. In particular, the maximum confidence score is usually adopted to evaluate the predictions inferred by the trained model [9, 10]. Note that a higher confidence score corresponds to better accuracy in detecting a lesion that exists inside the predicted bounding box [9, 10]. Regarding the numerical evaluation per cross-validation fold, weighted objective metrics, such as overall accuracy (ACC), specificity (SP), sensitivity (SE), Dice, the Matthews correlation coefficient (MCC), the positive predictive value (PPV), and the negative predictive value (NPV) [9, 10] are employed. A weighted class strategy [32] is adopted to avoid test sets of class-imbalanced images. Specifically, the ratios of coefficients for atelectasis, infiltration, pneumothorax, masses, effusion, pneumonia, cardiomegaly, nodules, and COVID-19 are set to 0.14, 0.10, 0.08, 0.06, 0.12, 0.09, 0.11, 0.06, and 0.25, respectively. Accordingly, multiclass confusion matrices are used to represent the experimental results for each validation fold [9, 10].

7.4 Experimental results

7.4.1 Extraction of suspicious lung ROIs

7.4.1.1 Optimization of the appropriate values of the IoU threshold and the confidence score

The presented AI-based CAD system has a good ability to extract five different boxes with respect to each grid cell across the whole CXR image. To ignore or suppress unwanted extracted boxes, we use the non-max suppression (NMS) technique [9, 26, 33]. An example of the boxes detected after the application of NMS is shown in figure 7.3 in section 7.4. Meanwhile, the IoU between the final extracted box and the GT should be greater than 0.005. This is to ensure that the detected box contains an object (e.g. COVID-19). For this study, we experimentally conclude that the appropriate threshold for the IoU is 45%. The study results show that the final detected ROIs from most test CXR images have IoU > 90%. In contrast, the final extracted boxes with IOU < 45% are assigned as false detection results. To control the number of boxes detected in each CXR image, we experimentally set the confidence score threshold to be 10%. This then excludes or ignores unwanted boxes with smaller conditional class probabilities. Figure 7.3 in section 7.4 shows an example of the number of detected boxes with respect to threshold values of 0.005, 0.02, 0.10, and 0.20.

7.4.1.2 Lung ROI extraction results

Table 7.2 shows the average detection results using fivefold cross-validation for all test CXR images in all classes. Detected lung ROIs with IoU = 45% are considered to be correct results, while the other ROIs with IoU < 45% are assigned as false results. Based on the average of the fivefold tests, the proposed AI-based CAD system is shown to be capable of extracting COVID-19 abnormalities from the test CXR images with an overall accuracy of 96.31%. Generally, our AI-based CAD

Table 7.2. Lung ROI detection results for the proposed AI-based CAD system for COVID-19 detection vs. all other eight lung respiratory diseases as an average over fivefold tests using the test data sets.

	Lung ROI extraction results	
Class of disease	Correct detection accuracy (%)	False detection accuracy (%)
1. COVID-19	96.309	3.688
2. Atelectasis	88.889	11.112
3. Infiltration	97.602	2.405
4. Pneumothorax	71.520	28.50
5. Mass	90.585	9.419
6. Effusion	91.612	8.387
7. Pneumonia	86.669	13.339
8. Cardiomegaly	97.245	2.756
9. Nodule	78.749	21.250

system is shown to be reliable for the extraction of abnormalities in all classes with an overall accuracy of 90.67%. In addition, the achieved detection accuracies are found to lie between 71.50% for the case of pneumothorax and ~ 97.60% for the case of infiltration diseases.

Qualitatively, Figure 7.4 shows some examples of the detected ROI regions for COVID-19 cases. The extracted boxes and class labels are also depicted on each CXR image indicating whether the detected region is correct or not. The correct detected regions usually have high IoU values, while the false detection cases have near-zero values.

7.4.2 Classification results

The AI-based CAD system can simultaneously diagnose the detected suspicious regions end-to-end into nine different classes (i.e., COVID-19, pneumonia, lung mass, etc). The classification task is done using two dense layers (i.e. a neural network). Figure 7.4 shows some examples of COVID-19 classification in which the class label is displayed beside the IoU and confidence score. Figures 7.4 (a)–(b) represent the best detection and classification results, in which the detected lung regions are a good fit for their GTs and the classification labels are correctly matched with the original ones. The detected lung regions shown in Figures 7.4 (c)–(d) are falsely detected, but they are diagnosed correctly. Such results may help physicians to focus and investigate again for the potential effects of COVID-19. Moreover, since we set the confidence score threshold to 10%, multiple lung ROIs are sometimes detected and classified as a COVID-19, as shown in figure 7.3 in section 7.4. Such results could also be helpful for physicians, because COVID-19 has the ability to affect both lungs (right and left). Figure 7.4 (e) shows a false prediction case for COVID-19, since the detected lung ROI has an IoU of 0.0%, a confidence score of 75.39%, and an incorrect classification label. The false prediction results are also important to evaluate patient cases in a rapid manner. For quantitative evaluation results, multiclass confusion matrices are used for nine different classes. Figure 7.5 shows the derived confusion matrices for each of Fold1 to Fold5, respectively. As clearly shown in table 7.3, the COVID-19 cases are correctly classified from among all the other lung diseases with an average classification accuracy of 97.401%. The presented AI-based CAD system achieves overall

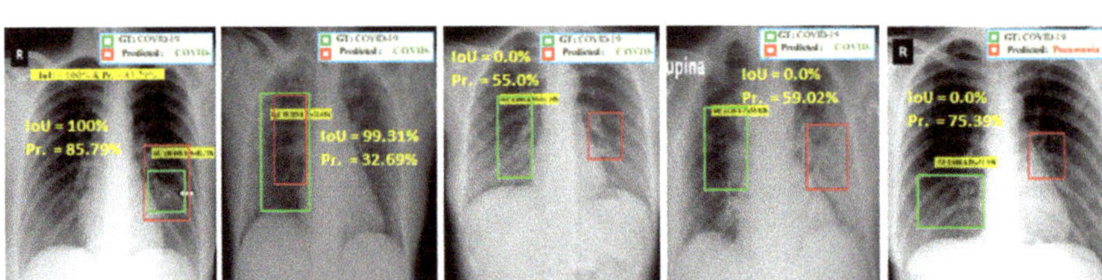

(a) (b) (c) (d) (e)

Figure 7.4. Examples of the COVID-19 detection results. The GT information (green) and the corresponding detected boxes (red), IoUs, and their confidence scores are depicted on the input CXR images.

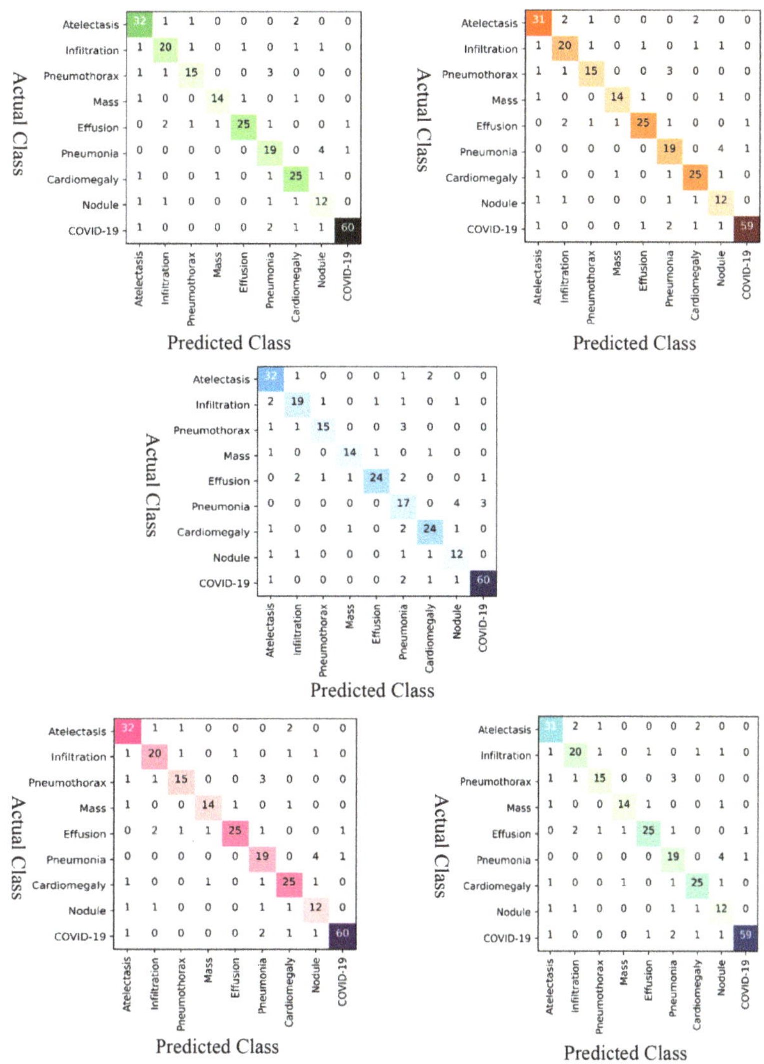

Figure 7.5. Classification evaluation results in terms of multiclass confusion matrices for Fold1 ~ Fold5, respectively.

classification accuracies of between 94.60% and 97.401% for pneumonia and COVID-19, respectively.

In general, our AI-based CAD system has demonstrated its reliability and its ability to assist hospital physicians by providing a second opinion to make the final decision in an easy and more accurate way. This is the most advantageous aspect of the proposed CAD system. In addition, the proposed system does not need a high level of attention or user intervention to achieve the final prediction results. Although admirable prediction results are achieved for COVID-19 diagnosis, some limitations and challenges are still present. The GT information is not yet

Table 7.3. Classification evaluation results (%) of the proposed AI-based CAD system for all nine lung diseases as an average using fivefold tests with the test sets.

Folds	SE	SP	ACC	Dice	MCC	PPV	NPV
Fold1	88.249	99.155	97.590	85.466	83.601	86.012	98.905
Fold2	84.470	99.091	97.368	84.751	82.750	85.330	98.721
Fold3	83.334	98.784	97.082	83.635	81.504	84.401	98.679
Fold4	85.251	99.1581	97.587	85.467	83.601	86.023	98.901
Fold5	84.470	99.091	97.370	84.752	82.751	85.328	98.718
Avg.(%)	**85.152**	**99.056**	**97.401**	**84.811**	**82.842**	**85.412**	**98.784**

fully available to help researchers to perform deep investigations using supervised learning. The process of annotation by experts is also a very exhausting and difficult process.

In the future, deep reinforcement learning (DRL) should find a way to process medical images in real time to fight COVID-19 or any other pandemic that may arise. We also plan to build an intelligent medical platform to be a real-time support for physicians by providing them with a practical solution in a more accurate and rapid way.

7.4.3 Prediction time

The proposed AI-based CAD system needs 2.441 seconds to predict all the test CXR images from nine classes. This means that our presented CAD system has the ability to process 108 frames per second. This is the key to making our system practically available, especially in a pandemic or epidemic situation.

7.5 Conclusions

An AI-based CAD framework is presented in this chapter that can simultaneously predict COVID-19 from among eight other lung respiratory diseases. It provides its prediction results using two consecutive steps. First, lung ROIs containing suspicious diseases are extracted from the whole CXR image. Second, each detected ROI is simultaneously passed into dense layers or fully connected layers to perform the classification task. Our framework is validated with respect to nine different lung respiratory diseases. It achieves impressive results in terms of ROI prediction, for which it achieves an SE of 85.152%, an SP of 99.056%, an ACC of 97.401%, a Dice score of 84.811%, an MCC of 82.842%, a PPV of 85.412%, and an NPV of 98.784%. Rapid results and high prediction scores are key to deploying a CAD system that can be useful in practice and building a smart triage system for patients in hospital and healthcare systems.

Acknowledgement

This research was supported by the MSIT (Ministry of Science and ICT), Korea, under the ITRC (Information Technology Research Center) support program (IITP-2017-0-01629) supervised by the IITP (Institute for Information & communications Technology Promotion), by Institute for Information & communications Technology Promotion (IITP) grant funded by the Korea government (MSIT) (No. 2017-0-00655), by the MSIT (Ministry of Science and ICT), Korea, under the Grand Information Technology Research Center support program (IITP-2020-0-01489), (IITP-2021-0-00979) supervised by the IITP (Institute for Information & communications Technology Planning & Evaluation) and NRF2019R1A2C2090504.

References

[1] Alimadadi A, Aryal S, Manandhar I, Munroe P B, Joe B and Cheng X 2020 *Artificial Intelligence and Machine Learning to Fight COVID-19.* (Bethesda, MD: American Physiological Society)

[2] Wu F, Zhao S, Yu B, Chen Y-M, Wang W, Song Z-G, Hu Y, Tao Z-W, Tian J-H and Pei Y-Y 2020 A new coronavirus associated with human respiratory disease in China *Nature* **579** 265–9

[3] Chinazzi M, Davis J T, Ajelli M, Gioannini C, Litvinova M, Merler S, Piontti A P, Mu K, Rossi L and Sun K 2020 The effect of travel restrictions on the spread of the 2019 novel coronavirus (COVID-19) outbreak *Science* **368** 395–400

[4] Robson B 2020 Computers and viral diseases. Preliminary bioinformatics studies on the design of a synthetic vaccine and a preventative peptidomimetic antagonist against the SARS-CoV-2 (2019-nCoV, COVID-19) coronavirus *Comput. Biol. Med.* **119** 103670

[5] Zhao S, Lin Q, Ran J, Musa S S, Yang G, Wang W, Lou Y, Gao D, Yang L and He D 2020 Preliminary estimation of the basic reproduction number of novel coronavirus (2019-nCoV) in China, from 2019 to 2020: A data-driven analysis in the early phase of the outbreak *Int. J. Infect. Dis.* **92** 214–7

[6] Coronavirus disease (COVID-19) 2020 World Health Organization https://who.int/emergencies/diseases/novel-coronavirus-2019

[7] Pereira R M, Bertolini D, Teixeira L O, Silla C N Jr and Costa Y M 2020 COVID-19 identification in chest x-ray images on flat and hierarchical classification scenarios *Comput. Methods Programs Biomed.* **194** 105532

[8] Ozturk T, Talo M, Yildirim E A, Baloglu U B, Yildirim O and Acharya U R 2020 Automated detection of COVID-19 cases using deep neural networks with x-ray images *Comput. Biol. Med.* **121** 103792

[9] Al-Antari M A, Al-Masni M A, Choi M T, Han S M and Kim T S 2018 A fully integrated computer-aided diagnosis system for digital x-ray mammograms via deep learning detection, segmentation, and classification *Int. J. Med. Inform.* **117** 44–54

[10] Al-Masni M A, Al-Antari M A, Park J M, Gi G, Kim T Y, Rivera P, Valarezo E, Choi M T, Han S M and Kim T S 2018 Simultaneous detection and classification of breast masses in digital mammograms via a deep learning YOLO-based CAD system *Comput. Methods Programs Biomed.* **157** 85–94

[11] Al-Masni M A, Al-Antari M A, Choi M T, Han S M and Kim T S 2018 Skin lesion segmentation in dermoscopy images via deep full resolution convolutional networks *Comput. Methods Programs Biomed.* **162** 221–31

[12] Al-Masni M A, Kim D-H and Kim T-S 2020 Multiple skin lesions diagnostics via integrated deep convolutional networks for segmentation and classification *Comput. Methods Programs Biomed.* **190** 105351
[13] Cohen J P, Morrison P and Dao L 2020 COVID-19 image data collection https://githubcom/ieee8023/covid-chestxray-dataset
[14] Chowdhury M, Rahman T, Khandakar A, Kadir R, Mahbub Z, Islam K, Khan M, Iqbal A, Emadi N and Reaz M 2020 Can AI help in screening viral and COVID-19 pneumonia? https://wwwkagglecom/tawsifurrahman/covid19-radiography-database
[15] Wang X, Peng Y, Lu L, Lu Z, Bagheri M and Summers R M 2017 Chestx-ray8: hospital-scale chest x-ray database and benchmarks on weakly-supervised classification and localization of common thorax diseases *Proc. of the IEEE Conference on Computer Vision and Pattern Recognition* pp 2097–106
[16] Oh Y, Park S and Ye J C 2020 Deep learning covid-19 features on cxr using limited training data sets *IEEE Trans. Med. Imaging* **39** 2688–700
[17] Wang L, Lin Z Q and Wong A 2020 COVID-Net: a tailored deep convolutional neural network design for detection of COVID-19 cases from chest radiography images *Sci. Rep.* **10** 19549
[18] Hemdan E E-D, Shouman M A and Karar M E 2020 Covidx-net: a framework of deep learning classifiers to diagnose covid-19 in x-ray images arXiv:2003.11055
[19] Ardakani A A, Kanafi A R, Acharya U R, Khadem N and Mohammadi A 2020 Application of deep learning technique to manage COVID-19 in routine clinical practice using CT images: results of 10 convolutional neural networks *Comput. Biol. Med.* **121** 103795
[20] Apostolopoulos I and Mpesiana T 2020 Covid-19: automatic detection from x-ray images utilizing transfer learning with convolutional neural networks *Phys. Eng. Sci. Med.* **43** 635–40
[21] Khan A I, Shah J L and Bhat M 2020 Coronet: a deep neural network for detection and diagnosis of COVID-19 from chest x-ray images *Comput. Methods Programs Biomed.* **196** 105581
[22] Mohamadou Y, Halidou A and Kapen P T 2020 A review of mathematical modeling, artificial intelligence and datasets used in the study, prediction and management of COVID-19 *Appl. Intell.* **50** 3913–25
[23] Shoeibi A, Khodatars M, Alizadehsani R, Ghassemi N, Jafari M, Moridian P, Khadem A, Sadeghi D, Hussain S and Zare A 2020 Automated detection and forecasting of COVID-19 using deep learning techniques: a review arXiv:2007.10785
[24] Krizhevsky A, Sutskever I and Hinton G E 2012 ImageNet classification with deep convolutional neural networks *25th Int. Conf. on Neural Information Processing Systems, USA* 1097–105
[25] Al-antari M A, Hua C-H, Bang J, Choi D-J, Kang S M and Lee S A 2021 Rapid deep learning computer-aided diagnosis to simultaneously detect and classify the novel COVID-19 pandemic *2020 IEEE-EMBS Conf. on Biomedical Engineering and Sciences (IECBES)* (Piscataway, NJ: IEEE) pp 585–8
[26] Al-antari M A, Hua C-H, Bang J and Lee S 2021 Fast deep learning computer-aided diagnosis of COVID-19 based on digital chest x-ray images *Appl. Intell.* **51** 2890–907
[27] Takahashi R and Kajikawa Y 2017 Computer-aided diagnosis: a survey with bibliometric analysis *Int. J. Med. Informatics* **101** 58–67

[28] Chougrad H, Zouaki H and Alheyane O 2018 Deep convolutional neural networks for breast cancer screening *Comput. Methods Programs Biomed.* **157** 19–30
[29] Celik Y, Talo M, Yildirim O, Karabatak M and Acharya U R 2020 Automated invasive ductal carcinoma detection based using deep transfer learning with whole-slide images *Pattern Recognit. Lett.* **133** 232–9
[30] Girshick R 2015 Fast R-CNN *Proc. of the IEEE International Conference on Computer Vision* 1440–8
[31] Felzenszwalb P F, Girshick R B, McAllester D and Ramanan D 2010 Object detection with discriminatively trained part-based models *IEEE Trans. Pattern Anal. Mach. Intell.* **32** 1627–45
[32] Al-Antari M A and Kim T-S 2020 Evaluation of deep learning detection and classification towards computer-aided diagnosis of breast lesions in digital x-ray mammograms *Comput. Methods Programs Biomed.*
[33] Redmon J and Farhadi A 2017 *YOLO9000: Better, Faster, Stronger, 2017 IEEE Conference on Computer Vision and Pattern Recognition (CVPR)* (Piscataway, NJ: IEEE) 6517–25
[34] Al-Antari M A, Al-Masni M A and Kim T-S 2020 Deep learning computer-aided diagnosis for breast lesion in digital mammogram *Deep Learning in Medical Image Analysis.* (Berlin: Springer) pp 59–72

IOP Publishing

Artificial Intelligence Strategies for Analyzing COVID-19 Pneumonia Lung Imaging, Volume 1
Characterization approaches
Ayman El-Baz and Jasjit S Suri

Chapter 8

Diagnosis of COVID-19 by feature selection techniques using support vector machine

Amira M Hasan, Hala M Abd El-Kader and Aya Hossam

8.1 Introduction

The COVID-19 disease was discovered in the Wuhan region of China at the end of 2019. This viral disease causes fever, cough, and fatigue, eventually leading to patient death [1]. Medical imaging is a technique which is used to study the human body. Image processing methods for image interpretation are necessary for the analysis of images and accurate diagnosis. Computed tomography (CT) images are accurate and effective tools for the detection of COVID-19. Physicians need a precise and reliable diagnosis procedure that allows them to distinguish cases of COVID-19 and reduce the burden on clinicians [2]. As a result, it is critical to create a computer aided diagnosis (CAD) system based on machine learning (ML) algorithms to detect cases of COVID-19. CAD systems have various stages, such as image collection, image enhancement, and image segmentation [3]. The first stage begins by extracting the best images from a data set. To obtain the highest levels of quality and clarity, the second stage employs image enhancement techniques. In the the third stage, image segmentation algorithms are applied to extract the region of interest (ROI). The fourth stage extracts the original features from the ROI, which provides indicators of COVID-19 and non-COVID-19 conditions in CT images [4]. The data set that was used in [5] contains about 32 features. CAD systems face the challenges caused by large numbers of features in data sets, because not all of these features are required. The selected features have useful information and play an important role in building the COVID-19 detection model [6]. The data reduction process aids in the removal of irrelevant or noisy data as well as the reduction of the features. When a predictive model is developed, feature selection (FS) reduces the input variables and the data's dimensionality. FS allows learning algorithms to operate more quickly and efficiently. FS is very essential for the detection of the

doi:10.1088/978-0-7503-3795-3ch8

feature subset which describes the data of the learning task, which should be better than the original data set. Therefore it is necessary to construct an automated model which is based on ML and follows the decisions made by clinical physicians. ML techniques are gaining traction for medical diagnosis because of their high accuracy rates in classification. The accuracy of classification algorithms depends on using the appropriate feature selection algorithms to reduce the dimensions of the data set. It is necessary to construct an automated model based on the ML approach to initiate corrective action, following the decision of the treating physician. This chapter proposes two effective FS models, based on the wrapper approach and the filter approach, respectively, as evaluators for the detection of COVID-19 using chest CT images. A support vector machine (SVM) classifier was used with the evaluators to optimize the feature subset using the 'best first' search method. The experimental results show that the proposed FS filter model is more intelligent than the wrapper FS method and outperforms it.

8.2 Computer aided diagnosis

A CAD system consists of many stages of medical diagnosis. The first stage is the detection of images in the data set. Several image enhancement techniques are used in second stage to realize the highest levels of quality and clarity. Segmentation algorithms are used in the third stage, the original features are extracted from the ROIs of the image in the fourth stage, and feature selection takes place in the fifth stage. Finally, classification is the final stage in the construction of the classification model, as shown in figure 8.1.

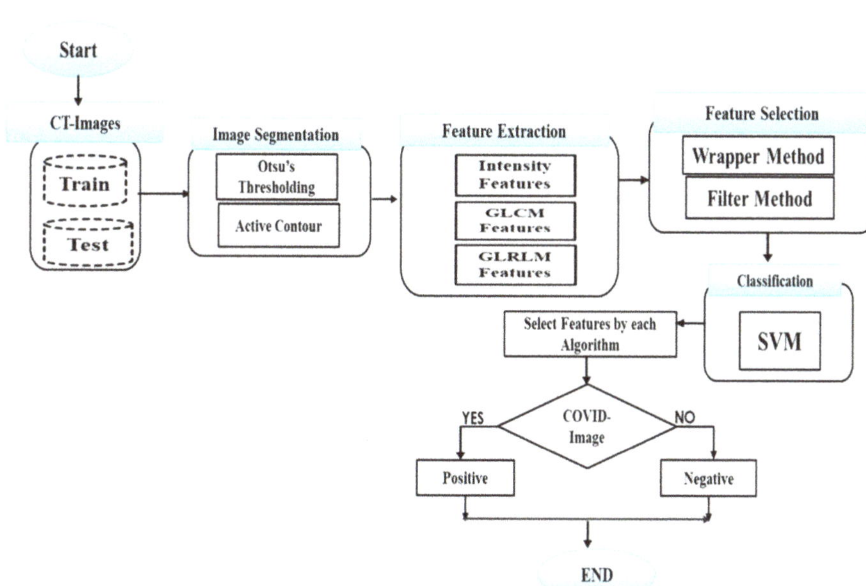

Figure 8.1. Graphical diagram of the proposed model.

8.2.1 Feature selection (FS)

FS is an essential preprocessing task in data mining. By removing the irrelevant features, it leads to more efficient and accurate classification. This technique simplifies the visualization and understanding of data, as well as the time and storage required for the data-mining process. By avoiding an explosion of dimensionality, it improves algorithmic performance [7].

8.2.2 Feature selection process

FS techniques strive to select the smallest number of features that preserve a data set's most important information. FS is used as a preprocessing step in data-mining tasks to remove irrelevant or redundant features. As a result, classification, clustering, and similarity searching processes become more efficient and accurate (in terms of computational cost and memory requirement) [8]. Consequently, the image processing community has developed a plethora of techniques for selecting the 'optimal' subset of features from a larger set of potential features. Images have a wide range of characteristics, from which it is critical to distinguish and extract the interesting features. The FS process consists of subset generation, subset evaluation, a stopping criterion, and result validation, as shown in figure 8.2.

1. **Subset Generation**: subsets of features are produced for the evaluation based on a specific search strategy (which starts with either an empty subset of features, with all features, or with a random subset of features).
2. **Subset Evaluation**: the quality of the subset, as generated by a generation criterion, is measured using an evaluation task. The generated subset is compared to the previous best subset and, if found to be superior, replaces it.
3. **Stopping Criterion**: because the selection process may continue to generate feature subsets, a stopping criterion is essential for this process. This can be achieved, for example, by stopping at a set number of features/iterations,

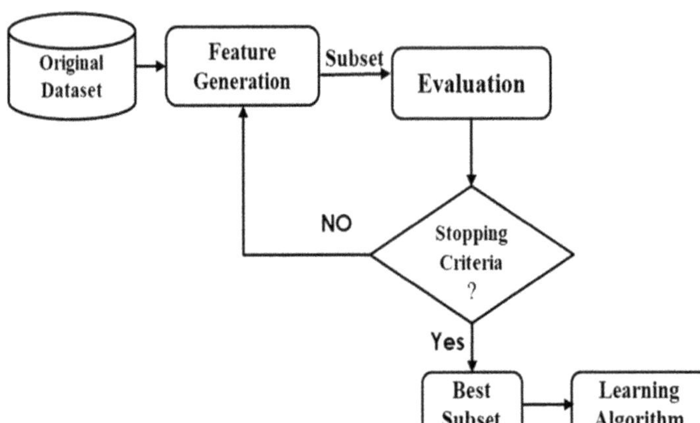

Figure 8.2. A flowchart of the FS process.

when adding or removing a feature reduces performance, or when an optimal subset of features is obtained.

4. **Result Validation**: different examinations are carried out to verify the validity of the subset of the selected features.

8.2.3 Feature selection methods

Feature selection methods are grouped into two types, namely, filter and wrapper methods. Wrapper methods are more accurate and more computationally intensive; so we used wrapper methods to build the classification models.

8.2.3.1 The filter approach

The filter approach evaluates feature subsets based on the general characteristics of the data set. This is done without taking any mining algorithm into account. It is typically applied to data sets with high dimensionality. This approach employs ranking and space search methods based on a strategy to select the best subset of features [9]. Figure 8.3 shows the flowchart of the filter approach.

8.2.3.2 The wrapper approach

Due to the disadvantages of the filter approach, the wrapper approach was proposed in 1997. The evaluation of the best feature subset in the wrapper approach necessitates using a specified data-mining algorithm. In this approach, an analytical model is used to score the feature subset. This means there is no need to have any knowledge about the algorithm used; only an interface is required. The feature

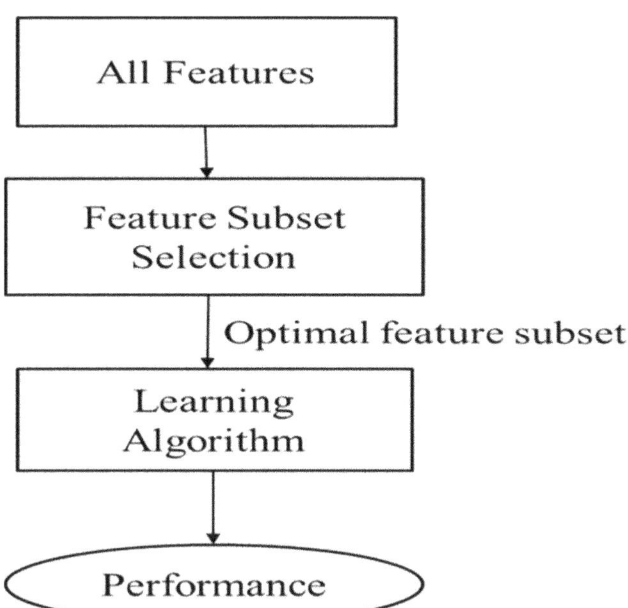

Figure 8.3. The flowchart of the filter approach.

subsets can be evaluated based on the accuracy of the classifier using the interface to obtain the optimal feature subset. A full search in the wrapper method necessitates $2n$ (where n is the number of features) assessments. While the ability to deal with correlated features and the discovery of relevant associations are advantages of this approach, it may lead to overfitting issues. Figure 8.4 shows a flowchart of the wrapper approach. Finally, table 8.1 provides a comparison between the filter and wrapper approaches.

8.2.4 Feature subset selection evaluators

To create the best subset of the data set, each method of feature selection makes use of feature subset evaluators and search algorithms [11]. We provide brief descriptions of the evaluators and the search methods used for feature selection:

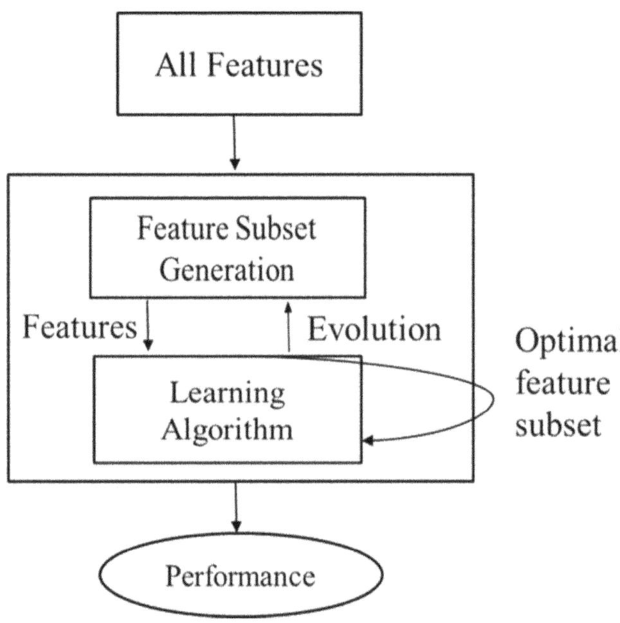

Figure 8.4. A flowchart of the wrapper approach.

Table 8.1. Comparison between the filter and wrapper approaches.

	Filter approach	Wrapper approach
Speed	Simple and fast	Complex and lower
Attribute dependencies	Only to some degree	Fully incorporated
Cost	Less expensive	Expensive
Performance	Lower performance	Better performance
Overfitting	Avoids overfitting	Better avoidance

8.2.4.1 Wrapper subset evaluator (WrapperSubsetEval)

To evaluate variable sets, a classifier is used, and cross-validation is used to estimate the learning scheme's accuracy for each set [12].

8.2.4.2 Filtered subset evaluator (FilterSubsetEval)

The filtered subset evaluator evaluates the values of feature subsets by predicting the degree of redundancy among them to choose the most suitable subset of features [13].

8.2.4.3 Best first search method

Selects the node with the highest score using hill climbing and a backtracking facility. Using an evaluation function, it assigns a score to each candidate node. There are two node lists. One list contains the nodes which will be explored (open nodes), and another list contains the nodes which are visited (close nodes). The search can begin with a forward search using an empty attribute set, a backward search using a full attribute set, or a backward and forward search from any node. When open nodes are close to the goal, they are prioritised. Rather than using a small subset of neighbour nodes, the best first algorithm searches unvisited nodes to find the best node among all nodes. The search is resumed when the algorithm reaches a dead-end node. As a result, it seeks out the best node from all the others [14].

8.2.5 Data set

In COVID-19 applications, data collection is the primary and first step. The authors used a data set of 2,110 CT scans, including 1,110 CT images of people infected with COVID-19 and 1,000 images of uninfected people. The data set used was collected from the open-source data repositories GitHub and Kaggle [15, 16].

8.2.6 Classification using support vector machine (SVM)

Classification is the final step in building the COVID-19 detection model by using Waikato Environment for Knowledge Analysis (WEKA) which is a collection of machine learning algorithms for data mining tasks [17]. WEKA contains tools for classification, regression, clustering, association rules mining, and visualization. There are classification algorithms which are capable of performing the required task, such as SVM. SVM is a powerful classification algorithm that performs classification tasks by constructing hyperplanes in a space that splits the values of several class labels. The aim of SVM is to obtain a hyperplane which optimally separate the classes from each other. Classification is usually represented by class labels, such as $\{-1, +1\}$. The data to be classified can be separated linearly. Referring to figure 8.5, let $\{x_1 \ldots x_m\}$ be the values of the data set and $y_i \in \{1, -1\}$ is the class label of x_i. Suppose that a pair of variables (v, b) defines a hyperplane which has the following equation:

$$v.\ x_i + b = 0, \tag{8.1}$$

where v is the normal weight vector which is perpendicular to the hyperplane and b is an intercept term that represents a shift of the hyperplane from the origin of the

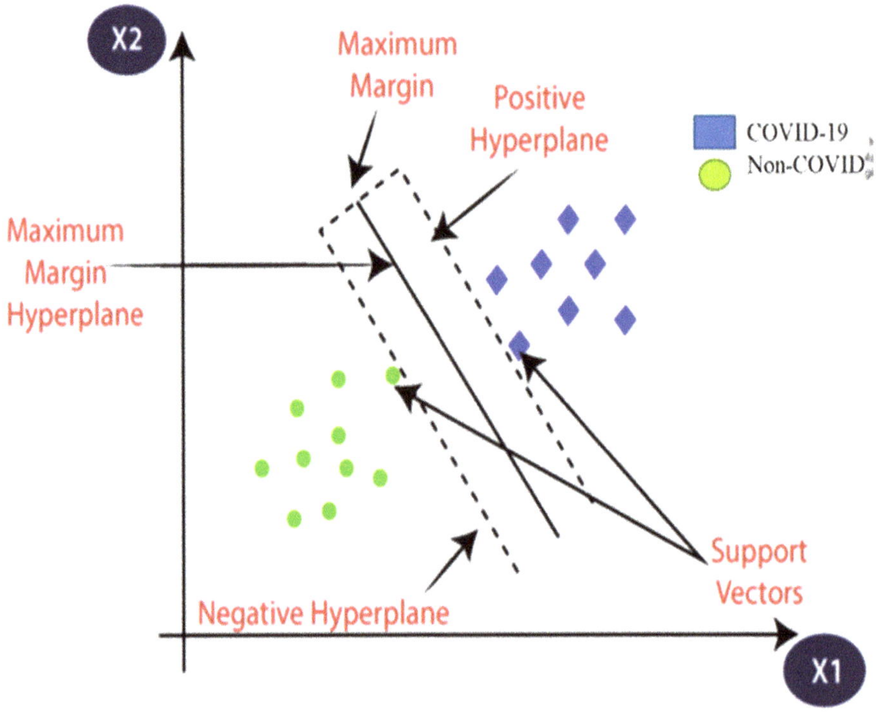

Figure 8.5. The concept of support vector machine operation.

coordinate system. In addition, the training data can be described by the following equations:

$$v.\ x_i + b \geqslant +1 \ \text{If}\ y_i = +1 \tag{8.2}$$

$$v.\ x_i + b \leqslant -1 \ \text{If}\ y_i = -1 \tag{8.3}$$

where R^d represents the d-dimensional space of the input patterns, xi, yi represent the labels that classify the inputs as $\{-1, +1\}$, v represents the normal value of multiple planes, and b represents the tendency (bias) value. In order to detect the optimal separation plane, the boundaries that are parallel to this correction must be determined. That is, support vectors are required. This procedure is expressed as $v.\ xi + b = \pm 1$. In figure 8.5, a typical example of a support vector machine is depicted. By mapping the inputs to high-dimensional areas and solving the quadratic programming optimization problem, SVM improve the generalisation performance, so it was used in conjunction with the FS method to create a classification model for identifying cases of COVID-19 [18].

8.3 Performance metrics

WEKA is a software tool which is used for data-mining tasks. In WEKA, FS methods have two components: a feature evaluator, which evaluates feature subsets,

Table 8.2. Evaluation criteria used for the proposed model.

Metrics	Formula
Accuracy	$Accuracy = \frac{TP + TN}{TP + TN + FP + FN}$
Specificity	$FP\text{-}Rate = \frac{TN}{TN + FP}$
Sensitivity (Recall)	$TP - Rate = \frac{TP}{TP + FN}$

Table 8.3. Confusion matrix.

		Prediction	
Confusion matrix		Positive	Negative
Actual	**Positive**	**TP**	**FN**
	Negative	**FP**	**TN**

and a search method, which searches the space of the feature subsets. The data set is separated into training and testing portions, which are allocated percentages of 70 and 30, respectively, with tenfold cross-validation. Performance is described in terms of accuracy, specificity, and sensitivity by applying a confusion matrix. This matrix contains of four indices: true positive (TP), true negative (TN), false positive (FP), and false negative (FN). TP and TN represent the numbers of correctly predicted positive and negative samples, respectively, whereas FP and FN correspond to numbers of incorrectly predicted positive and negative samples, respectively. All metrics are listed in table 8.2. Additionally, the receiver operating characteristic (ROC) is a 2D graph in which the true positive rate (TPR) is plotted against the false negative rate (FNR). Also, to compare different classifiers, the area under the curve (AUC) is calculated [19, 20].

8.4 Evaluation model

The data set was used to identify cases of COVID-19 using the SVM classifier. The original features were contained in the COVID-19 data set which was prepared in [5]. A total of 32 features were extracted from each image, as shown in figure 8.6, but not all of these features were provided to the classifiers, because the number of features was large [21]. Afterwards, the wrapper approach and the filter approach were used for feature selection. These methods can reduce a data set's dimensionality while achieving higher classification accuracy in less time. For each subset obtained through the feature selection methods, the SVM algorithm was used to detect COVID-19. The ROC curves of the proposed FS models are shown in figure 8.7. A comparison of the results is presented in detail in figure 8.8. The goal of each evaluator and searching method used was detection of the best method to obtain the

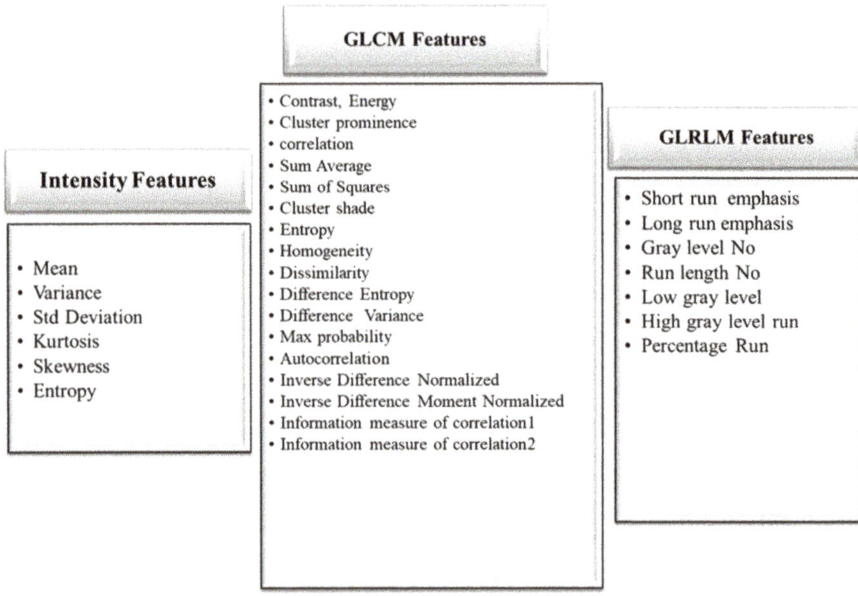

Figure 8.6. The feature extraction techniques.

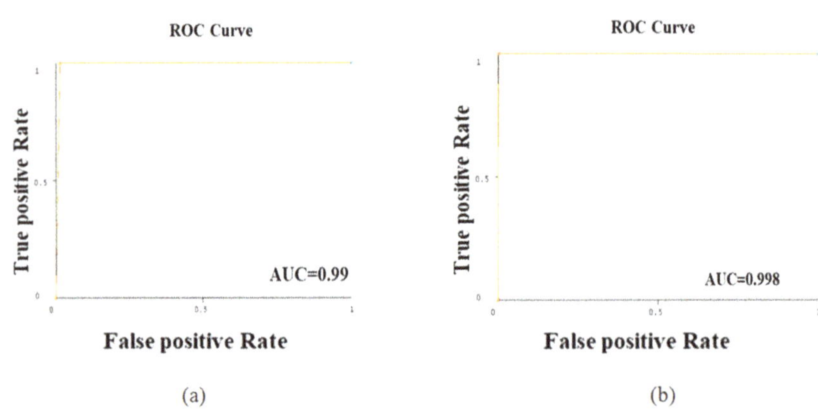

Figure 8.7. ROC curves of the FS models: (a) wrapper model; (b) filter model.

best results for the best COVID-19 diagnosis. WrapperSubsetEval with a 'best first' search was used on the training data set for the wrapper method, and FilterSubsetEval with a 'best first' search was used on the entire training data set for the filter method. The SVM algorithm was used to classify the cases of COVID-19 after the feature selection methods were used and the dimensionality of the data set was reduced. In the training phase of the classification algorithm, the WEKA tool (version 3.6.13) and tenfold cross-validation were used for feature selection and classification.

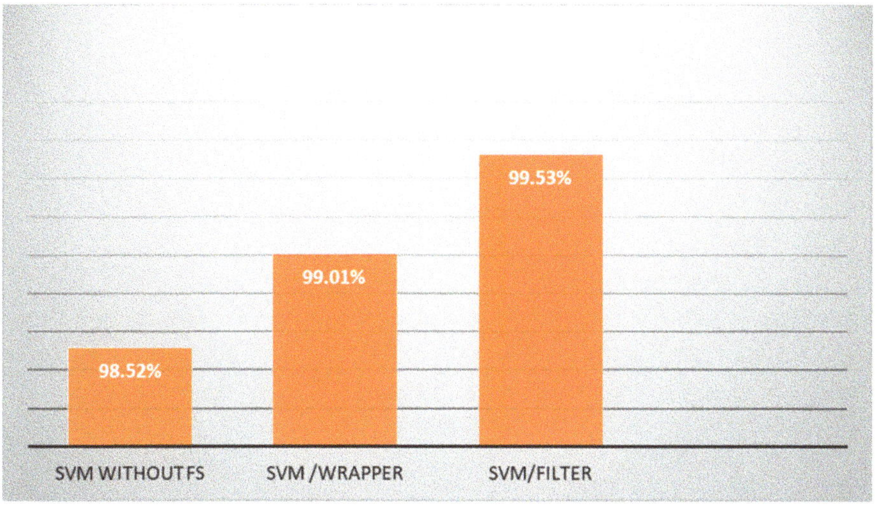

Figure 8.8. Comparison between the SVM classifiers before and after FS.

Table 8.4. Confusion matrix of the SVM before and after the FS methods were used.

		Prediction	
Confusion matrix	Actual	COVID-19	Non-COVID-19
SVM without feature selection	***COVID-19***	210	1
	Non-COVID-19	8	392
SVM with WrapperSubsetEval with best first	***COVID-19***	211	0
	Non-COVID-19	6	394
SVM with FilterSubsetEval with best first	***COVID-19***	211	0
	Non-COVID-19	1	399

Table 8.5. Performance of SVM classification with feature selection methods.

Classifier	TP Rate	FP Rate	Precision	Recall	ROC Area	Class
SVM	0.995	0.020	0.963	0.995	0.988	COVID-19
without FS	0.980	0.005	0.997	0.980	0.988	Non-COVID-19
SVM with	1.000	0.015	0.972	1.000	0.993	COVID-19
WrapperSubsetEval	0.985	0.000	1.000	0.985	0.993	Non-COVID-19
SVM with	1.000	0.003	0.995	1.000	0.999	COVID-19
FilterSubsetEval with	0.998	0.000	1.000	0.998	0.999	Non-COVID

Table 8.6. Performance of the SVM classifier before and after FSA.

Classifier	Method Used	Time Test	Correctly/ Incorrectly Instances	Number Features	Sensitivity (%)	Specificity (%)	AUC (%)	Accuracy (%)
SVM without FS	Without FS	2.48 s	602/9	32	99.5%	98%	98.7%	98.52%
SVM with WrapperSubsetEval	Wrapper	1.31 s	605/5	17	100%	98.5%	99.2%	99.01%
SVM with FilterSubsetEval	Filter	1.22 s	610/1	4	100%	99.7%	99.8%	99.53%

8.5 Test results

FS approaches, such as the filter and wrapper methods were employed to minimise the dimensionality of the data set and improve the accuracy of the classifier. These methods generated a new data set that had lower dimensionality than the original data set. The COVID-19 data set used had 32 attributes. The first wrapper method, WrapperSubsetEval, an evaluator with Best First search, reduced the data set dimensions to 17 attributes. The data set dimension was reduced to four attributes using the second filter approach, FilterSubsetEval with Best First search. Table 8.4 shows the confusion matrices of the SVM classifiers for the COVID-19 data set without any feature selection methods and following the use of all feature selection methods. Furthermore, tables 8.5 and 8.6 compare various classification algorithms and feature subset evaluators. It was shown that multiple strategies might be utilised to select the optimal subset from the data set. The usage of an accurate feature selection strategy improved the classification algorithm's accuracy.

8.6 Conclusions

In conclusion, feature selection is a multi-objective step which helped us to investigate two main objectives, namely, decreasing the features and improving the classification performance. Recently, researchers introduced FS methods to increase accuracy and reduce the model building time of ML classifiers. Such methods can significantly reduce the model building time without sacrificing detection accuracy. FS plays an important role in data-mining processes; it chooses the significant features by removing redundant features from the COVID-19 data set to improve performance, e.g. prediction accuracy and to reduce the build time. In this chapter, the wrapper and filter methods were utilized on the COVID-19 data set. Two different evaluators were used for each method. FilterSubsetEval with the 'best first' search was used for the filter method, and the wrapper method used WrapperSubsetEval with the 'best first' search method. The SVM classifier's accuracy rate on the training set was compared to the accuracy rate obtained using feature selection methods. The findings show that when the dimensions of the COVID-19 data set were reduced, the accuracy rate of diagnosis improved for all methods. Finally, SVM classification of the reduced data set using FilterSubsetEval with 'best first' search had a higher accuracy rate (99.53%) than the other methods used. Furthermore, classification results can differ in accuracy rates when using different methods of feature selection and classification algorithms on different disease data sets.

References and further reading

[1] Huang C, Wang Y, Li X, Ren L, Zhao J, Hu Y and Cao B 2020 Clinical features of patients infected with 2019 novel coronavirus in Wuhan, China *Lancet* **395** 497–506

[2] Chen N, Zhou M, Dong X, Qu J, Gong F, Han Y and Zhang L 2020 Epidemiological and clinical characteristics of 99 cases of 2019 novel coronavirus pneumonia in Wuhan, China: a descriptive study *Lancet* **395** 507–13

[3] Hui D S, Azhar E I, Madani T A, Ntoumi F, Kock R, Dar O and Petersen E 2020 The continuing 2019-nCoV epidemic threat of novel coronaviruses to global health—the latest 2019 novel coronavirus outbreak in Wuhan, China *Int. J. Infect. Dis.* **91** 264–6
[4] Rahman M M, Talukder A, Chowdhury M M H, Talukder R and Akter R 2020 Coronaviruses in wild birds–a potential and suitable vector for global distribution *Vet. Med. Sci.* **7** 264–72
[5] Hasan A M, Hala M, El Kader A and Hossam A 2021 An intelligent detection system for Covid-19 diagnosis using CT-images *J. Eng. Sci.* **49** 476–508
[6] Li K, Fang Y, Li W, Pan C, Qin P, Zhong Y and Li S 2020 CT image visual quantitative evaluation and clinical classification of coronavirus disease (COVID-19) *Eur. Radiol.* **30** 4407–16
[7] Nour M, Cömert Z and Polat K 2020 A novel medical diagnosis model for COVID-19 infection detection based on deep features and Bayesian optimization *Appl. Soft Comput.* **97** 106580
[8] Yang R, Li X, Liu H, Zhen Y, Zhang X, Xiong Q and Zeng W 2020 Chest CT severity score: an imaging tool for assessing severe COVID-19 *Radiol.: Cardiothorac. Imaging* **2** e200047
[9] El-Kenawy E S M, Ibrahim A, Mirjalili S, Eid M M and Hussein S E 2020 Novel feature selection and voting classifier algorithms for COVID-19 classification in CT images *IEEE Access* **8** 179317–35
[10] Nouri-Moghaddam B, Ghazanfari M and Fathian M 2021 A novel multi-objective forest optimization algorithm for wrapper feature selection *Expert Syst. Appl.* **175** 114737
[11] Brezočnik L, Fister I and Podgorelec V 2018 Swarm intelligence algorithms for feature selection: a review *Appl. Sci.* **8** 1521
[12] Ariani A and Samsuryadi S 2021 Classification of kidney disease using genetic modified KNN and artificial BEE colony algorithm *Sinergi.* **25** 177–84
[13] Abdulkareem N M, Abdulazeez A M, Zeebaree D Q and Hasan D A 2021 COVID-19 world vaccination progress using machine learning classification algorithms *Qubahan Acad. J.* **1** 100–5
[14] Hossam A, Magdy A, Fawzy A and Abd El-Kader S M 2020 An Integrated IoT System to Control the Spread of COVID-19 *Egypt Int. Conf. on Advanced Intelligent Systems and Informatics V* 336–46
[15] https://kaggle.com/luisblanche/covidct?select=CT_NonCOVID
[16] COVID-CT/Images-processed at master · UCSD-AI4H/COVID-CT GitHub
[17] Wang L, Lin Z Q and Wong A 2020 Covid-net: a tailored deep convolutional neural network design for detection of covid-19 cases from chest x-ray images *Sci. Rep.* **10** 1–12
[18] Singh V, Poonia R C, Kumar S, Dass P, Agarwal P, Bhatnagar V and Raja L 2020 Prediction of COVID-19 corona virus pandemic based on time series data using Support Vector Machine *J. Discr. Math. Sci. Cryptog.* **23** 1583–97
[19] Garg P and Jain T 2017 A comparative study on histogram equalization and cumulative histogram equalization *Int. J. New Technol. Res.* **3** 263242
[20] Apostolopoulos I D and Mpesiana T A 2020 Covid-19: automatic detection from x-ray images utilizing transfer learning with convolutional neural networks *Phys. Eng. Sci. Med.* **43** 635–40
[21] Alqudah A M, Qazan S, Alquran H, Qasmieh I A and Alqudah A 2020 Covid-19 detection from x-ray images using different artificial intelligence hybrid models Jordan *J. Elec. Eng.* **6** 168–78

IOP Publishing

Artificial Intelligence Strategies for Analyzing COVID-19 Pneumonia Lung Imaging, Volume 1
Characterization approaches
Ayman El-Baz and Jasjit S Suri

Chapter 9

Post-analysis of COVID-19 pneumonia based on chest CT images using AI algorithms: a clinical point of view

M Parimala Devi, G Boopathi Raja, T Sathya and V Gowrishankar

COVID-19 has placed the human world in a vulnerable position, suspending life and taking thousands of lives all over the world. At the beginning of 2020, SARS-CoV-2 spread all over the globe. Artificial intelligence (AI) can help in the accelerated assessment of CT scans by distinguishing COVID-19 from other clinical conditions. It would be helpful if COVID-19 could be detected automatically and accurately using chest Computed Tomography (CT) images. Therefore, researchers should aim to develop and validate a fully automatic COVID-19 diagnostic framework using chest CT images. COVID-19 can be diagnosed and community-acquired COVID-19 pneumonia can be distinguished from all other lung diseases using a deep learning approach.

9.1 Introduction

During November 2019, a novel coronavirus, SARS-CoV-2, started to emerge, causing a respiratory-related illness known as COVID-19. This illness has been proved to cause complicated health issues with symptoms starting from moderate to severe illness and the possibility of organ failure and death. It ranges from a moderate self-limiting respiratory infection to extreme progressive pneumonia, causing multiple organ loss and death [1, 2]. There are strong reasons to be concerned about the virus's symptoms as the pandemic progresses, causing a growing number of reported cases. In addition, COVID-19 patients can suffer from severe respiratory illness and cardiovascular complications [3]. The importance of determining effective approaches to solving COVID-19-related problems has gained a lot of press coverage. However, an important and challenging problem

doi:10.1088/978-0-7503-3795-3ch9

faced by researchers and health experts is the huge amount of available data, which may increase exponentially. This is known as big data, which in turn complicates the battle against the coronavirus. However, artificial intelligence (AI) can play a role in the growth and advancement of global healthcare systems [4]. AI has recently sparked increased study in several fields, including economics [5], medicine [6], engineering [7], and psychology [8]. It is important to coordinate and manage medical, logistical, and human resources in a disaster such as this outbreak. AI can play an important role in these areas; thus, it not only helps with diagnostics but also saves time in a situation in which even an hour saved could save lives in all areas where the COVID-19 virus is a severe problem. As a result of AI's increasing performance in clinical environments, it can help to reduce the number of undesirable effects while also improving productivity and efficiency in large-scale trials [9], and higher levels of prediction and diagnosis precision are predicted [10]. Using big data to model viral behavior will help researchers in every country. Outcome analysis allows healthcare authorities to prepare their countries for an epidemic and make well-informed choices [11]. Even though AI has the potential to help healthcare providers combat COVID-19 by helping with recovery plans, emergency detection, enhancement, and improvement monitoring approaches, such as image processing algorithms and advanced medical analytics, it has not been widely adopted. Image-based medical diagnosis is one domain that can benefit from AI's useful feedback, as it can provide fast and precise COVID-19 diagnosis and save lives [12]. AI therapies might bridge the gap between machine-learning-based solutions and medical standards and protocols in the field of COVID-19-related problems. AI specialists will utilize these platforms to help the relationships between various criteria to be established and speed up processes to attain optimal performance.

This chapter mainly discusses the results of recent studies focused on COVID-19 and its numerous problems in order to generalize and propose a range of methods applicable to vulnerable populations, epidemiology, radiology, and other fields. Section 9.2 examines and addresses the potentials of AI methods to solve COVID-19-related problems as research progresses. Artificial Neural Network (ANN)-based methods for large data processing are presented in section 9.3. The platform is described in section 9.4, and a discussion is offered in section 9.5.

9.2 COVID-19 testing

The analysis of samples to check whether SARS-CoV-2 is present or has ever been present is included in the COVID-19 testing process. The two major categories of testing are detection of the coronavirus and detection of SARS-CoV-2 antibodies produced in response to pathogens. Molecular tests based on molecular components are used to classify particular patients as well as to help public health officials track down and monitor outbreaks. Alternatively, antibody tests (serology immuno-assays) can determine whether an individual has ever had the disease. Antibodies are much less efficient in the identification of infections related to COVID-19 because they take weeks to develop after infection. However, they may be utilized to determine the prevalence of a disease, which aids in determining the infection fatality rate.

Individual governments have implemented a variety of research procedures, including who should be tested, how much they should be tested, the review protocols, sample selection, and how the test findings should be used. This variability is likely to have had a substantial impact on the number of incidents and records.

Medical laboratory scientists also conduct test research in advanced, high-throughput medical laboratories. Point-of-care monitoring is also performed in doctors' offices and parking lots, as well as schools, institutional environments, and transit centres.

9.2.1 Detection of the virus

Viruses are often identified by analyzing the inner DNA of the virus or protein fragments on the surface of the virus. Antigen scans are procedures that look for viral antigens (parts of the virus).

A variety of techniques may be developed to screen for the virus by detecting its DNA. These are classified as molecular studies in molecular biology terms. In 2021, the reverse transcription-polymerase chain reaction (RT-PCR) was the most favorable and widely used molecular test. Other molecular testing methods include microarray analysis, digital polymerase chain reactions, CRISPR, and next-generation sequencing.

9.2.1.1 Reverse transcription polymerase chain reaction test

The polymerase chain reaction (PCR) is a technique that amplifies (replicates) a small, well-defined DNA fragment hundreds of thousands of times to produce enough material for research. Certain chemicals are used to prepare test samples, allowing the DNA to be removed. Reverse transcription is the process of converting RNA to DNA.

The reverse transcription-polymerase chain reaction (RT-PCR) begins with reverse transcription, which is used to obtain DNA; this is then amplified by the PCR to produce enough DNA for analysis. SARS-CoV-2 contains RNA which can be detected using RT-PCR. The RT-PCR procedure takes a few hours on average. Molecular or genetic assays are other names for these techniques.

Automation, better throughput, and more efficient instrumentation are all benefits of real-time PCR (qPCR), which has been the tool of choice. The combined technique is known as quantitative RT-PCR or real-time RT-PCR. It is commonly abbreviated as RT-qPCR, rRT-PCR, or qRT-PCR, but RT-PCR and PCR are also used.

The probability of identifying the virus is determined by the sampling process and the elapsed time after infection. Throat swab examinations, according to Drosten, are only valid for the first week. The virus may then migrate to the lungs after leaving the throat. Sputum or deep airway selection is favored in the second week.

Saliva collection might be just as successful as nose and throat swabs, although this has yet to be confirmed. The use of saliva samples may decrease the danger to medical personnel by allowing close physical contact to be avoided. It also makes the patient feel more at ease. Using this approach, individuals who have been quarantined are allowed to take their own samples. The diagnostic value of a saliva test is determined by the location of the sample (deep throat, oral cavity, or salivary glands). Compared to swab tests, saliva has been shown to have higher sensitivity and reliability. After the onset of symptoms, the viral load estimated to be present in upper respiratory specimens decreases.

9.2.1.2 Other molecular tests

The virus's genome is also amplified by isothermal nucleic acid amplification studies. Since they do not need regular heating and cooling cycles, they are faster than PCR. Fluorescent tags are used to detect DNA in these samples, which are read out by advanced devices.

9.2.1.2.1 Antigen tests

An antigen is a pathogen component which triggers an immune response. Antigen studies always aim to identify antigen proteins on the surface of the virus. In the case of SARS-CoV-2, these are generally proteins found on the surface spikes. Although this method is less sensitive than viral PCR testing, SARS-CoV-2 antigens can be detected before the first COVID-19 symptoms appear.

Antigen testing might be a way to scale up testing even further. In this method, only one sample can be processed at a time by isothermal nucleic acid amplification machines. RT-PCR procedures are accurate, but they take a lot of time and effort and they require specialized staff.

Samples may be taken using a nasopharyngeal swab, an anterior nares swab, or saliva. After that, the swab is exposed to paper strips that contain coronavirus antigen-binding synthetic antibodies. Antigens attach to the strips, causing an effect that can be seen. The testing time is less than 30 min and the results can be obtained quickly; this method does not need any special equipment or preparation.

Respiratory virus swabs always lack adequate antigen content for detection. This is particularly true for patients who are asymptomatic with little to no nasal discharge. In an antigen examination, viral proteins are not multiplied. According to the WHO, related antigen scans for infectious illnesses such as flu have sensitivities of between 34% and 80%. Antigen testing can easily determine whether asymptomatic individuals are infectious, and PCR testing can be used to validate the diagnosis if more information is needed.

9.2.1.2.2 Sniff tests

The sudden loss of smell can be utilized in frequent patient testing for COVID-19. According to research published by the National Institutes of Health, those infected with COVID-19 were unable to identify a 25% combination of ethanol and water. A sniff test would not be definitive, since a loss of sense of smell can have several causes, so it would lead to the need for a PCR test. There has been a demand for systematic sniff tests because the absence of the sense of smell appears before any other signs. Sniff tests have been largely overlooked by healthcare bureaucracies, even though they are quick, easy, and self-administrable daily. As a result, several medical journals have published editorials in favor of sniff research.

9.2.1.2.3 Imaging

Bilateral multilobar ground-glass opacities with peripheral or posterior distributions are quite common visible features on early CT scans. CT allows for a more precise identification of COVID-19 than RT-PCR.

As the disease progresses, subpleural domination, 'crazy paving', and convergence can appear. COVID-19 should not be diagnosed using chest CT scans or chest x-rays. The radiological results of COVID-19 are not very clear.

9.2.1.2.4 Antibody tests

Antibodies are produced by the body when it is exposed to viral infection to help neutralize the virus. Antibodies can be detected in blood samples. Antibody monitoring can be used to determine what proportion of a population has already been infected by a disease, and then the disease's mortality rate can be determined. It can also be used to determine whether a unit of convalescent plasma contains antibodies that can treat COVID-19 and whether a vaccination has evoked a healthy immune response.

The efficacy and duration of defense against SARS-CoV-2 provided by antibodies have yet to be determined. As a result, a positive antibody test cannot guarantee immunity from infection in the future. Furthermore, it is unknown whether mild or asymptomatic infections result in enough antibodies to be detected by a test. Antibodies to certain pathogens can last for years in the body, while antibodies to others fade away.

IgM and IgG are the most well-known antibodies. IgM antibodies are usually found several days after diagnosis, but the number of antibodies produced during the infection and afterward is uncertain. IgG antibodies are usually observed 10–14 days after infection and peak at about 28 days. SARS-CoV-2 follows a different pattern of antibody production than other viruses, with IgM occurring after IgG, in conjunction with IgG, or not at all. The median IgM detection time is five days after the onset of symptoms, while the median IgG detection time is 14 days. IgG levels are significantly reduced after two to three months.

Antibody tests are more reliable than genetic tests in confirming infection. On day seven of their illness, only 30% of patients who had a positive genetic test also had a positive antibody test.

9.2.2 Types of test

9.2.2.1 Rapid diagnostic test (RDT)

A positive/negative lateral flow assay that can be done at the point of therapy is widely used in RDTs. Blood, saliva, or fluids from a nasal swab can be processed by RDTs. RDTs show whether the results are positive or negative using colored lines.

9.2.2.2 Enzyme-linked immunosorbent assay (ELISA)

ELISAs may be qualitative or quantitative, and almost all of them necessitate the use of a lab. These tests typically use whole blood, plasma, or serum extracts. A viral protein, such as the SARS-CoV-2 spike protein, is coated onto a plate. The samples are incubated with the antigen, allowing some antibodies to react to it. A second wash of antibodies is then used to detect the antibody–protein complex, which produces a color/fluorescent readout.

9.2.2.3 Neutralization assay

Neutralization assays are used to establish whether sample antibodies can protect test cells from viral infection. Blood, plasma, or serum can be used as samples in these tests. Cells that allow for viral replication are cultured in the test. By changing antibody concentrations, researchers can analyze how many test antibodies inhibit viral reproduction.

9.2.2.4 Chemiluminescent immunoassay

Chemiluminescent immunoassays are used in quantitative lab samples. They use blood, plasma, or serum samples. The samples contain a known viral protein, buffer reagents, and uncommon, enzyme-labeled antibodies. The final product is luminous. In a chemiluminescent microparticle immunoassay, magnetic protein-coated microparticles are employed.

Antibodies that bind to viral proteins result in a complex. Antibodies with secondary enzyme labels are bound to these complexes. As a result of the chemical reaction, light is emitted. The number of antibodies is calculated using the radiance. This test can detect antibodies of various types, including IgG, IgM, and IgA.

9.2.2.5 Neutralizing antibodies versus binding antibodies

The vast majority of large-scale COVID-19 antibody research, if not all, focuses exclusively on binding antibodies, ignoring the more significant neutralizing antibodies (NAb). An NAb is an antibody that shields a cell against infection by neutralizing an infectious particle's biological effects.

After neutralization, the particle is no longer infectious or harmful. A binding antibody's purpose is to bind to the pathogen while leaving it infectious, so that the immune system can kill it. It can also increase infectivity by interfering with macrophage receptors. Since most COVID-19 antibody tests are positive if only binding antibodies are present, they cannot tell if the subject has acquired defensive NAbs to prevent reinfection.

Binding antibodies are thought to indicate the presence of NAbs, and total antibody responses are thought to be related to NAb responses in many viral diseases, but this is not the case with COVID-19. According to a report, ten of the 175 recovering patients in China with minor symptoms had no detectable NAbs at the time of discharge or thereafter. It was not stated whether these patients recovered without the use of NAbs or were in danger of reinfection. Viruses such as HIV can evade NAb responses even when NAbs are present, adding to the uncertainty.

NAbs to the original SARS virus (the precursor of the contemporary SARS-CoV-2) remain active for two years before vanishing after six years, according to research. Memory cells, such as memory B and memory T cells, live far longer than most other cells and may be able to decrease the severity of reinfection.

9.2.2.6 Other tests

After regeneration, most patients' upper respiratory specimens no longer contain detectable viral RNA. Three days after regeneration, RNA concentrations are normally below the threshold required for successful isolation of replication-competent viruses from those that are not. There is no connection between the length of illness and the amount of viral RNA shed in upper respiratory specimens during recovery.

9.3 The role of artificial intelligence in the COVID-19 pandemic

The previous sections emphasized the implementation of several AI-based solutions that can supplement existing COVID-19-related conventional approaches in healthcare systems around the globe. These strategies and procedures were created in response to and depend on the most relevant AI-related published medical updates and the most recent COVID-19 updates to demonstrate strategies and techniques for improving efficacy.

Suggestions for enhancing and speeding up the development of ANN-based techniques to create recovery methods, patient care, identification, and diagnosis are discussed in this part. However, a certain amount of human input and coordination in various roles is required for AI tools to perform optimally during the COVID-19 pandemic. Data scientists, on the other hand, have a special perspective on AI's benefits and drawbacks, since they code AI systems [12].

The flowchart in figure 9.1 depicts the various stages in the implementation of AI-based approaches to solve the challenges related to COVID-19. The first step is to prepare the necessary information for data processing, which is required to understand, analyse, and store large amounts of data. Medical evidence, such as health notes, documentation, images, and other sources of knowledge that can be converted into data that a computer can understand, is the subject of this review. Some of the goals of data comprehension are to understand data characteristics and identify fundamental aspects, such as the volume of data and the total number of variables that characterise the data. Data preparation is required before the data can be processed and analyzed. This consists of refining and transforming raw data. In other words, it is a procedure for reformatting, correcting, and combining data to create enriched data. The collection, processing, and optimization of data such as patient, physical, consumer, and medical data result in big data. Experts review and assess data at this phase as part of machine learning approaches to acquire data with nested structures, patterns, and other properties.

Since human capabilities and abilities are not available to an ML approach, which, unlike humans, can interact with large data sets far beyond what humans can manage or observe at the same time, human input is crucial at this stage.

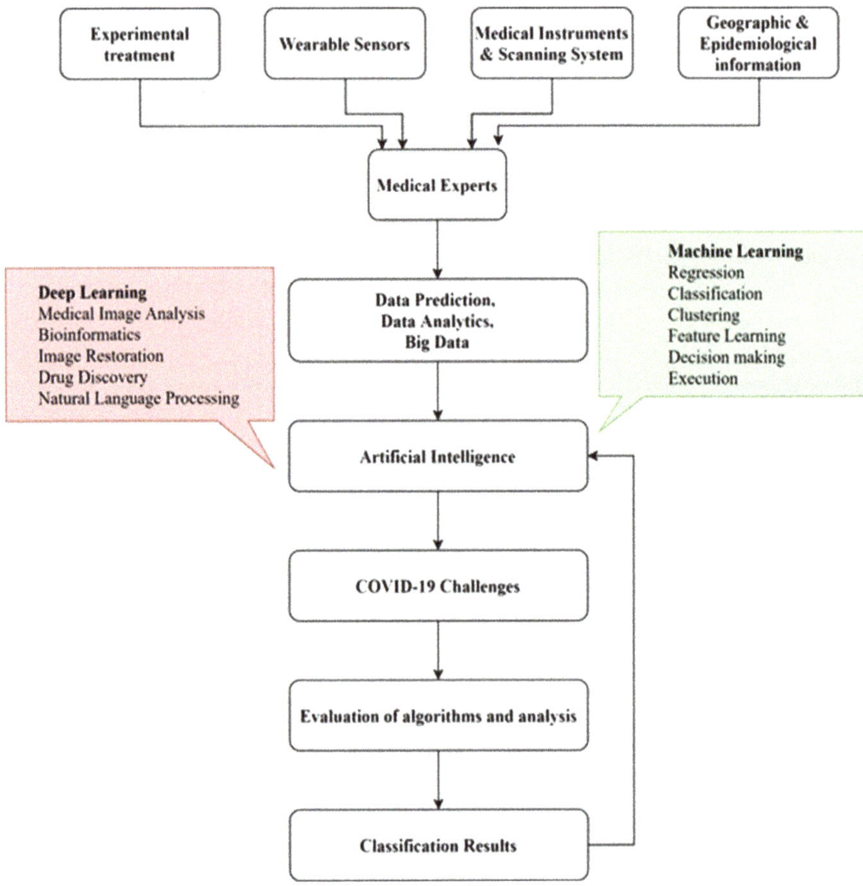

Figure 9.1. Various stages in the implementation of the AI-based approach for the diagnosis of COVID-19.

Deep learning (DL) techniques may also be used in cases in which large or complex data processing presents an obstacle for machine learning (ML) or traditional data processing methods. As can be seen in figure 9.1, DL approaches do not require human involvement. DL is a type of machine learning that comprises many layers of algorithms with diverse outcome interpretations. DL differs from ML in that it addresses data in a different way. Unsupervised learning, in contrast to supervised learning, is described as a kind of machine learning that seeks out undiscovered patterns in a data set with no previous labeling and is characterized by limited human intervention. Traditional medicine, also known as conventional medicine, orthodox medicine, allopathic medicine, biomedicine, and Western medicine, involves the use of medicines, surgery, or radiation to treat infections and prevent complications. AI has the potential to be widely employed in addressing COVID-19, and its objective is to discover the best possible solutions to the COVID-19-related issues that have posed the greatest obstacles to healthcare systems. As a result, (i) extremely vulnerable groups, (ii) illness, and (iii) monitoring, detection and diagnosis are treated as three separate categories.

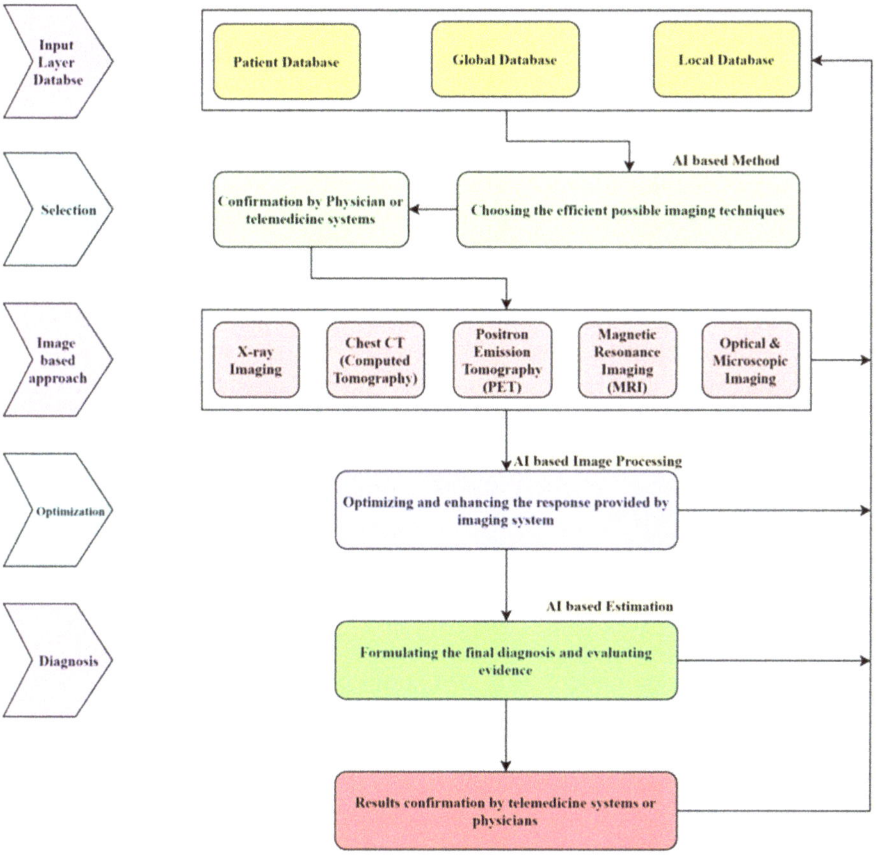

Figure 9.2. Classification, analysis, and improvement of medical imaging approaches using AI-based methods.

Figure 9.2 is a flowchart depicting the different uses of ANNs in diagnosis and symptom tracing in five layers. Although the protocol was created to address COVID-19-related issues, it can also be used for other medical imaging analyses. The first layer, the input layer, is connected to the database and is used to receive data from it. A high-speed channel connects this layer to the main (front-end) devices. The database server is loosely networked, whereas the storage processor is tightly coupled to the main CPU. Database machines can send large packets of data to the mainframe by integrating a large number of microprocessors with database programs.

The selection layer, which is created by an observational ANN-based selector, is responsible for applying the best imaging techniques available based on the system's previous experiences. If the decisions taken by this layer are confirmed by doctors, the third layer's prescribed procedures obtain the necessary images. As a consequence of the previously acquired findings, one or more imaging approaches can be proposed. X-ray imaging, magnetic resonance imaging (MRI), positron emission tomography (PET), CT scans, optical and digital microscopic imaging methods and applications in pathology can all be used in the treatment. In pathological tests, the traditional optical microscope has become the standard instrument. PET scans are useful imaging tests for determining the nature and consistency of body tissues and organ functions [13]. Under certain circumstances, PET scans can diagnose disease before other imaging tests can identify it. A radioactive drug (tracer) is used in the PET scan to provide this functionality [14].

The fourth layer manages image enhancement and optimization. The network configuration was created using DL technology, and features were extracted using the classic ResNet algorithm to construct a classification network that can distinguish between COVID-19 and influenza-A viral pneumonia [15]. The fifth layer is for optimal diagnosis based on saved data in the system, and it is a layer in which learning algorithms based on an ANN method may be used. Convolutional neural networks (CNNs) and other deep learning systems are thought to be the best way to achieve these objectives. The reason for this is that this kind of network is very good at nonlinear simulation and has a lot of applications in medical image analysis and diagnosis [16].

9.4 A possible platform for accelerating conventional methods

The main objective of this chapter is to identify therapies for COVID-19-infected highly vulnerable populations. We will aim to demonstrate how ANN-based approaches may be used in conjunction with older methods to achieve the best potential results. Patients must be kept active, as indicated by [17]. The COVID-19 database, which highlights health risks and cardiovascular conditions, aids in assessing the history of cardiovascular complications, developing a risk model for heart complications, and recognizing and/or forecasting the responses to different treatment modalities.

This section describes an extreme learning machine (ELM) model that uses data from studies published in [17] to forecast appropriate medications for people suffering from cardiovascular complications. Previous examples added to the model can be used by the ELM ANN to simulate optimal outputs. This implies that actual data is used to train the supervised model in the network. As a result, the ELM will recommend the best available medications for heart complications based on different types of viral infection in previous cases.

The learning speed of ELMs is significantly faster than that of traditional feedforward network learning algorithms such as the back-propagation (BP) algorithm, and it achieves improved generalization accuracy [18]. Traditional tuning-based algorithms, on the other hand, often require far fewer hidden neurons than ELM [19]. Several previous studies [18, 20, 21] looked at ELM with fixed network architectures. A research or verification protocol may be used to forecast new data during the training phase. SARS-CoV-2 can cause myocarditis, vascular inflammation, and cardiac arrhythmias, according to [17]. The proposed model is based on evidence provided that predicts how SARS-CoV-2 affects the cardiovascular system [17]. As a result, the proposed model has the potential to reduce the possibility of cardiovascular risks. It may also forecast the trend of cardiovascular complications, allowing it to predict reactions to various treatment modalities. As a result, ELMs are preferred for this type of problem due to their properties and many benefits.

Heart disruption is another COVID-19 problem within the older section of the community. It is important for cardiac clinicians to be vigilant and establish a systematic approach to these patients, as well as involve them in the development of algorithms for their diagnosis in the early stages of the disease, before definitive universal COVID-19 examinations and a better knowledge of the disease's final stages become available [21]. In elderly patients, the excessive use of fluids and medications such as NSAIDs should be avoided because they can disrupt the salt and water balance. In vulnerable elderly patients with underlying systemic cardiac disease, reference [22] and biomarkers should be used with caution.

The model was based on the long short-term memory (LSTM) network proposed in [22]. To forecast the optimal treatment as accurately as possible, this model depends on properly considered inputs. LSTM networks are particularly useful for learning sequences of longer-term patterns of undetermined length due to their capacity to store lengthy memories [23].

LSTMs manage constant error flow using the internal states of special memory cells with multiplicative gates [23]. In recurrent neural networks (RNNs), the problem of vanishing gradient is solved by LSTM neural networks [24]. Others who referred to and popularized LSTMs [25] followed Hochreiter and Schmidhuber, who were the first to present them [24]. Over the last ten years, LSTM NNs have become increasingly common and are widely used in human behavior recognition, face recognition, robot control, handwriting recognition, and other areas [26], and they have performed admirably in speech recognition [27] and text classification [28, 29]. According to reference [30], fault estimation is a central theme in nonlinear systems [31].

Alternative techniques for forecasting COVID-19 outbreaks are ANN-based approaches. An overview of the database areas can be found on Github[1]. Geographic information has been gathered in two ways: by referring to individual settlements and by referring to regions that are administrative units. Xu *et al* organized real-time epidemiological data to forecast illness transmission [32]. Using clinical and regional big data, a DL method driven by RNN forecasts the distribution of infection associated with COVID-19. Variations of RNNs can be used to forecast the propagation of infection based on regional and clinical evidence. However, it appears that LSTM networks [24], gated recurrent unit RNNs (GRURNNs) [33], and clockwork RNNs (CW-RNNs) [34] are the best structures for making predictions. The RNN, also known as the auto associative or feedback network, is a type of ANN that uses relations between units to create a guided cycle [35]. RNNs constitute a well-known DL family that has shown potential in several machine learning and computer vision tasks [36]. When using this model, though, the quantification of contextual inputs such as country and location is a significant challenge.

[1] https://github.com/ncbi-nlp/COVID-19-CT-CXR.

The proposed ANN model can be used to propose a virus epidemiological model for various locations. The key goal of the proposed structure is to use DL-based approaches to increase the precision and speed of recognizing and classifying the problems caused by SARS-CoV-2.

Although radiological tests such as CT scans and digital photography (DR) have been effective in screening, diagnosing, and monitoring COVID-19 patients [37], there has been no prior experience that can help radiologists and technologists to deal with COVID-19 patients. Negative RT-PCR results crosschecked against CT characteristics are important indicators of COVID-19 in areas affected by the epidemic, highlighting the importance of early diagnosis of the virus, which offers the population and clinicians a greater chance of controlling viral transmission [38]. Even though radiological examinations such as CT are helpful for screening and diagnosis, there is evidence that a large number of radiologists and technicians have become infected while working with COVID-19 patients [37]. CT scans reveal bilateral, subpleural, ground-glass opacities with air bronchograms, ill-defined borders, and a slight preponderance in the right lower lobe in pneumonia caused by COVID-19 [39]. The picture classification model makes it easier to distinguish between pathogens based on their presence and shape. The model uses relative distance-from-edge as an extra weight to learn the approximate position details of the patch in the pulmonary picture [15]. Although a large number of medical images can be collected for machine learning systems, radiologists are the only ones that can retrieve diagnostic information from images and make it available as structured test records [40].

COVID-19 infections damage human airway epithelial cells, as shown in [41]. A suggested neural network model, the generative adversarial network (GAN), is discussed below. The feature extraction technique can be used to examine electron microscopy images. GANs are a type of neural network model in which two networks, one of which is used for image formation and the other of which is used for discrimination, are trained at the same time [42]. GANs [43] can accurately model the latent distribution of the training data. Picture-to-image conversion [43], segmentation [44], and a host of other medical image computing subfields [45] have all made progress using GANs. The adversarial training scheme has recently enjoyed a lot of popularity due to its success in preventing domain transfer and producing new image samples. This model has achieved state-of-the-art efficiency in a variety of tasks, including text-to-image synthesis [46], super-resolution [47], and image-to-image conversion [48]. These are all linked to image development. Estimating the degree of cardiac activity is another issue that ANN-based methods can overcome. According to reference [49], the COVID-19 virus is a significant cause of myocarditis. Reference [49] examined the cardiac impact of a COVID-19 infection capable of causing severe acute respiratory syndrome and concluded that clinical recognition of the association between COVID-19 and acute myocarditis could aid in the close monitoring of compromised patients and could help public health officials to better understand such life-threatening abnormalities. An LSTM network has been proposed to assess COVID-19-related cardiac involvement as a result of these findings and suggestions [49]. Feedforward neural networks are restricted because they can only transmit signals in one direction, from input to output. RNNs are favored because they allow signals to flow in both directions, forming network loops and allowing hidden units to communicate internally [50]. Unlike a feedforward neural network, an RNN processes sequential inputs through a recurring hidden state in which each stage's activation is dependent on the activation of the one before it, allowing the network to exhibit complex temporal behavior [36].

Remdesivir's behavior, as well as some clinical parameters, can be predicted using an AI-based model. According to [51], patients with less chronic infections in the upper respiratory tract may require different therapeutic therapies compared to those with significant viral replication and systemic virus transmission, based on viral kinetics testing. However, since there are very few patients in this situation, data processing should be performed with caution. Reference [49] examines the clinical and biological evidence of five COVID-19 patients. The actions of Remdesivir (an antiviral drug for COVID-19 post-infection care used in therapies as well as in hospital stays), are estimated using these individuals' medical records, which include chronic disease or a history of chronic illness, signs, age, gender, and test findings on hospital entry. Nonetheless, the patient images from the ELM network were insufficient. ELM is a least-squares-based learning algorithm for generalized single-hidden-layer feedforward networks (SLFNs) that can be used to estimate regression problems or classify tasks [52].

Output weights (linking the hidden layer to the output layer) are determined analytically using a Moore–Penrose (MP) generalized inverse [19], in contrast to the random range of input weights (linking the input layer to the hidden layer) and hidden biases of ELM. As a result, the proposed model can be trained using the ELM technique.

In the last section of the diagnostic scheme, we suggest a model equipped with GAN to estimate the risk of viral gastrointestinal infection. Xiao *et al* present evidence for SARS-CoV-2 gastrointestinal illness as well as the possibility of fecal–oral transfer [53]. Because the virus spreads from infected to uninfected cells, identifying viral-specific target cells or organs is critical for defining viral transmission pathways.

Over 20% of SARS-CoV-2 patients had positive viral RNA in their feces even after negative viral RNA conversion in the respiratory tract, indicating viral gastrointestinal infection and the potential for fecal–oral transmission even after viral clearance in the respiratory tract [53].

Routine rRT-PCR monitoring for SARS-CoV-2 in feces is strongly suggested for SARS-CoV-2 patients. Furthermore, transmission-based treatments for hospitalized SARS-CoV-2 patients should be performed if rRT-PCR monitoring reveals a positive fecal test [53]. COVID-19-induced gastrointestinal infection is being researched. The histology and immunofluorescent staining of the duodenum, rectum, intestine, and oesophagus in the sample reveals a COVID-19-related gastrointestinal infection. These fluorescent staining images were created using laser scanning confocal microscopy [53]. The extraction of a function from these images will be used to build a GAN network to predict the likelihood of a viral gastrointestinal infection, which will aid patients in their recovery.

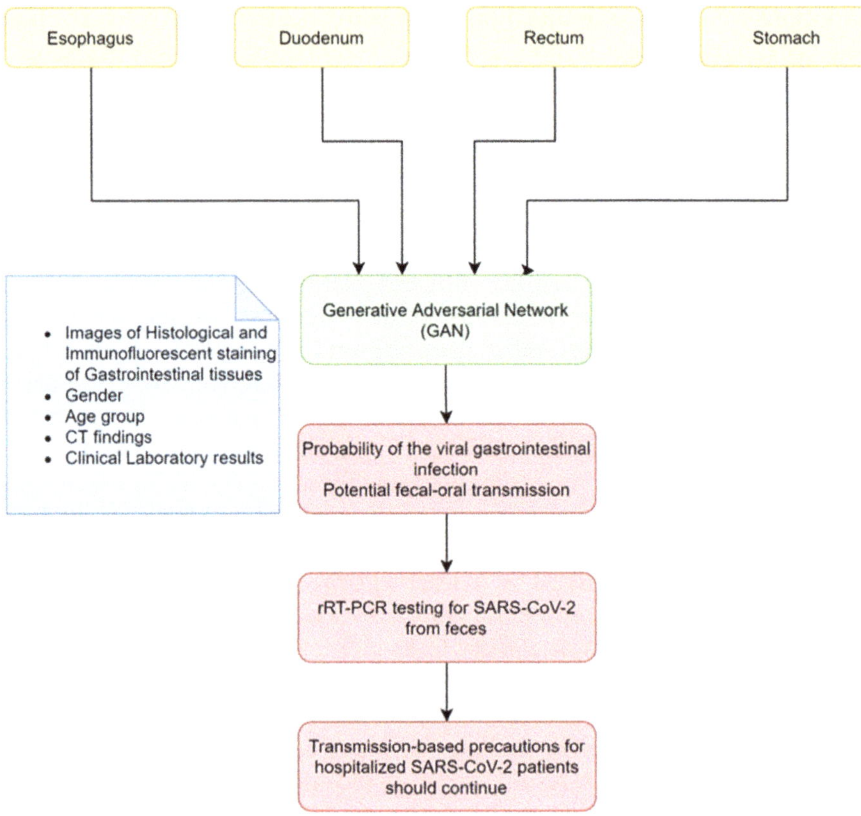

Figure 9.3. The technique for estimating the chance of viral gastrointestinal infection from feces using a combination of GAN and rRT-PCR testing for SARS-CoV-2 to establish transmission-based precautions for hospitalized SARS-CoV-2 patients.

Figure 9.3 shows how this model decides whether to continue or stop transmission-based precautions for hospitalized patients. SARS-CoV-2 patients are tested for SARS-CoV-2 using rRT-PCR. The GAN generation technique, which projects a conventional distribution onto complicated high-dimensional real-world data distributions, outperforms other discriminative tasks (e.g., classification and clustering) [54]. In addition to image creation, GANs have been utilized for tasks such as video generation, visual monitoring [55], domain adaptability, hash coding, and attribute learning [56].

In medical imaging, GANs have been used by two distinct types of consumer [42]. Due to their focus on the generative component, they encourage study and experimentation with the underlying nature of the training data, as well as being able to learn how to generate new images. Advanced diagnoses of COVID-19 patients can be successfully performed using DL models, as shown in this report, which can be a useful supplemental diagnostic tool for clinical doctors who regularly work with patients [57].

9.5 Discussion

Advanced machine learning algorithms (LSTM, GAN, RNN, and ELM) combine and interpret large-scale data from COVID-19 patients to help researchers better understand the virus's propagation pattern, increase detection speed and precision, create new, innovative therapeutic methods, and even classify the individuals who are most vulnerable to the disease based on their genetic and physiological characteristics [58]. Despite the great recognition AI has gained for its role in enhancing performance, competitiveness, and procedures in various industries, it has been criticized because of the limited number of consumers who capture, store, handle, and access the data [59]. However, since it tracks and gathers data from social media, newsfeeds, and airline ticketing services, AI, according to Heyman, makes it easy to know whether bad things are happening or when COVID-19 needs to be addressed.

The techniques suggested will encompass a substantial quantity of distinct knowledge collected from recent breakthroughs and publications in the field. Even though there are many other inputs, clinical evidence is the one that almost all medicines rely on. In high-risk communities, it is especially crucial to keep track of COVID-19 patients' clinical features during pregnancy or the disease cycle. The model described here can be used by patients with heart failure who are at the hyper-inflammation stage of the disease, as well as those who have systemic clinical indicators and cardiovascular symptoms.

For the second instance, which is the optimal treatment style, we advise an LSTM-equipped model. Because lags of varying lengths can occur between major events in a time series, LSTM networks appear to be promising candidates for time series data classification, processing, and prediction. The difficulties of exploding and disappearing gradients that can arise while training traditional RNNs can be readily handled by LSTMs, which are therefore a good suggestion. Another topic that we covered in this chapter was AI's ability to predict epidemiology and outbreaks. The model we propose is based on an RNN with a large number of inputs that can be augmented with data from the database listed in [32]. RNNs are a type of ANN in which the connections between nodes form a directed graph along a temporal chain, allowing for the display of temporal dynamic actions. RNNs run in a loop while attempting to reach the unseen layers, and their future predictions are based on prior experiences before the underlying relationship governing the outcome is understood. Given the importance of the early diagnosis of viral infection, which may aid in more successful viral containment, the clinical and social ramifications of this point cannot be overlooked [38]. Radiological exams, such as computed tomography CT, have been explored as useful ways to test for infection and diagnose it. It was also noted that a large number of radiologists and technologists have become contaminated while examining COVID-19 patients [37]. COVID19 pneumonia is characterized by bilateral, subpleural, ground-glass opacities with air bronchograms, ill-defined margins, and a marginal predominance in the right lower lobe on lung CT scans [39].

COVID-19 is noted for quickly declining respiratory system function, which generally happens in the second week of the disease; thus, current patient wellness cannot guarantee that a patient will not be affected by the disease, and safeguarding recommendations must be followed [60]. This emphasizes the necessity of visualizing and classifying novel human coronaviruses using an ANN-based method. This approach learns how to create new data using the same statistics as those of the training set when it is given a training set. GANs have also been shown to be useful for semi-supervised, completely supervised, and reinforcement learning [61]. In several architectures, LSTM units are used. Inside an LSTM device, one typical architecture includes a cell and three 'regulators' or information flow gates: an input layer, an output layer, and a hidden layer. The cell keeps track of the dependencies between the elements in the input list. The input gate is responsible for determining how much new data flows into the cell, the activation function determines how long a value stays in the cell, and the output gate is in charge of determining the extent to which the value in the cell is utilized to compute the LSTM unit's output activation.

Several techniques are available for reducing the reliance on random feedback [62]. A GAN can forecast the likelihood of contagious gastrointestinal infection in the last event. The generative network is in charge of candidate generation, while the discriminative network is in charge of candidate evaluation [43]. Data distributions are the basis for the competition. The discriminative network separates the generator's candidates from the true data delivery, showing the utility of this feature in an estimated viral gastrointestinal infection.

While the suggested procedures have still not been tested for efficacy, there are several published studies and reliable sources of evidence that demonstrate the efficacy and accuracy of these approaches in a variety of diseases. The most interesting finding is that such powerful approaches based on COVID-19 characteristics can be extended.

9.6 Experimental setup

The proposed network's performance is assessed by utilizing an optimized GAN to produce CT images of COVID-19 and non-COVID-19 patients; tests are carried out to measure classification performance using various DL networks, [63]. Figures 9.4 and 9.5 illustrate examples of COVID-19 and non-COVID-19 training images, respectively.

The SARS-CoV-2 CT scan data set was used to gather COVID-19 and non-COVID-19 chest CT images. There are 2482 COVID-19 CT scan images in the

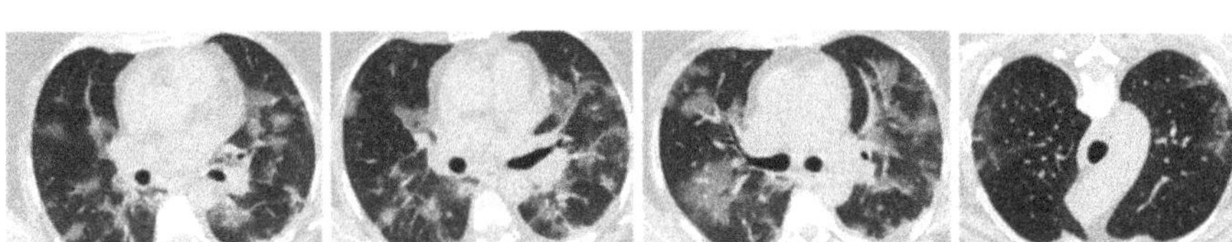

Figure 9.4. Sample COVID-19 training images.

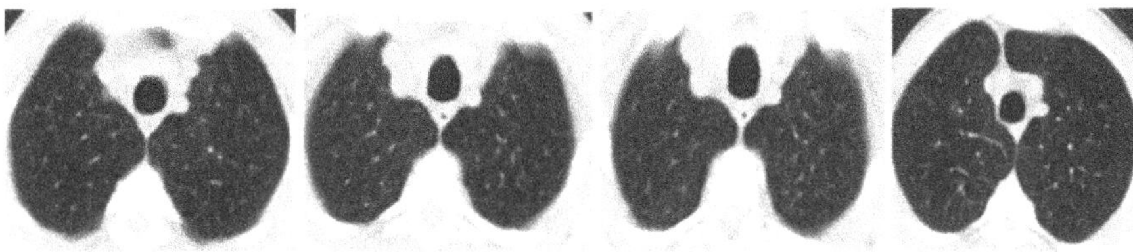

Figure 9.5. Sample non-COVID-19 training images.

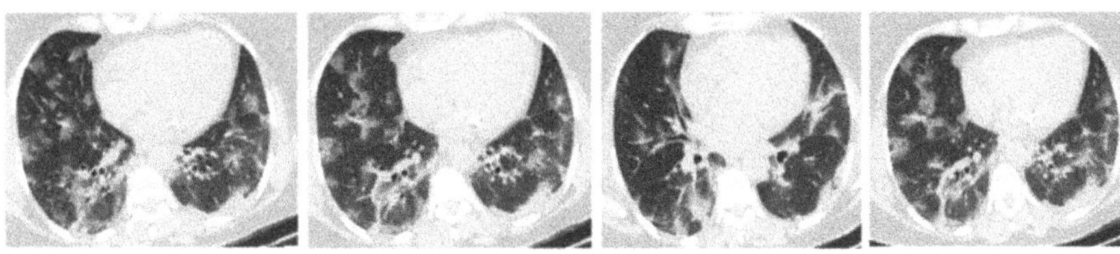

Figure 9.6. Sample COVID-19 test images.

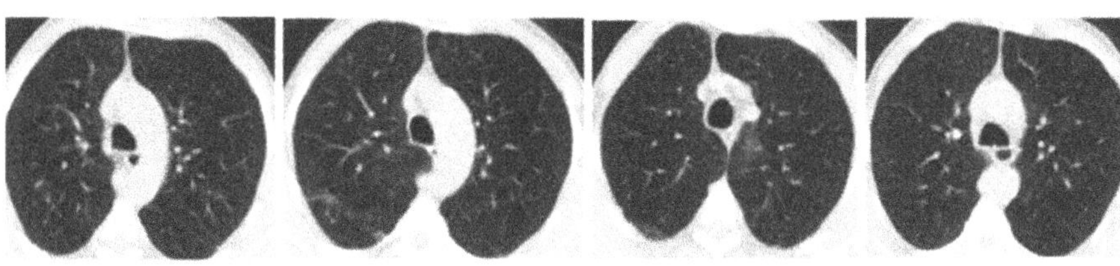

Figure 9.7. Sample non-COVID-19 test images.

collection, including 1230 non-COVID-19 and 1252 COVID-19 images. Figures 9.6 and 9.7 show sample COVID-19 and non-COVID-19 test images, respectively.

The major goal of this study was to autonomously diagnose COVID-19 using CT images that have been analyzed. Therefore, performance metrics, such as accuracy, F1 score, specificity, sensitivity, negative predictive value (NPV), and positive predictive value (PPV) are used to assess the algorithm's performance. Out of all false positive and true negative COVID-19 instances, the NPV determines how many actual negative cases were categorized as negative. The F1 score is a single number that represents the algorithm's accuracy and recall.

9.7 Results and discussion

For the automated diagnosis of COVID-19 using CT scan images, the network efficiency is evaluated; a comparison study is performed for three distinct situations as follows. Table 9.1 and figure 9.8 compare the performance of the DL network with optimized and non-optimized data augmentation, demonstrating the proposed network's benefit.

Table 9.1. Performance comparison of optimized and non-optimized GANs.

Parameter	COVID-19 non-optimized GAN	COVID-19 optimized GAN
Accuracy (%)	91.60	98.78
Sensitivity (%)	84.80	99.78
Specificity (%)	98.40	97.78
F1 Score (%)	90.99	98.79
PPV (%)	84.8	97.82
NPV (%)	98.4	99.77

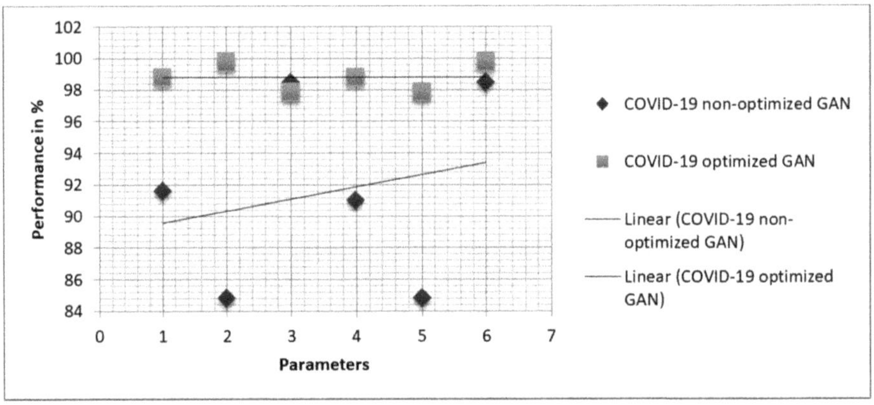

Figure 9.8. Performance metrics of optimized and non-optimized GANs.

9.8 Conclusions

This chapter has focused on recently developed models in the field of AI-based strategies that can be used to solve COVID-19 problems. LSTM, GAN, RNN, and ELM are some of the strategies that have been introduced to integrate COVID-19 diagnostic systems. COVID-19 diagnosis has faced several major problems, including spatial issues, identification and radiology, and highly vulnerable people, all of which have been explored and resolved in this study. We demonstrated a mechanism that chooses suitable models for parameter estimation and prediction using a variety of clinical and non-clinical databases. These platforms can assist AI specialists to analyze large data sets; they can also help clinicians to train computers, develop algorithms, and optimize the acquired data for faster and more precise virus detection. We addressed how attractive these platforms are, which is the case because they can provide a workspace where AI experts and physicians can collaborate. While AI improves the pace at which COVID-19 can be conquered, a further real-world study is needed to gain a full understanding of the benefits and drawbacks of AI-based COVID-19 approaches. Building an array of channels, strategies, tactics, and techniques that combine to accomplish the desired targets and save more lives is critical to success in the fight against COVID-19 and achieving its inevitable demise.

References

[1] Jamshidi M (B) *et al* 2020 Artificial intelligence and COVID-19: deep learning approaches for diagnosis and treatment *IEEE Access* **8** 109581–95

[2] Wang D *et al* 2020 Clinical characteristics of 138 hospitalized patients with 2019 novel coronavirus infected pneumonia in Wuhan, China *JAMA* **323** 1061–9

[3] Guo T *et al* 2020 Cardiovascular implications of fatal outcomes of patients with coronavirus disease 2019 (COVID-19) *JAMA Cardiol.* **5** 811–818

[4] Hamet P and Tremblay J 2017 Artificial intelligence in medicine *Metabolism* **69** S36–S40

[5] Jamshidi M B, Gorjiankhanzad M, Lalbakhsh A and Roshani S 2019 A novel multiobjective approach for detecting money laundering with a neuro-fuzzy technique *Proc. IEEE 16th Int. Conf. Netw., Sens. Control (ICNSC)* 454–8

[6] Mintz Y and Brodie R 2019 Introduction to artificial intelligence in medicine *Minim. Invasive Ther. Allied Technol.* **28** 73–81

[7] Jamshidi M, Lalbakhsh A, Mohamadzade B, Siahkamari H and Mousavi S M H 2019 A novel neural-based approach for design of microstrip filters *AEU-Int. J. Electron. Commun.* **110** 152847

[8] Jamshidi M B, Alibeigi N, Rabbani N, Oryani B and Lalbakhsh A 2018 Artificial neural networks: a powerful tool for cognitive science *Proc. IEEE 9th Annu. Inf. Technol., Electron. Mobile Commun. Conf. (IEMCON)* 674–9

[9] Huang S, Yang J, Fong S and Zhao Q 2019 Mining prognosis index of brain metastases using artificial intelligence *Cancers* **11** 1140

[10] Rashidi P and Bihorac A 2020 Artificial intelligence approaches to improve kidney care *Nature Rev. Nephrol.* **16** 71–2

[11] Ting D S W, Carin L, Dzau V and Wong T Y 2020 Digital technology and COVID-19 *Nature Med.* **26** 459–61

[12] Naudé W 2020 *Artificial intelligence against COVID-19: an early review* 13110 IZA Inst. Labor Econ., Maastricht, The Netherlands

[13] Trotman J *et al* 2014 Prognostic value of PET-CT after first-line therapy in patients with follicular lymphoma:Apooled analysis of central scan review in three multicentre studies *Lancet Haematol.* **1** e17–27

[14] Meignan M, Gallamini A, Meignan M, Gallamini A and Haioun C 2009 Report on the first international workshop on interim-PET scan in lymphoma *Leuk. Lymphoma* **50** 1257–60

[15] Butt C, Gill J, Chun D and Babu B A 2020 Deep learning system to screen coronavirus disease 2019 pneumonia *Appl. Intell.* 1

[16] Hesamian M H, Jia W, He X and Kennedy P 2019 Deep learning techniques for medical image segmentation: achievements and challenges *J. Digit. Imag.* **32** 582–96

[17] Madjid M, Safavi-Naeini P, Solomon S D and Vardeny O 2020 Potential effects of coronaviruses on the cardiovascular system: a review *JAMA Cardiol.* **5** 831–840

[18] Liang N-Y, Huang G-B, Saratchandran P and Sundararajan N 2006 A fast and accurate online sequential learning algorithm for feedforward networks *IEEE Trans. Neural Netw.* **17** 1411–23

[19] Zhu E, Yin J and Zhang G 2005 Fingerprint matching based on global alignment of multiple reference minutiae *Pattern Recognit.* **38** 1685–94

[20] Huang G-B and Siew C-K 2004 Extreme learning machine: RBF network case *Proc. ICARCV 8th Control, Autom., Robot. Vis. Conf.* **2** 1029–36
[21] Zong W, Huang G-B and Chen Y 2013 Weighted extreme learning machine for imbalance learning *Neurocomputing* **101** 229–42
[22] Cunningham J W *et al* 2020 Natriuretic peptide-based inclusion criteria in a heart failure clinical trial: insights from COMMANDER HF *JACC, Heart Failure* **8** 359–68
[23] Malhotra P, Vig L, Shroff G and Agarwal P 2015 Long short term memory networks for anomaly detection in time series *Proc.l 23rd European Symp. on Artificial Neural Networks, (ESANN) (Bruges, Belgium, April 22-24)* 89 (Louvain-la-Neuve, Belgium: Presses Univ. de Louvain)
[24] Hochreiter S and Schmidhuber J 1997 Long short-term memory *Neural Comput.* **9** 1735–80
[25] Kawakami K 2008 Supervised sequence labelling with recurrent neural networks *PhD Dissertation* Carnegie Mellon University Pittsburgh, PA
[26] Ma X, Tao Z, Wang Y, Yu H and Wang Y 2015 Long short-term memory neural network for traffic speed prediction using remote microwave sensor data *Transp. Res. Part C, Emerg. Technol.* **54** 187–97
[27] Cai M and Liu J 2016 Maxout neurons for deep convolutional and LSTM neural networks in speech recognition *Speech Commun.* **77** 53–64
[28] Farzad A, Mashayekhi H and Hassanpour H 2019 A comparative performance analysis of different activation functions in LSTM networks for classification *Neural Comput. Appl.* **31** 2507–21
[29] Rao A and Spasojevic N 2016 Actionable and political text classification using word embeddings and LSTM arXiv:1607.02501
[30] Yuan M, Wu Y and Lin L 2016 Fault diagnosis and remaining useful life estimation of aero engine using LSTM neural network *2016 IEEE Int. Conf. on Aircraft Utility Systems (AUS)* 135–40
[31] Yang J, Guo Y and Zhao W 2019 Long short-term memory neural network based fault detection and isolation for electro-mechanical actuators *Neurocomputing* **360** 85–96
[32] Xu B *et al* 2020 Epidemiological data from the COVID-19 outbreak, realtime case information *Sci. Data* **7** 1–6
[33] Cho K, van Merrienboer B, Gulcehre C, Bahdanau D, Bougares F, Schwenk H and Bengio Y 2014 Learning phrase representations using RNN encoder-decoder for statistical machine translation arXiv:1406.1078
[34] Hsieh C-J, Si S and Dhillon I 2014 A divide-and-conquer solver for kernel support vector machines *Proc. of the 31st Int. Conf. on Machine Learning ICML'14: 31st International Conference on Machine Learning* 566–74
[35] Poznyak T I, Oria I C and Poznyak A S 2019 *Ozonation and Biodegradation in Environmental Engineering.* (Amsterdam: Elsevier)
[36] Mou L, Ghamisi P and Zhu X X 2017 Deep recurrent neural networks for hyperspectral image classification *IEEE Trans. Geosci. Remote Sens.* **55** 3639–55
[37] Dinga J *et al* 2020 Experience on radiological examinations and infection prevention for COVID-19 in radiology department *Radiol. Infect. Dis.* early access, Mar. 13
[38] Ai T, Yang Z, Zhan C, Chen C, Lv W, Tao Q, Sun Z, Xia L and Hou H 2020 Correlation of chest CT and RT-PCR testing in coronavirus disease 2019 (COVID-19) in China: a report of 1014 cases *Radiology* **296** E32-E40

[39] Shi H, Han X, Jiang N, Cao Y, Alwalid O, Gu J, Fan Y and Zheng C 2020 Radiological findings from 81 patients with COVID-19 pneumonia in Wuhan, China: a descriptive study *Lancet Infect. Dis.* **20** 425–34
[40] Banerjee I *et al* 2019 Comparative effectiveness of convolutional neural network (CNN) and recurrent neural network (RNN) architectures for radiology text report classication *Artif. Intell. Med.* **97** 79–88
[41] Zhu N *et al* 2020 China novel coronavirus investigating and research team. A novel coronavirus from patients with pneumonia in China, 2019 *New England J. Med.* **382** 727–33
[42] Yi X, Walia E and Babyn P 2019 Generative adversarial network in medical imaging: a review *Med. Image Anal.* **58** 101552
[43] Goodfellow I, Pouget-Abadie J, Mirza M, Xu B, Warde-Farley D, Ozair S, Courville A and Bengio Y 2014 Generative adversarial nets *Advances in Neural Information Processing Systems 27 (NIPS 2014)* 27Z ed Ghahramani *et al* 2672–80
[44] Wolterink J M, Leiner T, Viergever M A and Isgum I 2017 Generative adversarial networks for noise reduction in low-dose CT *IEEE Trans. Med. Imag.* **36** 2536–45
[45] Kohl S, Bonekamp D, Schlemmer H-P, Yaqubi K, Hohenfellner M, Hadaschik B, Radtke J-P and Maier-Hein K 2017 Adversarial networks for the detection of aggressive prostate cancer arXiv:1702.0801
[46] Xu T, Zhang P, Huang Q, Zhang H, Gan Z, Huang X and He X 2018 AttnGAN: Fine-grained text to image generation with attentional generative adversarial networks *2018 IEEE/CVF Conf. on Computer Vision and Pattern Recognition* 1316–24
[47] Ledig C *et al* 2017 Photo-realistic single image super-resolution using a generative adversarial network *2017 IEEE Conf. on Computer Vision and Pattern Recognition (CVPR)* 105-14
[48] Zhu J-Y, Park T, Isola P and Efros A A 2017 Unpaired image-to-image translation using cycle-consistent adversarial networks *2017 IEEE Int. Conf. on Computer Vision (ICCV)* 2242–51
[49] Inciardi R M *et al* 2020 Cardiac involvement in a patient with coronavirus disease 2019 (COVID-19) *JAMA Cardiol.* **5** 819–824
[50] Zheng J, Xu C, Zhang Z and Li X 2017 Electric load forecasting in smart grids using long-short-term-memory based recurrent neural network *2017 51st Annual Conference on Information Sciences and Systems (CISS)* 1–6
[51] Gupta S, Parker J, Smits S, Underwood J and Dolwani S 2020 Persistent viral shedding of SARS-CoV-2 in faeces—a rapid review *Colorectal Dis.* **22** 611-620
[52] Wang N, Er M J and Han M 2015 Generalized single-hidden layer feedforward networks for regression problems *IEEE Trans Neural Netw. Learn. Syst.* **26** 1161–76
[53] Xiao F, Tang M, Zheng X, Liu Y, Li X and Shan H 2020 Evidence for gastrointestinal infection of SARS-CoV-2 *Gastroenterology* **158** 1831–3
[54] Wang C, Xu C, Yao X and Tao D 2019 Evolutionary generative adversarial networks *IEEE Trans. Evol. Comput.* **23** 921–34
[55] Song Y, Ma C, Wu X, Gong L, Bao L, Zuo W, Shen C, Lau R W H and Yang M-H 2018 Vital: vIsual tracking via adversarial learning *2018 IEEE/CVF Conf. on Computer Vision and Pattern Recognition* 8990–9
[56] Donahue J, Krähenbühl P and Darrell T 2017 Adversarial feature learning arXiv:1605.09782
[57] Xu X *et al* 2020 Deep learning system to screen coronavirus disease 2019 pneumonia *Engineering* **6** 1122–9

[58] Alimadadi A, Aryal S, Manandhar I, Munroe P B, Joe B and Cheng X 2020 Artificial intelligence and machine learning to fight COVID-19 *Physiol. Genomics* **52** 200–2
[59] Allam Z and Jones D S 2020 On the Coronavirus (COVID-19) Outbreak and the Smart City Network: Universal Data Sharing Standards Coupled with Artificial Intelligence (AI) to Benefit Urban Health Monitoring and Management *Healthcare* **8** 46
[60] Greenhalgh T, Koh G C H and Car J 2020 Covid-19: a remote assessment in primary care *Brit. Med.* J. **368** m1182
[61] Fu T-C, Liu Y-C, Chiu W-C, Wang S-D and Wang Y-C F 2017 Learning cross-domain disentangled deep representation with supervision from a single domain arXiv:1705.01314
[62] Neumann K and Steil J J 2013 Optimizing extreme learning machines via ridge regression and batch intrinsic plasticity *Neurocomputing* **102** 23–30
[63] Goel T, Murugan R and Mirjalili S *et al* 2021 Automatic screening of COVID-19 using an optimized generative adversarial network *Cogn. Comput.* https://doi.org/10.1007/s12559-020-09785-7

IOP Publishing

Artificial Intelligence Strategies for Analyzing COVID-19 Pneumonia Lung Imaging, Volume 1
Characterization approaches
Ayman El-Baz and Jasjit S Suri

Chapter 10

Lung CT scans for the management of COVID-19 pneumonitis and the diagnosis of COVID-19

Lakshna Mahajan, Nitin K Puri and Mukesh Kumar

Lung CT scans have proved extremely useful in the management of COVID-19. COVID-19 pneumonitis scans depict typical features, such as unilateral or bilateral ground-glass opacities in the lower lobes, consolidation, reticulation, thickening of the adjacent pleura, pleural effusion, honeycombing, bronchiectasis, the presence of nodules or masses, interlobular pleural traction, etc. These features, which allow the severity of the pneumonitis to be characterised, are observed in patients that require admission to hospital and intensive care. CT scans have also been employed in checking for COVID-19 complications, such as acute respiratory distress syndrome, pulmonary embolism, etc. The diagnostic aspect of CT scans is helpful in symptomatic patients with negative RT-PCR results, or in areas where RT-PCR availability is limited. However, there are many inherent limitations to CT imaging, due to the need to follow standard operating procedures and for scanning to follow the 'as low as reasonably achievable' (ALARA) principle, avoiding extensive patient exposure to high levels of radiation. In addition, proper decontamination after each use of the CT scanning facility is recommended, which limits the output per facility. An issue of false positives arises due to the existence of diseases with overlapping features; and non-involvement or non-reactive immune responses in the lung parenchyma can yield false negative results. This chapter is an attempt to compile these findings and to present the possibilities and limitations associated with this approach.

doi:10.1088/978-0-7503-3795-3ch10

10.1 Novel coronavirus, COVID-19

The novel coronavirus disease generally known as 'covid', specifically, COVID-19, first identified in 2019 (Wuhan, China), is the seventh coronavirus known to infect humans [1]. The name 'corona' is derived from the typical feature of this enveloped virus showing crown-like spikes on its outer surface with a size ranging from 65–125 nm in diameter and is a single stranded RNA virus with 26–32 kbs. [2, 3]. The Corona family of viruses has diverse hosts; some cause illness in humans, and others cause illness in animals, such as bats, camels, and civets; they have the ability to develop strains that jump from a different host species to humans in a spillover event. In two major incidents coronavirus infected human populations. One of these was caused by SARS-CoV (Severe Acute Respiratory Syndrome-coronavirus), which also began in China and infected around 8000 people (with 774 cases of mortality) in 29 different countries, and the other by MERS-CoV (Middle East Respiratory Syndrome—coronavirus), which originated in Saudi Arabia in July 2019 and caused 2458 infections and 848 deaths [2, 3].

COVID-19 was previously named SARS-CoV-2, as it is genetically related to the SARS-CoV outbreak of 2003, however, it was later specifically renamed as COVID-19, renamed by the World Health Organization (WHO) [4]. COVID-19, the organism of interest, is known to cause illness ranging from that of the common cold to pneumonitis, blood clots, and other severe forms of disease.

10.1.1 Modes of transmission: respiratory droplets, the airborne mode, and lung involvement

Human-to-human transmission is most likely to take place by respiratory droplets among individuals in close contact. Aerosol-mediated transmission has also been demonstrated, though it requires a higher dose of viral exposure for longer periods of time [5]. A wide range of clinical manifestations have been observed in COVID-19 patients. The most common symptoms are fever, dry cough, and fatigue, which affect the majority of the infected population. Other symptoms include shortness of breath, difficulty in breathing, and in severe cases, this can result in pneumonitis of the lung and can be fatal. A considerable number of patients have also reported olfactory and gustatory dysfunction, diarrhea, shivering (10.9%), nausea and vomiting (10.2%), and abdominal pain; in some people these developed into major clinical symptoms [5].

10.2 Preventive strategies—lessons to be learnt and implemented

The contagious nature of the disease demands preventive strategies such as strict state-wide travel rules, the isolation of travellers on arrival, urgent patient segregation, contact tracing and control, disease diagnosis, proper clinical care, careful infection management, etc. Airway protection mechanisms that restrict droplet contact are the basis of the protective mechanisms adopted to control the spread of infection. Thermal screening is helpful in symptomatic patients, however the fever can easily be suppressed by paracetamol; the cases have been recorded in which

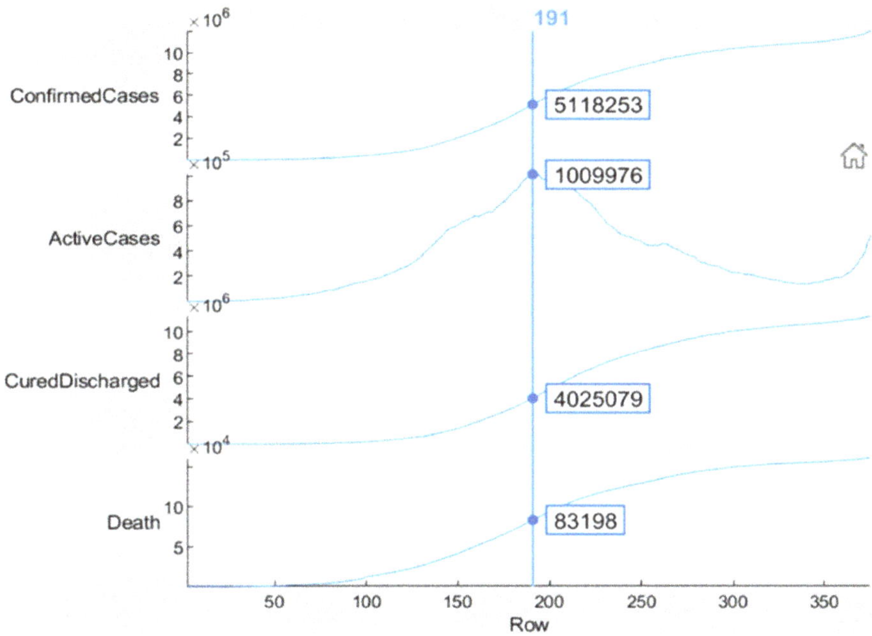

Figure 10.1. COVID-19 infection status in India [CBCP].

travellers took such medications. Further, the window period from exposure to the development of disease can vary from three days and up to a week or so. Many passengers in the vicinity of a patient can be exposed to COVID-19 and will only start to suffer after few days. The use of thermal screening is thus not a very successful way to control the spread of infection [6]. Bans on travel or strict quarantines for a suitable length of time thus remain the major alternatives for curbing the international/interstate spread of infection.

The first instances of COVID-19 in India were seen in the state of Kerala among three medical students who had returned from Wuhan in January 2020. Soon afterwards, COVID-19 expansion was reported by other states, which then spread to different parts of the country by the end of March 2020. Since then, it displayed a ‘leaps and bounds’ trend, as shown in figure 10.1. In mid-September, 2020, the number of COVID-19 cases rose to over 90 000; a decreasing trend of less than 15 000 cases per day followed later. The devastating second wave started in March 2021, which resulted in a shortage of medical resources throughout the country, in the form of limited hospital beds, oxygen cylinders, and other medicines. On 30 April 2021, over 400 000 new cases were reported in a 24 h period.

India took significant action, implementing various coordinated strategies in order to limit the spread of infection, these efforts were only successful on the implementation of lockdown, owing to the highly contagious nature of this disease. Numerous efforts have been made to prevent/fight this deadly epidemic, including patient sampling, testing, and isolation, provision of personal protective equipment (PPE) to the caregivers and people managing bio-medical waste, life-sustaining drugs, and therapies such as yoga, Ayush guidelines for caregivers and patients, and strict implementation of personal precautions such as social distancing, masks and gloves, regular hand washing, and so on.

10.3 The golden test—RT-PCR—and its limitations

COVID-19 is heterogeneous in clinical presentation, course, and outcome. Potential symptoms in individuals also vary, and there have also been reports of asymptomatic individuals with hardly any signs of infection [7]. The golden test for the diagnosis of COVID-19 is the real-time reverse transcription-polymerase chain reaction (RT-PCR). The RT-PCR test can be performed using nasopharyngeal swabs to obtain nasopharyngeal specimens or by obtaining other upper respiratory tract specimens using a throat or saliva swab [8, 9]. Although it is considered to be the 'golden test' for COVID-19, the sensitivity of the RT-PCR test is not absolute; a pooled estimate for RT-PCR sensitivity is 89% (95% CI: 81%, 94%), and thus one or more negative results do not rule out COVID-19 [10]. In the second wave of COVID-19, there were many cases in which patients showed respiratory symptoms and fever, etc., however RT-PCR tests showed false negative results. On the basis of RT-PCR results, clinical symptoms, and a person's exposure history, the WHO has provided criteria that define the possibility that a person is infected, which will help to enhance surveillance and limit the spread of this infectious pandemic, in particular, as observed during its second wave. Tested persons are categorized into suspect, probable, and confirmed cases of COVID-19 [11]. A *suspect case* is one who shows clinical symptoms but for whom laboratory reports and RT-PCR test results are negative. A *probable case* is defined as a suspected case for whom certain lab tests show a positive report, or who has been exposed to an established confirmed case. A *confirmed case* is defined as a patient with RT-PCR test-confirmed COVID-19, irrespective of clinical signs and symptoms [11].

A number of factors can result in the problem of false negative results; these include: *(a)* poor/inadequate sample collection; *(b)* early collection of the specimen, i.e. the time window between the exposure to COVID-19 and symptom onset may be up to one week and sample collection before the onset of symptoms will yield a negative result; *(c)* late collection of the sample, i.e. a specimen taken ~4 weeks after symptom onset and beyond; *(d)* inappropriate handling and shipping of the specimen; and *(e)* technical errors or contamination of the test [12]. If this is taken into account, additional specimens should be collected and tested even if a patient with a high suspicion index for COVID-19 has a negative result. Occasional false positive results may also occur because the RT-PCR test detects the viral RNA only, irrespective of whether it is viable and infectious [8, 12].

Another drawback of the RT-PCR test is that it takes between 50 min and 4 h for machines that are semi automated or fully automated, and around 6–14 h for manually performed assays [8, 13]. Various rapid lateral flow immunodiagnostic tests have also been developed now, though their efficiency with respect to different variants is yet to be validated and therefore no recommendations can be made for their use in patient care.

Chest radiographs and CT scans become a useful resort for diagnostics.

10.4 CT scans for COVID-19 detection

Disease Progression to lung involvement–CT scan findings in COVID-19 patients without severe respiratory distress

Typical radiological images of COVID-19 from recently published literature for patients who did not develop severe respiratory distress and thus did not require hospitalization, demonstrated a clear distinction between the different stages of lung involvement in the CT findings. In mild early COVID-19 infections at 0–4 days, described as stage 1, CT scans demonstrated small ground-glass opacities in the lower lobes unilaterally or bilaterally in the subpleural region. During the progressive stage 2, lasting from around 8th–9th day from the first day of infection, the infection is aggravated and extends to bilateral multilobes showing diffuse ground glass opacities with crazy paving patterns and this is usually followed by subsequent consolidation and stage 3, sometimes with a rounded morphology and peripheral lung distribution. In mild to moderate cases who recovered from COVID-19, these changes gradually resolved in another two weeks; residual glass ground opacities and a few subpleural parenchymal bands were generally seen. In stage 4 (the absorption stage) the infection control is obtained in 14 days or could be extended to more than 26 days from the onset of initial symptoms. These stages can easily be distinguished from CT scan analyses. The CT scans clearly depicted that most patients that recovered from COVID-19 showed the maximum severity at around the tenth day, and improvement in the chest CT scans began at around the fourteenth day after the onset of initial symptoms [14].

10.5 Findings of CT scans for patients with severe Covid-19 pneumonitis

Apart from the pattern observed in the recovered patients, lung pathology in patients with severe pneumonitis has been studied. In a study by Han *et al* (2021), 65% of COVID−19 patients who developed severe pneumonitis and had fibrotic changes, the pathology was resolved in six months, while 35% of the patients continued to show typical fibrotic-like changes in a six-month follow-up study [15].

The severity of pneumonitis in patients of COVID-19 was defined by CT-scan findings according to the Fleischner Society glossary for ground-glass opacities, consolidation, reticulation, thickening of the adjacent pleura, pleural effusion, honeycombing, bronchiectasis, presence of nodules or masses, and interlobar pleural traction, etc [16].

The typical findings related to COVID-19 include round multifocal ground-glass opacities with a peripheral and basal distribution with non-sharp demarcations, crazy paving, and consolidations, as described above. The atypical findings include central, peri-bronchial, or apical distributions or cavitation, while very atypical observations include cavitation, pleural thickening, nodular patterns, etc. Follow-up studies to measure the severity have been helpful, as they included CT scans; these showed fibrotic changes in the lungs of patients who survived severe COVID pneumonia [15].

The diagnosis of COVID-19-mediated changes in lung tissue using CT scan analyses in severe pneumonia patients has been concluded to be 80%–90% sensitive and ~82%–96% specific, which is better than the performance of RT-PCR diagnosis [16]. This has been a reason for the boom in CT-scan-mediated diagnosis of COVID-19 related to the lungs. As discussed earlier, findings such as consolidation in lungs, bronchial wall thickening, crazy paving, etc. are associated with raised CT severity scores; the worst prognoses indicate a requirement for intensive care support. However, imaging findings for COVID-19 and other infectious diseases considerably overlap, especially seasonal pandemics, such as influenza. This remains, however, an effective method of analysis in pandemic-hit areas when other seasonal viral diseases are minimally present or absent from the population. However, it remains to be mentioned that the CT findings for COVID-19 display an overlap with other lung diseases, such as acute interstitial pneumonitis and other viral pneumonias, etc.

10.5.1 Important requisites for the implementation of CT scan facilities

The prerequisites for a CT scanning facility should include the implementation of precautionary safety measures, standard protocols for chest CT optimization, and a standard reporting structure for pulmonary findings [17].

Safety measures for radiological personnel and patients is of the utmost importance to prevent the spread of disease. In the MERS-CoV infection outbreak of 2014 in Saudi Arabia, which had a similar outcome to that of COVID-19, radiological technicians were most frequently infected among all healthcare personnel [18]. This fact emphasize the requirement to take precautionary measures seriously, e.g. the use of PPE equipment, gloves, N95 face masks with appropriate eye protection, etc., with appropriate procedures for use, removal, disinfection, and disposal. Furthermore, cleaning and disinfection would require proper decontamination of the room and passive air exchange after use by each patient. This could be achieved by increasing air exchange per hour or by high-efficiency particulate air (HEPA) filtering to limit the infection. This would require a halt of CT-Scan facility for 30 minutes to 1 hour after each use, resulting in limiting patient throughput [17]. The failure to follow these precautionary measures has resulted in some of these diagnostic centres being a source of infection, as observed in the second wave of COVID-19 [19].

The results obtained by chest CT analysis can provide added value in making diagnostic decisions with the help of available RT-PCR tests. Knowledge of the prevalence of COVID-19 and/or overlapping or similar chest CT diseases is also helpful. Chest CT exams can also produce false negative and false positive results. However, the sensitivity and specificity of tests increases if both RT-PCR tests and CT scans supplement each other.

10.5.2 Protocol for chest CT

Chest CT has been helpful in the diagnosis and risk stratification of patients. However, a standard protocol defined on the basis of the research studies should be kept under consideration. A Fleischner Society consensus statement does not recommend chest imaging for the screening of COVID-19 asymptomatic patients or mildly symptomatic patients with respiratory symptoms (i.e. patients who do not show significant pulmonary dysfunction) [20]. This is mainly because of the confinement of the virus to the upper respiratory tract, low viral loads, or the absence of a pulmonary inflammatory response to the virus (thus, no lung injury) that would result in false negative chest CT findings in these patients [17]. CT chest imaging is, however, helpful in screening and categorizing patients with moderate to severe respiratory symptoms and in patients with such symptoms but showing negative RT-PCR test result, or also in case RT-PCR is not readily available/ performed [20]. These patients may frequently need to undergo chest CT scans to check on lung involvement and to help in deciding on an appropriate treatment. In addition, patients of all ages may need to have chest imaging performed [17]. It is therefore highly recommended that low-radiation-dose CT scans rather than full-radiation-dose be performed for the evaluation of the lung parenchyma on the basis of the ALARA principle. This is achieved using lower kilovoltage settings, noise reduction, etc., which takes advantage of recent developments in scanning methodology, depending on local availability [17]. Furthermore, patients should be subjected to non-contrast chest CT scans unless CT pulmonary angiography is recommended for the detection of pulmonary embolism.

There are, however, certain challenges that need to be addressed, even when using CT scans for the diagnosis of symptomatic patients. The issue becomes very important while differentiating between different types of viral pneumonia using chest CT scans. While a few studies suggest presence of a peripheral distribution of ground-glass opacities as a more typical observation in COVID-19 pneumonia, other studies state that this feature is not useful in perceiving the differences between COVID-19 pneumonia and influenzal pneumonia [21–23].

Furthermore, specific disease conditions, such as alveolar hemorrhages, acute interstitial pneumonitis, etc. may cause false positive findings and thus limit the specificity of chest CT scans for COVID-19 [17]. Various other factors, such as the population under observation, may also have variable findings and responses at the tissue level. While a negative chest CT examination result certainly does not exclude COVID-19, the number of false positive chest CT examination results is also substantial, due to the overlap between COVID-19 imaging features and those of numerous other diseases, including other viral pneumonias [17].

10.5.3 Reporting chest CT findings

A few observations related to typical findings in COVID-19 lung scans have been discussed earlier. The American College of Radiology Practice Parameter for Communication of Diagnostic Imaging Findings is used for standardised communications related to COVID-19 cases. The findings essentially use four categories,

Table 10.1. Imaging classification and CT features of COVID-19 pneumonia. Adapted and reprinted under the CCBY 4.0 license from reference 25.

Imaging classification	Rationale	CT features
Typical appearance	Commonly reported imaging features of greater specificity for COVID-19 pneumonia	Peripheral, bilateral, ground-glass opacities with or without consolidation or visible intralobular lines ("crazy paving" pattern) Multifocal ground-glass opacities of rounded morphology, with or without consolidation or visible interlobular lines (crazy paving pattern) Reverse halo sign or other findings of organizing pneumonia (seen later in the disease)
Indeterminate appearance	Nonspecific imaging features of COVID-19 pneumonia	Absence of typical features AND the presence of the following features: multifocal, diffuse, perihilar, or unilateral ground-glass opacity with or without consolidation lacking a specific distribution and that are nonrounded or nonperipheral Few small ground-glass opacities. with a nonrounded and nonperipheral distribution
Atypical appearance	Uncommonly or not reported features of COVID-I9 pneumonia	Absence of typical or indeterminate features AND the presence of the following features: isolated lobar or segmental consolidation without ground-glass opacities; discrete small nodules (centrilobular, "tree-in-bud" appearance); lung cavitation; smooth interlobular septal thickening with pleural effusion
Negative for pneumonia	No features of pneumonia	No CT features to suggest pneumonia.

with the aims of fully defining each observation, reducing reporting variability, easing communication with physicians, etc. The four categories are named: (i) typical appearance, (2) indeterminate appearance, (iii) atypical appearance, and (iv) negative for pneumonia [24] (table 10.1).

The 'typical appearance' imaging classification recommends CT features such as peripheral, bilateral ground-glass with interlobular lines, appearing as a 'crazy paving' pattern with or without consolidation and the reverse halo signs found in the later stages of disease. The 'indeterminate appearance' category includes those cases showing the absence of the typical features as described above, but instead, ground-glass opacity with or without consolidation is observed without a specific distribution, along with the typical rounded structure considered to be a nonspecific imaging feature of COVID-19 pneumonitis. 'Atypical appearance' is an imaging classification with features that are not reported for COVID-19 pneumonia, showing segmental or lobar consolidation without ground-glass opacities, lung cavitation, discrete small nodules, etc. The fourth category is 'negative for pneumonia', in which no CT scan features suggest pneumonia [25].

10.5.4 Chest CT scans of COVID-19 complications

To understand the severity of complications involved, a chest CT is advisable to keep a check on the progression of COVID-19 or to check any other cardiopulmonary complications, such as acute respiratory distress syndrome, superimposed pneumonia, or COVID-19-induced cardiac injury [20].

10.5.4.1 Acute respiratory distress syndrome (ARDS)

ARDS is observed in COVID-19 patients and to a large extent is due to the release of large amounts of proinflammatory cytokines by immune and non-immune cells. It results in the acute onset of pulmonary edema and hypoxemia without cardiac involvement. COVID-19 patients may rapidly develop ARDS [26]. ARDS is a common reason for the use of mechanical ventilation and the need for the patient to receive intensive care, as well as a major cause of death in COVID-19 patients. ARDS is diagnosed using bilateral opacities in the lung scan imaging, according to the Berlin definition. COVID-19-mediated ARDS develops 8–12 days after the onset of symptoms [27]. This is a distinguishing factor that differentiates ARDS developed as a result of COVID-19.

10.5.4.2 Pulmonary embolism

SARS-CoV-2 activates a coagulation cascade in the patient, which is initiated by local or systemic inflammation. Patients who have thromboembolic complications are exposed to a fivefold higher risk of mortality [28]. Pulmonary embolisms are reported in around 2.6%–8.9% of COVID-19 patients who needed hospitalization and have been observed in ~30% of patients in intensive care units (ICUs). CT pulmonary angiography has been recommended for COVID-19 patients with hemoptysis, the signs and symptoms of deep venous thrombosis, and/or unexplained tachycardia, etc [28].

Increased D-dimer cutoff levels have been associated with pulmonary embolism and pulmonary artery obstruction in COVID-19 patients and thus recommended as another parameter to help in risk stratification of patients along with CT scans. Thromboprophylaxis has been thus recommended to all suspected and confirmed COVID-19 patients who require admission to hospital [29].

10.5.4.3 Superimposed pneumonia

Superimposed pneumonia due to secondary bacterial and fungal infections has been a threat to roughly 10% of the hospitalized patients. It is highly recommended that lower respiratory tract samples should be obtained for culturing and that chest imaging should be performed to detect any superimposed bacterial pneumonia [30].

10.5.5 Role of chest CT for prognostication

The Fleischner Society recommends that imaging should be performed *(a)* to establish a baseline pulmonary status; *(b)* to identify underlying cardiopulmonary abnormalities (to facilitate risk stratification for clinical worsening in patients with mild symptoms of COVID-19) ; and *(c)* to identify risk factors for disease progression (e.g. age >65 years, comorbidities, such as cardiovascular disease, diabetes, chronic respiratory disease, hypertension, and immunocompromised status); and *(d)* in patients with moderate to severe symptoms of COVID-19 [20]. Again, the consensus statement from the Fleischner Society does not indicate whether radiography or CT is preferred in this environment.

The use of a chest CT severity score may be useful for a standardized assessment of the degree of pulmonary involvement in COVID-19 for prognostication purposes [31]. However, currently proposed prediction models for COVID-19, including those that include chest CT features, are poorly reported and are exposed to a high risk of bias; their reported performance is probably optimistic [32]. Therefore, it is currently not recommended to use any of the reported prediction models in clinical practice [32]. More research is required, including correlation with the patient outcome, to further validate the use of chest CT scans for the prognosis of COVID-19.

However, a potential value for the rapid triage of CT has been suggested in resource-constrained environments in which COVID-19 is very prevalent for patients with moderate to severe respiratory symptoms. Moreover, if an alternative diagnosis is suspected, a chest CT may be performed. CT scans carried out for other reasons may incidentally detect the typical or indeterminate features of COVID-19 pneumonia. In these cases, the interpreting radiologist should talk to the referring doctor in a timely fashion about the possibility of COVID-19. Standardized reporting according to guidelines such as those proposed by the RSNA can facilitate this information transfer [20]. In the course of COVID-19 advancement or secondary cardiopulmonary complications, such as ARDS, PE, superimposed pneumonia and heart failure, chest CT scans could also be helpful in evaluating the clinical deterioration of patients. Future studies are required to define the predictive role of CT in COVID-19.

10.6 Implementation of artificial intelligence in CT-scan-mediated COVID-19 diagnosis

An article in Nature (2021) suggested that a diverse multinational data set of COVID-19 patients should be compiled and analyzed using advanced machine learning algorithms to better understand viral spread, improve diagnosis speed and

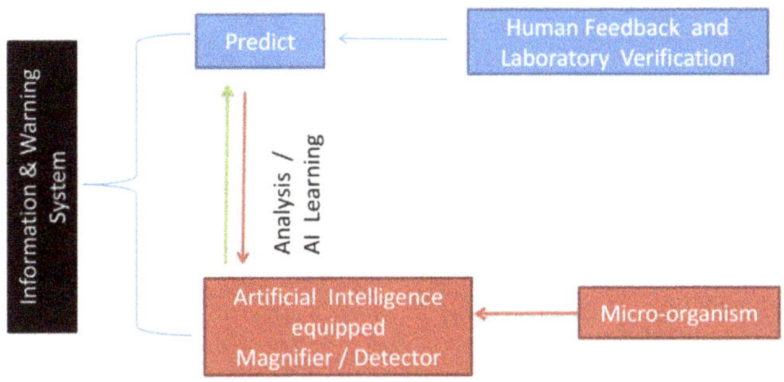

Figure 10.2. AI COVID-19 infection detection using optical reflection.

efficiency, monitor patients, and develop novel therapeutic approaches [33]. This has also been proposed to identify the most susceptible people based on personalized genetic and physiological characteristics and to provide personalized therapy. Algorithm-trained programs and advanced machine learning techniques are already being employed for the taxonomic classification of COVID-19 genomes. Several groups have demonstrated the AI-based diagnosis of COVID-19 lung pathology with detection accuracies as high as 95% [33, 34]. The latest learning version referred to as COVID-19 to reap a neural network (COVNet) was developed to capture the precise features of COVID-19 diagnostic characteristics using X-ray chest images and help medical experts to distinguish between the characteristics of pneumonia and different lung diseases [35]. AI models primarily based on existing statistics can help scarce healthcare resources to be used better, offer personalized patient management programs, inform policy, and speed up medical trials (figure 10.2).

A vital role has been suggested for the use of AI algorithms in diagnosis. First, predicted results, such as versions of optical patterns or field variations for given objects are used for training purposes. Finally, we look in advance and compare the future possibilities of smart healthcare. Other detected images or video could provide further medical data, such as heartbeat, blood pressure, blood oxygen saturation, etc. and also help to differentiate between healthy and infected people; to progress this, scanning data are needed for different stages [36–38]. AI models rely upon historical facts to make predictions from external observations. The size of the observation will increase accuracy and improve the analysis level. AI learns using trial and error to achieve a complicated objective. Reducing the wide variety of variables in a data set, such as the detection of a particular microorganism, may lead to a greater accuracy of prediction. One needs access to remote/local server data and AI field sensors for prediction and warnings. Here, hospitals or governments need to be assigned secure remote servers for storage and analysis, similar to those used for banking or secure information [36–39] (figure 10.3).

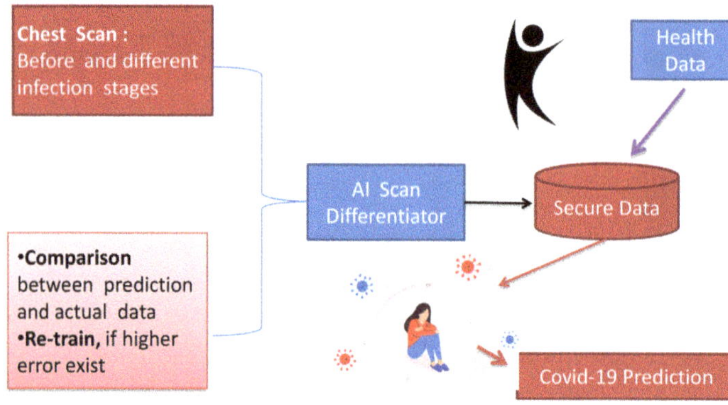

Figure 10.3. AI supported detection of field variations.

10.7 Conclusions

Chest CT scans cannot be considered the standard test for the diagnosis of COVID-19 patients who are asymptomatic, or those who do not severe lung involvement; however the correlation between lung scans, clinical presentation, and epidemiologic history remains crucial for monitoring and managing the severity of COVID-19 patients who develop lung pneumonitis. These findings suggest the use of CT scans for diagnosis in appropriate settings. It would not be an over exaggeration to say that chest CT scanning is good approach when an alternative diagnosis is required to provide appropriate healthcare to a patient, while its role for prognostication requires further investigation. AI models that are primarily based on existing statistics can help better use to be made of scarce health resources. This can be utilized in various ways by training machine learning systems through the use of historical facts and making predictions from current external observations. The classification and prediction of COVID-19 variants and spikes in cases, the analysis of x-ray and CT scan images with greater accuracy, the implementation of COVID-19-appropriate behaviours in the population, etc. are few ways in which artificial intelligence can help us to overcome any imminent viral surge. It is mainly the responsibility of the populace to be more responsible, efficiently isolate themselves in case of infection, report infections to the health authorities, follow COVID-19-appropriate behaviour, and get vaccinated (jabs are free in India); only then will the disease be curbed.

References

[1] https://who.int/docs/default-source/coronaviruse/situation-reports/20200121-sitrep-1-2019-ncov.pdf

[2] Shereen M A, Khan S, Kazmi A, Bashir N and Siddique R 2020 COVID-19 infection: Origin, transmission, and characteristics of human coronaviruses *J. Adv. Res.* **24** 91–8

[3] Hu B, Guo H, Zhou P and Shi Z L 2021 Characteristics of SARS-CoV-2 and COVID-19 *Nat. Rev. Microbiol.* **19** 141–54

[4] https://who.int/emergencies/diseases/novel-coronavirus-2019/technical-guidance/naming-the-coronavirus-disease-(covid-2019)-and-the-virus-that-causes-it

[5] Bao L *et al* 2020 Transmission of severe acute respiratory syndrome coronavirus 2 via close contact and respiratory droplets among human angiotensin-converting enzyme 2 mice *J. Infect. Dis.* **222** 551–5

[6] https://thehindu.com/news/national/telangana/hiding-covid-19-symptoms-is-homicide/article 31141393.ece

[7] Oran D P and Topol E J 2020 Prevalence of asymptomatic SARS-CoV-2 infection: a narrative review *Ann. Intern. Med.* **173** 362–7

[8] Tahamtan A and Ardebili A 2020 Real-time RT-PCR in COVID-19 detection: issues affecting the results *Expert Rev. Mol. Diagn.* **20** 453–4

[9] https://fda.gov/media/136151/download#:~:text=The%20COVID%2D19%20RT%2DPCR %20Test%20is%20a%20real%2D,tract%20aspirates%2C%20bronchoalveolar%20lavage% 2C%20and

[10] Kim H, Hong H and Yoon S H 2020 Diagnostic performance of CT and reverse transcriptase polymerase chain reaction for coronavirus disease 2019: a meta-analysis *Radiology* **296** E145–55

[11] https://who.int/hac/techguidance/training/case%20definitions_en.pdf

[12] Kucirka L M, Lauer S A, Laeyendecker O, Boon D and Lessler J 2020 Variation in false-negative rate of reverse transcriptase polymerase chain reaction-based SARS-CoV-2 tests by time since exposure *Ann. Intern. Med.* **173** 262–7

[13] Ching L, Chang S P and Nerurkar V R 2020 COVID-19 special column: principles behind the technology for detecting SARS-CoV-2, the cause of COVID-19 *Hawai'i J. Health Soc. Welf.* **79** 136–42

[14] Pan F *et al* 2020 Time course of lung changes at chest CT during recovery from coronavirus disease 2019 (COVID-19) *Radiology* **295** 715–21

[15] Han X *et al* 2021 Six-month follow-up chest CT findings after severe COVID-19 pneumonia *Radiology* **299** E177–86

[16] Penha D, Pinto E G, Matos F, Hochhegger B, Monaghan C, Taborda-Barata L, Irion K and Marchiori E 2021 CO-RADS: coronavirus classification review *J. Clin. Imaging Sci.* **11** 9

[17] Kwee T C and Kwee R M 2020 Chest CT in COVID-19: what the radiologist needs to know *Radiographics* **40** 1848–65

[18] Alraddadi B M *et al* 2016 Risk factors for middle east respiratory syndrome coronavirus infection among healthcare personnel *Emerg. Infect. Dis.* **22** 1915–20

[19] https://timesofindia.indiatimes.com/city/aurangabad/ct-scan-behind-spread-of-covid-19-says-civil-surgeon/articleshow/82220088.cms

[20] Rubin G D, Ryerson C J and Haramati L B *et al* 2020 The role of chest imaging in patient management during the COVID-19 pandemic: a multinational consensus statement from the Fleischner society *Chest.* **158** 106–16

[21] Bai H X, Hsieh B and Xiong Z *et al* 2020 Performance of radiologists in differentiating COVID-19 from Non-COVID-19 viral pneumonia at Chest CT *Radiology* **296** E46–54

[22] Wang H, Wei R, Rao G, Zhu J and Song B 2019 Characteristic CT findings distinguishing 2019 novel coronavirus disease (COVID-19) from influenza pneumonia *Eur. Radiol.* **30** 4910–7

[23] Liu M, Zeng W, Wen Y, Zheng Y, Lv F and Xiao K 2020 COVID-19 pneumonia: CT findings of 122 patients and differentiation from influenza pneumonia *Eur. Radiol.* **30** 5463–9

[24] Chung M *et al* 2020 CT imaging features of 2019 novel coronavirus (2019-nCoV) *Radiology* **295** 202–7

[25] Simpson S, Kay F Y and Abbara S *et al* 2020 Radiological Society of North America expert consensus statement on reporting chest CT findings related to COVID-19: Endorsed by the Society of Thoracic Radiology, the American College of Radiology, and RSNA *Radiol. Cardiothorac. Imaging* **2** e200152

[26] Matthay M A, Zemans R L and Zimmerman G A *et al* 2019 Acute respiratory distress syndrome *Nat. Rev. Dis. Primers* **5** 18

[27] ARDS Definition Task ForceRanieri V M and Rubenfeld G D *et al* 2012 Acute respiratory distress syndrome: the Berlin Definition *JAMA* **307** 2526–33

[28] Oudkerk M, Büller H R and Kuijpers D *et al* 2020 Diagnosis, prevention, and treatment of thromboembolic complications in COVID-19: report of the National Institute for Public Health of the Netherlands *Radiology* **297** E216–22

[29] Sakr Y, Giovini M and Leone M *et al* 2020 Pulmonary embolism in patients with coronavirus disease-2019 (COVID-19) pneumonia: a narrative review *Ann. Intensive Care* **10** 124

[30] Huttner B D, Catho G, Pano-Pardo J R, Pulcini C and Schouten J 2020 COVID-19: don't neglect antimicrobial stewardship principles! *Clin. Microbiol. Infect.* **26** 808–10

[31] Yang R, Li X and Liu H *et al* 2020 Chest CT severity score: an imaging tool for assessing severe COVID-19 *Radiol. Cardiothorac. Imaging* **2** e200047

[32] Wynants L, Van Calster B and Collins G S *et al* 2020 Prediction models for diagnosis and prognosis of covid-19 infection: systematic review and critical appraisal *Brit. Med.* J. **369** m1328

[33] Harmon S A, Sanford T H and Xu S *et al* 2020 Artificial intelligence for the detection of COVID-19 pneumonia on chest CT using multinational datasets *Nat. Commun.* **11** 4080

[34] Bai H X *et al* 2020 Performance of radiologists in differentiating COVID-19 from non-COVID-19 viral pneumonia at chest CT *Radiology* **296** E46–54

[35] Kedia P, Anjum and Katarya R 2021 CoVNet-19: A Deep Learning model for the detection and analysis of COVID-19 patients *Appl. Soft Comput.* **104** 107184

[36] Kumar M 2020 Smart eye technology: a tool for microorganism *Int. J. Innov. Sci. Res. Rev.* **02** 455–8

[37] Kumar M and Rana L 2020 Artificial intelligence: a tool for COVID-19 surface detection *Int. J. Sci. Res. Multidiscip. Stud.* **6** 60–3

[38] Singh S K, Nidhi, Srivastav A, Lohia A and Yadav N 2020 A study on biomedical solid waste management in Delhi with emphasis on corona waste from hospitals *Int. J. Adv. Sci. Technol.* **29** 4114–22

[40] Singh P *et al* 2020 COVID-19, the novel coronavirus 2019: current updates and the future *Int. J. Res. Med. Sci.* **8** 1939–49

IOP Publishing

Artificial Intelligence Strategies for Analyzing COVID-19 Pneumonia Lung Imaging, Volume 1
Characterization approaches
Ayman El-Baz and Jasjit S Suri

Chapter 11

Applications of machine learning in the COVID-19 pandemic: a scoping review

M A Jabbar, Syed Saba raoof and Sonia Sharma

The use of machine learning (ML) methods to support medical decision-making has become critical. Due to the uneven and complex structures of CT lung images, it is often difficult to diagnose vessels and nodules in CT images of COVID-19-affected patients. ML methods are significant in decision-making. ML methods have great potential to improve disease prediction. ML-based decision support systems will help physicians to make fast and efficient decisions. The purpose of this scoping review is to systematically assess and summarize the literature describing the ML models used for the prediction of the COVID-19 pandemic. ML-based tools can be designed and developed to tackle COVID-19. Various ML and deep-learning methods can be employed to analyze COVID-19-related data.

11.1 Introduction

COVID-19 is a communicable disease—it spreads from person to person. It has a zoonotic origin; it spreads from animals or insects to human beings. The WHO has recognized it as a pandemic disease. The name of the virus strain responsible for COVID-19 is severe acute respiratory syndrome coronavirus-2 (SARS-CoV-2). It spreads through respiratory droplets with diameters of >5–10 μm by direct or indirect contact. The incubation period of this virus is 2–14 days. Different tests are used to diagnose it, but serological testing is widely used and detects the presence of infection. Plasma therapy is used to treat COVID-19, which passively increases the immunity of the body; hence, it is artificial method of immunization. Clinical trials are under way to discover medicines for COVID-19. Health can gain anything, but nothing can gain health, so follow precautions, stay safe at home and stay happy.

doi:10.1088/978-0-7503-3795-3ch11

The coronavirus disease named 'COVID-19' is an infectious disease caused by the exposure of the human body to a type of virus strain named 'severe acute respiratory syndrome coronavirus-2' (SARS-CoV-2). It belongs to the family *Coronoviridae* and the genus *Betacoronavirus*. It is considered to have a zoonotic origin, which means that it spreads from animals and insects to human beings. Zoonotic diseases are also known as zoonoses. These diseases ranges from short-term illnesses to long-term (chronic) illnesses, which may even lead to death of organisms (human beings).

The human coronaviruses other than COVID-19 are:

1. Sars-CoV.
2. HCoV-NL63.
3. HCoV-HKU1.
4. MERS-CoV.

SARS-CoV-2 emerged from a live seafood market in Wuhan, China, in December 2019; it then spread vigorously across the whole country, taking the lives of thousands of people; from there, it spread rapidly to Japan, South Korea, and worldwide. On January 30, 2020, the WHO declared it a serious health issue and a pandemic disease (which spreads from person to person quickly and globally).

It is widely known that SARS-CoV-2 arose in bats; and there is an intermediate mammal, which looks similar to an ant eater called a pangolin, which may act as a host between humans and bats; however, this is not confirmed. Scientists are researching the origin of SARS-CoV-2, which is important to stop the spread of this kind of virus.

11.1.1 Ways in which COVID-19 spreads

COVID-19 is a 'communicable disease' which spreads infection from one person to another in different ways, such as by physical contact, contact with contaminated surface areas, contact with body fluids, and blood from the bites of insects or animals.

COVID-19 spreads mainly by contact with droplets caused by coughs and sneezes. This contact can be divided into two types:

1. Direct contact—people and animals.
2. Indirect contact—objects and surfaces.

Direct Contact: when a person is in close contact with the infected person without maintaining a suitable distance, and if the infected person does not cover his nose and mouth, he ejects the virus through coughs and sneezes as droplets, which are contagious and may affect the healthy person as well. Direct contact also includes contact with animal saliva, blood, milk, flesh, urine, and faeces, which are responsible for the transmission of disease.

Indirect Contact: in this type of contact, a person need not be in contact with an infected person. Droplets containing infectious viruses can remain active for many days. If the affected person sneezes or coughs without covering his nose and mouth, droplets may fall onto the surfaces of objects, clothes, etc.; without knowing this, the other person comes into contact with them and may be infected. The virus can also spread indirectly through contaminated areas where animals sleep. The droplet size varies; if it is more than 5–10 μm in diameter, droplets are categorized as respiratory droplets, and if the size is less than 5–10 μm in diameter, they are known as droplet nuclei. In the case of COVID-19, respiratory droplets > 5–10 μm in diameter are responsible for transmission of the disease. Hence, it is not airborne, which requires droplets with diameters of < 5–10 μm.

Diagnosis: any disease can be diagnosed after a person shows the appropriate symptoms or signs. The symptoms of COVID-19 are fever, cough, sore throat, headache, tiredness, and difficulty in breathing.

For every action, there is a reaction; when viral particles enter the body, they become active and multiply. Our body recognizes them as foreign particles and tries to develop antibodies; in the case of weak immunity, the microorganisms (viral particles) will dominate, leading to infection. The incubation period of COVID-19 is 2–14 days. During this incubation period, a few may show the symptoms but others may not, depending on the immune response of each individual.

11.1.2 Tests used to diagnose COVID-19

1. Swab test: A six-inch-long swab with an absorbent tip is used to collect sputum from the cavity between the nose and the mouth. Swabbing is carried out for 15 s by rotating the swab several times. The sputum sample is collected and sent to a laboratory for diagnosis.
2. Nasal aspirate: Sputum from the inside of the nose or the upper portion of throat is collected with the help of a swab. In some cases, a device known as a suction tube is preferred. After the sample is collected, the secretions are sent to a laboratory, where they are incubated, grown in a culture medium, and then tested.
3. Sputum test: A thick substance is secreted (i.e. mucus) and accumulated in the lungs; it is ejected by a cough. During this test, sputum is collected when the person coughs onto a swab or into a cup; the sample is sent for culture testing.
4. Blood, antibody, or serology test: when the body becomes infected with any microorganisms, it produces antibodies to fight against them; these antibodies can be observed using a blood test. The blood test is performed by collecting blood from a vein; it is a widely used test in the diagnosis of disease and gives accurate results.

Treatment/Medication: COVID-19 vaccines are widely accessible throughout the globe. Many doctors, retail pharmacies, hospitals, offices and clinics offer COVID-19 vaccinations. COVID-19 vaccines can reduce the risk of spreading the virus that causes COVID-19.

Plasma therapy: this therapy was first discovered by German physiologist Emil Von Behring and was used in 1890. In 2009, it was used to cure the H1N1 infection. In 2014, the WHO suggested using this therapy to treat the Ebola virus. Plasma therapy is a passive form of immunization, in which antibodies from the plasma of recovered patients are injected into the bodies of infected persons. This therapy is also being used to treat the patients of COVID-19. The All India Institute of Medical Sciences (AIMS) is conducting plasma therapy in its centers. This passive way of introducing antibodies into a patient's body is a kind of 'artificial immunization'.

Plasma therapy might currently be advantageous, but it has negative effect as well; this artificial method of immunization may suppress the patient's natural immunity, which further affects the patient's ability to fight disease.

Drugs such as hydroxychloroquine, favipiravir, remdesivir, and lopinavir-ritonavir are used to treat COVID-19.

1. Hydroxychloroquine: this is actually an anti-malarial drug; it is also used for several inflammatory diseases, such as rheumatoid arthritis and lupus. During laboratory trials, this drug was shown to be effective in killing viruses.

   Its mechanism of action has two steps:

   i. The drug affects the virus by making it harder for the virion to adhere to the cell, which stops the entry of the virus into a cell; as a result, there is no multiplication
   ii. Even if the virus succeeds in entering a cell, the drug kills it before multiplication takes place.

   This drug is readily available and inexpensive, but it has side-effects i.e. an abnormal heart rhythm; it is also unsafe for cardiac patients. It is being used under emergency conditions with the prescribed dosage.
2. Favipiravir: this drug retails under the brand name Avigan, which is an antiviral drug licensed in Japan in 2014 to treat viral influenza infections. This drug was certified by the Japanese PM to be used in mild to moderate COVID-19 cases; along with China and Japan, Italy also has also performed clinical trials for its use.

   Its mechanism of action is the inhibition of a viral RNA polymer enzyme. RNA polymerase is an enzyme that helps to make new viral RNA. Favipiravir targets this enzyme, which inhibits the multiplication of the virus in the body. Therefore, the reproduction of the virus is stopped, as no new RNA is synthesized.
3. Remdesivir: this is an antiviral drug. The United States Food and Drug Administration (FDA) approved its use as an RNA polymerase inhibitor. It was first used to treat the Ebola virus. This drug is also effective in the case of COVID-19; it resulted in improved breathing, improved oxygen levels, and it also inhibits the RNA polymerase reaction, as it is an RNA inhibitor. In case of this drug, the US FDA has declared an 'emergency use authorization'. The manufacture of this drug is complex, and it is given in the form of an injection.

4. Lopinavir-ritonavir: These drugs were previously used to treat HIV infections by inhibiting the HIV protease enzyme. These drugs are given in combination with each other; ritonavir helps to boost the power of lopinavir.

Mechanism of action: these drugs increase the body's immunity by reducing the viral infection.

11.1.3 Myths and traditional treatments

- The addition of pepper to food may not cure COVID-19 patients.
- Eating garlic may not prevent people from being infected.
- The use of alcohol does not help in treating COVID-19; instead, it increases other health problems.
- The use of methanol, ethanol, bleach, or other disinfectants is very harmful to the human body and is of no use against COVID-19.
- The use of UV lamps as a disinfectant increases the risk of skin diseases and may affect the eyes.
- The use of hand driers to eradicate the virus.
- This virus cannot be spread by mosquito bites or by houseflies.
- Hot weather conditions of more than 25 °C are not effective in preventing the disease.
- Even cold weather and snow do not prevent infection.
- The ability to hold one's breath for more than 10 s without any discomfort is not an indication that one is free of coronavirus.

Preventive measures: 'Prevention is better than cure'; if there are no specific medications, prevention is the only cure.

1. Maintain social distance

    i. Avoid gatherings at religious meetings, marriage ceremonies, funerals, markets, etc.
    ii. Avoid physical contact such as hugs, holding and shaking hands, kissing, etc.
    iii. Maintain a distance of at least 1 meter or 3 feet between one person and another.

2. Maintain good hygiene
    i. Wash your hands with soap or alcohol-based liquids after
        a. Public meetings
        b. Contact with any metal surface or objects
        c. After coughs and sneezes
        d. Before preparing food and eating
        e. Coming indoors from the market or outside
3. Wear a face mask in public places.
4. Don't spit on roads.

5. Clean the house on a daily basis (windows, door knobs etc.) with a good detergent.
6. Children and elderly people at high risk from Covid-19 should avoid leaving the house during the pandemic.
7. Do not organize any unnecessary functions or gather for entertainment during lockdown.
8. Quarantine people who show symptoms or illness for 14 days.
9. Do not share your belongings with anyone.

'Newly emerged diseases need newly discovered medicine'. Clinical trials are ongoing worldwide to discover antiviral drugs for COVID-19. Due to the current emergency, scientists are using antiviral drugs that are already available in the hope that they may help to control the current situation.

The rest of this chapter is organised as follows. Section 2 presents related work. Section 3 describes machine learning methods and tools used for the prediction of pandemic diseases. Section 4 discusses the data sets available for COVID-19 predictions. Section 6 offers the conclusions and discusses future work.

11.2 Related work

Toğaçar M *et al* [5] implemented deep-learning models such as MobileNetV2 and SqueezeNet to detect coronavirus, and various other techniques were used, viz. SVM for classification and the social mimic optimization method for feature extraction. An accuracy rate of 99.27% was achieved for classification. F Ucar *et al* [6], proposed an AI-based model using SqueezeNet and additional Bayesian optimization to diagnose COVID-19.

Most researchers adopted machine learning techniques to detect, classify, and diagnose the epidemic outbreak using chest x-ray images, such as those described in [1–4, and 7], whose authors implemented SVM classifiers to classify COVID-19-infected patients and recorded accuracies in between 77% and 95%. An XGBoost classifier was used for the same purpose in [8–13, and 14].

Y Zifeng *et al* [15] utilized AI techniques to predict COVID-19 in China; citizen migration data pre- and post-January 23 were integrated to analyze the model and to obtain the epidemic curve. S S Yadav *et al* [16] implemented an algorithm to classify pneumonia; various classifiers, such as SVM, Inception V3, and VGG16 were utilized and an accuracy of 96.6% was recorded.

Benvenuto *et al* [17] developed an autoregressive integrated moving average (ARIMA) model to detect the spread of COVID-19. ARIMA and a correlogram prediction graph were used to predict epidemic prevalence. M Arpan *et al* [18] developed COVID-19 AI Detector (CovidAID) to classify patients for suitable therapy. The COVID Chest x-ray public data set was utilized for experimental analysis; an accuracy of 90.5% was obtained.

R H Abiyev *et al* [19] implemented two deep-learning models, namely the backpropagation neural network (B-NN) and the competitive neural network (C-NN) for pneumonia classification. Pneumonic and healthy chest x-ray scans were used for experimental analysis; a classification rate of about 89.5% was obtained.

J Chen *et al* [20] developed a deep-learning-based model to detect COVID pneumonia. The data set was collected from two hospitals, and included diseased images, healthy images, and images of control patients; an accuracy of 98% was achieved. Apart from the data collected, analysis was performed using an external data set; an accuracy of 96% was recorded.

F Shi *et al* [21] proposed an infection-size-aware random forest method (iSARF) to label infected images based on the size of the lesion; random forest (RF) was used as the classifier and an accuracy of 87.9% was achieved.

C Zheng *et al* [22] proposed a weakly-supervised DL-based model to automatically detect COVID-19. UNet was utilized to segment the lung regions, and chest CT scans were used to train the model, which recorded a high performance for the prediction of COVID-19.

E Hemdan *et al* [23] used different methods, such as VGG, DenseNet, ResNet, Inception, Inception-ResNet, Xception, and MobileNet to classify COVID-19.

11.3 Machine learning (Ml) algorithms

This section will discuss various machine learning algorithms that are used for the prediction of COVID-19.

11.3.1 K-nearest neighbours (K-NN)

K-nearest neighbours is a supervised ML algorithm which can be implemented to solve classification and regression problems. The working principle of K-NN is that nearby data are considered to fall into one class, which means that classification in K-NN is performed according to similarity by calculating the distance or space between the data points in a plane. There are different methods for calculating distance, but the most accepted is Euclidean distance; the mathematical expression for Euclidean distance is shown in (11.1).

$$\sqrt{(X_2 - X_1)^2 + (Y_2 - Y_1)^2} \qquad (11.1)$$

This algorithm saves the entire input data and uses it to classify new data according to the similarity metric. Thus, K-NN is also referred to as a 'lazy learner' algorithm, since it learns from the stored data set instead of learning from a training data set; during classification, it works with the stored data set. As shown in figure 11.1, when new data arrives on the plane, K-NN first calculates the distance and then, based on similarity, it labels the data with a specific class label.

11.3.2 Random forest (RF)

Random forest is a supervised ML algorithm based on ensemble learning, which is a method of integrating several classifiers together to resolve complicated problems. It can be employed for regression and classification tasks. As the name implies, it consists of several decision tress in different subsets, as shown in figure 11.2. Every

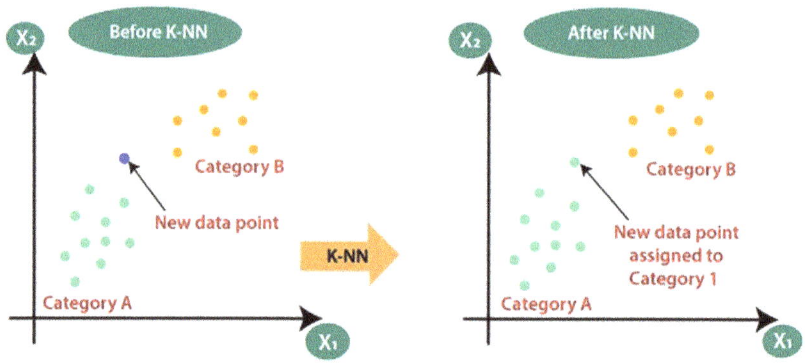

Figure 11.1. Representation of the classification performed by the K-NN algorithm [24].

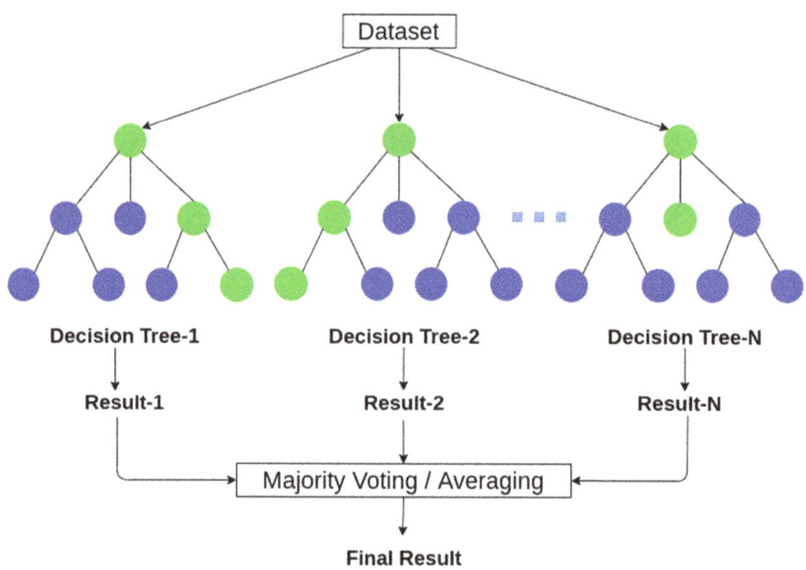

Figure 11.2. Random forest representation [25].

tree is used to predict the result, and the output is finalized by a majority decision. The more trees the forest contains, the more accuracy is enhanced and overfitting problems are precluded. Entropy and information gain are the two key concepts behind decision trees. The randomness of the system is known as entropy; its mathematical formula is shown in equation (11.2). Information gain, on the other hand, determines the amount of entropy reduction in the system; equation (11.3) shows its mathematical definition.

$$\text{Entropy E(S)} = -\sum p(x)_{*}\log_2(p(x)), \tag{11.2}$$

where $p(x)$ is the probability of obtaining class X.

$$\text{Gain}(S, A) = \text{Entropy}(S) - \sum_{v \in DA} \frac{|S_v|}{|S|} \text{Entropy}(S_v) \qquad (11.3)$$

11.3.3 Support vector machine (SVM)

SVM is supervised machine learning approach which works well for regression and classification tasks; however, in most cases, it is employed for classification. The key challenge of SVM is to originate a boundary or line (i.e. a hyperplane) which separates the different classes into *n*-dimensional space, allowing new data that arrive to be placed in the appropriate class. The hyperplane plays a major role in SVM classification; is is created by choosing extreme vectors in the plane, which are known as support vectors (leading to the name 'support vector machine'. Initially, data are plotted in an *n*-dimensional feature plane, in which each feature value is plotted at its specific coordinate value. After the data features are plotted, classification is carried out by determining the hyperplane which separates the different classes, as shown in figure 11.3. SVMs can be implemented for detection, classification, and recognition tasks.

11.3.4 Bayesian neural network (BNN)

A BNN is a combination of a neural network (NN) algorithm and probabilistic or statistical models; the objective of combining them is to exploit the advantages of both techniques. Here, the NN uses approximation techniques, whereas the probabilistic model governs model specifications through known parameters to generate data. The use of probabilistic models in the diagnosis phase creates a posterior distribution and generates probabilistic guarantees for its predictions. This algorithm is a good fit for small data sets and it possesses a robust nature which eradicates data overfitting problems.

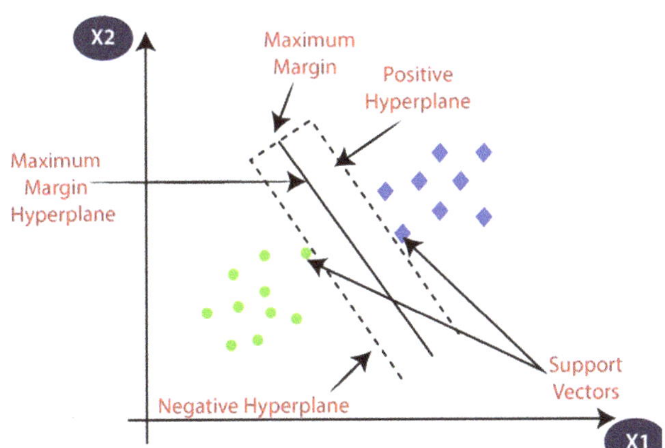

Figure 11.3. SVM classifier [24].

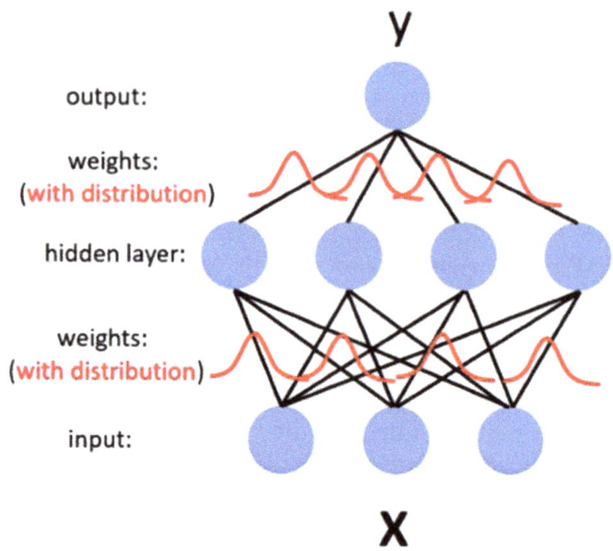

Figure 11.4. BNN architecture [26].

The working principle of BNNs is very simple: each entity in the network is accompanied by a weight, a bias, and a probability distribution, as shown in figure 11.4. The random variable of a Bayesian network generates different values whenever it is accessed. For example, consider X as a random variable; whenever we try to access it, it gives a different value. This technique of acquiring a different value for each access to X is known as sampling, and the value obtained from every sample relies on a probability distribution.

Unlike traditional NNs, which possess constant biases and weights that determine the output, BNNs contain a probability distribution connected to every layer. BNNs work well for classification tasks, as several forward passes are used; each one uses a new instance of biases and weights.

11.3.5 Convolutional neural network (CNN)

This widely implemented algorithm, which utilizes multiple perceptrons, aims to reduce preprocessing time; it is motivated by the workings of the human brain. It comprises one or more convolutional layers, including pooling layers, sampling layers, and fully connected layers. The convolutional layers are organized using feature maps which store image regions. All the feature map neurons are interconnected with the preceding layer's neurons, along with responsive fields to mask the image. Features are summarized in the convolutional layers, dimensionality reduction is performed in the pooling layer, and the fully connected layers are nothing more than hidden layers where labels are classified. The architecture of a CNN is shown in figure 11.5.

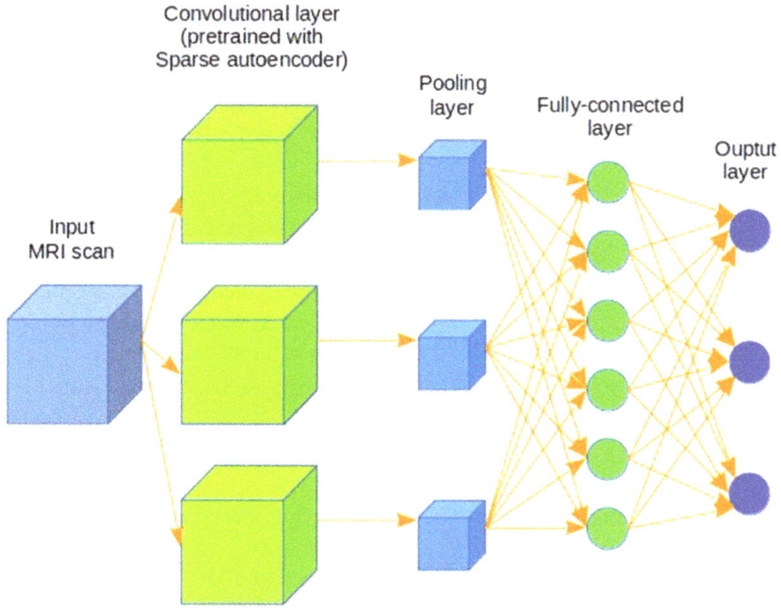

Figure 11.5. Architecture of a CNN [27].

In this section, the machine learning tools used to diagnose the COVID-19 were explained. Convolutional neural networks are widely used for the diagnosis of pandemic diseases. ML and deep-learning-based models are most suitable for the diagnosis of COVID-19. These methods are widely used to identify complications such as pneumonia based on the data augmentation of CT and x-ray images.

The use of ML methods will help to forecast the effect of COVID-19 by enabling efficient plans for timely treatment, early ICU support, and the allocation of resources for high-risk cases [51]. Popular machine learning methods used to identify COVID-19 are shown in table 11.1.

Various machine learning tools used for the diagnosis of COVID-19 are shown in table 11.2.

Table 11.3 highlights the various popular data sets used by the researchers in identifying the disease.

11.4 Conclusions

In this scoping review, we have analyzed the machine learning methods used to diagnose COVID-19. Our findings are based on various machine learning methods, in particular, supervised learning techniques that are used to make decision support systems for healthcare. Machine learning methods, such as SVM, logistic regression, Bayesian methods, and CNNs perform well for COVID-19 detection. More reliable and accurate ML methods have to be developed to reduce the risk of COVID-19.

Table 11.1. Machine learning methods used for the prediction of pandemic diseases.

Ref. No	ML methods used	Accuracy
[1]	LR, NN, RF, SVM	86.8% specificity and 82.4% sensitivity
[28–30]	RF	94.44% specificity and 100% sensitivity 81% accuracy, 82% specificity, and 60% sensitivity. 95.95% accuracy and 96.95% specificity
[31–34]	LR	86%–93% sensitivity and 35%–55% specificity 94.1% sensitivity and 90.2% specificity 73.7% specificity and 88.6% sensitivity 91.30% specificity and 95.24% sensitivity
[2–4, 7]	SVM	81.48% accuracy 91.38% accuracy, 90% sensitivity and 94% specificity 80% sensitivity and 96% specificity 77.5% accuracy and 78.4% specificity 87% to 95% accuracy
[8–14],	XGBoost	92.5% sensitivity and 97.9% specificity 86.4% accuracy, 86.8% specificity and 82.4% sensitivity 79% to 80% accuracy 93% accuracy 90% accuracy 95% specificity and 85% sensitivity 90% accuracy

Table 11.2. Machine-learning-based tools used for the diagnosis of COVID-19.

Ref. No.	Method used	Developed for	Performance measure (Accuracy)
[5]	SVM + CNN	Effective COVID-19 detection	99.27%
[35–40]	CNN	Automated diagnosis, automated screening, automated pneumonia differentiation	
[6]	Bayesian based network	Diagnostic tool to detect and diagnose COVID-19	100%
[41]	LR	COVID-19 progression prediction from CT scans	95%
[15]	Dense CNN	COVID-19 detection through chest CT scans	92%
[42]	LR, K-NN, DT, RF, SVM	COVID-19 severity detection at an early stage	50% to 80%

Table 11.3. Data sets for COVID-19.

Ref No	Data type	Availability
[42]	CT scans	Jiang *et al* [42]
[37]	CT scans	Liu *et al* [37]
[15]	CT scans	Yang *et al* [15]
[39]	CT scans	Sing *et al* [39]
[35]	CT scans	Li *et al* [35]
[40]	CT scans	Butt *et al* [40]
[5, 36, 38]	X-ray images	https://github.com/ieee8023/covidchestxray-dataset
[43]	CT scans and clinical information	Mei *et al* [44]
[45]	CT scans	Wu *et al* [46]
[44]	CT scans	Huang *et al* [47]
[46]	Genomes	https://data.mendeley.com/datasets/nvk5bf3m2f/1
[47]	CT scans	Sixteen-multidetector computed tomography (MDCT) scanner (Alexion, Toshiba Medical System, Japan)
[48]	X-rays	Oh *et al* [49]
[50]	Time series	https://ourworldindata.org/coronavirussource-data
[49]	Protein sequences	https://bigd.big.ac.cn/ncov
[14]	Time series	https://brasil.io/api/dataset/covid19/caso/data/?place_type=state
[52]	Genomes	https://sourceforge.net/projects/mldsp-gui/files/COVID19Dataset
[53]	Time series	Pirouz *et al* [17]

References

[1] Schwab P, Schütte A D, Dietz B and Bauer S 2020 Clinical predictive models for COVID-19: systematic study *J. Med. Internet Res.* **6** e21439

[2] Yao H, Zhang N, Zhang R, Duan M, Xie T, Pan J, Peng E, Huang J, Zhang Y and Xu X *et al* 2020 Severity detection for the coronavirus disease 2019 (covid-19) patients using a machine learning model based on the blood and urine tests *Front. Cell Develop. Biol.* **8** 683

[3] Zhao C, Bai Y, Wang C, Zhong Y, Lu N, Tian L, Cai F and Jin R 2021 Risk factors related to the severity of covid-19 in Wuhan *Int. J. Med. Sci.* **18** 120–7

[4] Sun L, Liu G, Song F, Shi N, Liu F, Li S and Shi Y 2020 Combination of four clinical indicators predicts the severe/critical symptom of patients infected COVID-19 *J. Clin. Virol.* **128** 104431

[5] Toğaçar M, Ergen B and Cömert Z 2020 COVID-19 detection using deep learning models to exploit social mimic optimization and structured chest X-ray images using fuzzy color and stacking approaches *Comput. Biol. Med.* **121** 103805

[6] Ucar F and Korkmaz D 2020 COVIDiagnosis-Net: deep Bayes-SqueezeNet based diagnostic of the coronavirus disease 2019 (COVID-19) from x-ray images *Med. Hypotheses* **140** 109761

[7] BBC: Coronavirus June 2020 Israel enables emergency spy powers https://bbc.com/news/technology-51930681
[8] Li W T *et al* 2020 Using machine learning of clinical data to diagnose covid-19: a systematic review and meta-analysis *BMC Med. Inf. Decis. Making* **20** 247
[9] Bayat V, Phelps S, Ryono R, Lee C, Parekh H and Mewton J *et al* 2020 A severe acute respiratory syndrome coronavirus 2 (SARS-CoV-2) prediction model from standard laboratory tests *Clin. Infect. Dis.* **73** e2901–7
[10] Vaid A, Somani S, Russak A J, De Freitas J K, Chaudhry F F and Paranjpe I *et al* 2020 Machine learning to predict mortality and critical events in covid-19 positive New York city patients: a cohort study *J. Med. Internet Res.;* **49** 1918–29
[11] Yan L, Zhang H-T, Xiao Y, Wang M, Sun C, Liang J, Li S, Zhang M, Guo Y and Xiao Y *et al* 2020 Prediction of criticality in patients with severe Covid-19 infection using three clinical features: a machine learning-based prognostic model with clinical data in Wuhan 2020.02.27.20028027v2 MedRxiv
[12] Yan L, Zhang H-T, Goncalves J, Xiao Y, Wang M, Guo Y, Sun C, Tang X, Jin L and Zhang M *et al* 2020 A machine learning-based model for survival prediction in patients with severe COVID-19 infection 2020.02.27.20028027 MedRxiv
[13] Guan X, Zhang B, Fu M, Li M, Yuan X, Zhu Y, Peng J, Guo H and Lu Y 2021 Clinical and inflammatory features based machine learning model for fatal risk prediction of hospitalized covid-19 patients: results from a retrospective cohort study *Ann. Med* **53** 257–66
[14] Ribeiro M H D M, da Silva R G, Mariani V C and Coelho L D S 2020 Short-term forecasting COVID-19 cumulative confirmed cases: perspectives for Brazil *Chaos, Solitons Fractals* **135** 109853
[15] Dogan O, Tiwari S and Jabbar M A *et al* 2021 A systematic review on AI/ML approaches against COVID-19 outbreak *Complex Intell. Syst.* **7** 2655–78
[16] Yadav S S and Jadhav S M 2019 Deep convolutional neural network based medical image classification for disease diagnosis *J. Big Data* **6** 113
[17] Benvenuto D, Giovanetti M, Vassallo L, Angeletti S and Ciccozzi M 2020 Application of the ARIMA model on the COVID-2019 epidemic dataset *Data Brief* **29** 105340
[18] Mangal A, Kalia S, Rajgopal H, Rangarajan K, Namboodiri V, Banerjee S and Arora C 2020 CovidAID: COVID-19 detection using chest x-ray arXiv:2004.09803v1
[19] Abiyev R H and Ma'aitah M K S 2018 Deep convolutional neural networks for chest diseases detection *J. Healthc. Eng.* **2018** 4168538
[20] Chen J, Wu L and Zhang J 2020 Deep learning-based model for detecting 2019 novel coronavirus pneumonia on high-resolution computed tomography *Sci. Rep.* **10** 1–11
[21] Shi F, Xia L, Shan F and Wu D 2021 Large-scale screening of covid-19 from community acquired pneumonia using infection size-aware classification *Phys. Med. Biol.* **66** 065031
[22] Zheng C, Deng X, Fu Q, Zhou Q and Feng J 2020 Deep learning-based detection for COVID-19 from chest CT using weak label *IEEE Trans. Med. Imag.* **39** 2615–25
[23] Hemdan E, Shouman M and Karar M 2020 COVIDX-Net: A framework of deep learning classifiers to diagnose COVID-19 in x-ray images arXiv:2003.11055
[24] https://javatpoint.com/machine-learning
[25] https://analyticsvidhya.com/blog/2020/12/lets-open-the-black-box-of-random-forests/
[26] https://researchgate.net/figure/A-Bayesian-neural-network-with-one-hidden-layer_fig1_328757994

[27] Khvostikova A, Aderghalb K, Benois-Pineaub J, Krylova A, Catheline G and for the Alzheimer's Disease Neuroimaging Initiative 2018 3D CNN-based classification using sMRI and MD-DTI images for Alzheimer disease studies arXiv:1801.05968

[28] Wu J *et al* 2020 Rapid and accurate identification of COVID-19 infection through machine learning based on clinical available blood test results 2020.04.02.20051136 medRxiv

[29] Brinati D, Campagner A, Ferrari D, Locatelli M, Banfi G and Cabitza F 2020 Detection of COVID-19 infection from routine blood exams with machine learning: a feasibility study *J. Med. Syst.* **44** 135

[30] Wu J *et al* 2020 Rapid and accurate identification of COVID-19 infection through machine learning based on clinical available blood test results 2020.04.02.20051136 medRxiv

[31] Joshi R P *et al* 2020 A predictive tool for identification of sars-cov-2 pcr-negative emergency department patients using routine test results *J. Clin. Virol.* **129** 104502

[32] Huang H *et al* 2020 Prognostic factors for covid-19 pneumonia progression to severe symptoms based on earlier clinical features: a retrospective analysis *Front. Med.* **7** 643

[33] Zhou Y, Yang Z, Guo Y, Geng S, Gao S, Ye S, Hu Y and Wang Y 2020 A new predictor of disease severity in patients with Covid-19 in Wuhan, China 2020.03.24.20042119 medRxiv

[34] Han Y, Zhang H, Mu S, Wei W, Jin C, Xue Y, Tong C, Zha Y, Song Z and Gu G 2020 Lactate dehydrogenase, a risk factor of severe COVID-19 patients: a retrospective and observational study 2020.03.24.20040162 medRxiv

[35] Li L *et al* 2020 Artificial intelligence distinguishes COVID-19 from community acquired pneumonia on chest CT *Radiology* **296** 200905

[36] Salman F M, Abu-Naser S S, Alajrami E, Abu-Nasser B S and Alashqar B A 2020 Covid-19 detection using artificial intelligence *Int. J. Acad. Eng. Res. (IJAER)* **4** 18–25

[37] Liu F *et al* 2020 CT quantification of pneumonia lesions in early days predicts progression to severe illness in a cohort of COVID-19 patients *Theranostics* **10** 5613–22

[38] Ozturk T, Talo M, Yildirim E A, Baloglu U B, Yildirim O and Acharya U R 2020 Automated detection of COVID-19 cases using deep neural networks with x-ray images *Comput. Biol. Med.* **121** 103792

[39] Singh D, Kumar V and Kaur M 2020 Classification of COVID-19 patients from chest CT images using multi-objective differential evolution-based convolutional neural networks *Eur. J. Clin. Microbiol. Infect. Dis.* **39** 1379–89

[40] Butt C, Gill J, Chun D and Babu B A 2020 Deep learning system to screen coronavirus disease 2019 pneumonia *Appl. Intell.* Epub ahead of print 22 April 2020

[41] Liu Z, Huang S, Lu W, Su Z, Yin X, Liang H and Zhang H 2020 Modeling the trend of coronavirus disease 2019 and restoration of operational capability of metropolitan medical service in China: a machine learning and mathematical model-based analysis *Global Health Res. Policy* **5** 1–11

[42] Jiang X *et al* 2020 Towards an artificial intelligence framework for data-driven prediction of coronavirus clinical severity *Comput. Mater. Contin.* **63** 537–51

[43] Mei X *et al* 2020 Artificial intelligence-enabled rapid diagnosis of patients with COVID-19 *Nat. Med.* **26** 1–5

[44] Huang L, Han R, Ai T, Yu P, Kang H, Tao Q and Xia L 2020 Serial quantitative chest ctassessment of covid-19: deep-learning approach *Radiol.: Cardiothor. Imaging* **2** e200075

[45] Wu X *et al* 2020 Deep learning-based multi-view fusion model for screening 2019 novel coronavirus pneumonia: a multicentre study *Eur. J. Radiol.* **128** 10904

[46] Barbosa R D M and Fernandes M A 2020 Chaos game representation dataset of SARS-CoV-2 genome *Data Brief* **30** 105618
[47] Ardakani A A, Kanafi A R, Acharya U R, Khadem N and Mohammadi A 2020 Application of deep learning technique to manage COVID-19 in routine clinical practice using CT images: results of 10 convolutional neural networks *Comput. Biol. Med.* **121** 103795
[48] Oh Y, Park S and Ye J C 2020 Deep learning covid-19 features on CXR using limited training data sets *IEEE Trans. Med. Imaging* **39** 2688–700
[49] Qiang X L, Xu P, Fang G, Liu W B and Kou Z 2020 Using the spike protein feature to predict infection risk and monitor the evolutionary dynamic of coronavirus *Infect. Dis. Poverty* **9** 1–8
[50] Tuli S, Tuli S, Tuli R and Gill S S 2020 Predicting the growth and trend of COVID-19 pandemic using machine learning and cloud computing *Internet Things* **11** 100222
[51] Randhawa G S, Soltysiak M P, El Roz H, De Souza C P, Hill K A and Kari L 2020 Machine learning using intrinsic genomic signatures for rapid classification of novel pathogens: COVID-19 case study *PLoS One* **15** e0232391
[52] Pirouz B, Shaffiee Haghshenas S, Shaffiee Haghshenas S and Piro P 2020 Investigating a serious challenge in the sustainable development process: analysis of confirmed cases of COVID-19 (new type of coronavirus) through a binary classification using artificial intelligence and regression analysis *Sustainability* **12** 2427
[53] Chen J, Wu L and Zhang J 2020 Deep learning-based model for detecting 2019 novel coronavirus pneumonia on high-resolution computed tomography *Sci. Rep.* **10** 1–11

www.ingramcontent.com/pod-product-compliance
Ingram Content Group UK Ltd.
Pitfield, Milton Keynes, MK11 3LW, UK
UKHW051855100926
8556IPUK00005B/643

9 780750 33793